INTRUSIVE THOUGHTS
IN CLINICAL DISORDERS

INTRUSIVE THOUGHTS
IN CLINICAL DISORDERS
Theory, Research, and Treatment

Edited by
DAVID A. CLARK

THE GUILFORD PRESS
New York   London

© 2005 The Guilford Press
A Division of Guilford Publications, Inc.
72 Spring Street, New York, NY 10012
www.guilford.com

Printed in the United States of America

This book is printed on acid-free paper.

Last digit is print number: 9   8   7   6   5   4   3   2   1

Library of Congress Cataloging-in-Publication Data

Intrusive thoughts in clinical disorders : theory, research, and treatment
/ edited by David A. Clark.
    p. cm.
  Includes bibliographical references and index.
  ISBN 1-59385-083-2 (hardcover : alk. paper)
  1. Cognition disorders.   2. Psychology, Pathological.   3. Thought
insertion.   I. Clark, David A., 1954–
  RC553.C64′55 2005
  616.89—dc22

                                      2004017740

In memory of
Richard "Rich" Wenzlaff

ABOUT THE EDITOR

David A. Clark, PhD, is a Professor in the Department of Psychology at the University of New Brunswick, Canada. He received his PhD from the Institute of Psychiatry, University of London, England. Dr. Clark has published numerous articles on cognitive theory and therapy of depression and obsessive–compulsive disorders, and is the author of *Cognitive-Behavioral Therapy for OCD* and the coauthor (with Aaron T. Beck and Brad A. Alford) of *Scientific Foundations of Cognitive Theory and Therapy of Depression*. Drs. Clark and Beck recently developed the Clark–Beck Obsessive–Compulsive Inventory to assess self-reported severity of obsessive and compulsive symptoms. Dr. Clark has received a number of research grants to study the cognitive basis of emotional disorders, the most recent being a Canadian federal grant to investigate intentional control of unwanted intrusive thoughts. He is a Founding Fellow of the Academy of Cognitive Therapy and an Associate Editor of *Cognitive Therapy and Research*.

CONTRIBUTORS

David A. Clark, PhD, Department of Psychology, University of New Brunswick, Fredericton, New Brunswick, Canada

Sherry A. Falsetti, PhD, Department of Family and Community Medicine, University of Illinois College of Medicine at Rockford, Rockford, Illinois

Allison G. Harvey, PhD, Department of Psychology, University of California, Berkeley, California

Calvin M. Langton, PhD, University of Toronto, Centre for Addiction and Mental Health, Toronto, Ontario, Canada

W. L. Marshall, PhD, Rockwood Psychological Services, Kingston, Ontario, Canada

Jeannine Monnier, PhD, Department of Psychiatry and Behavioral Sciences, Medical University of South Carolina, Charleston, South Carolina

Anthony P. Morrison, PhD, Department of Clinical Psychology, Mental Health Services of Salford, Salford, United Kingdom

Kieron O'Connor, PhD, Centre de recherche Fernand-Seguin, Université de Montréal, Montréal, Québec, Canada

Christine Purdon, PhD, Department of Psychology, University of Waterloo, Waterloo, Ontario, Canada

Heidi S. Resnick, PhD, Department of Psychiatry and Behavioral Sciences, Medical University of South Carolina, Charleston, South Carolina

Shelley Rhyno, BA, Department of Psychology, University
of New Brunswick, Fredericton, New Brunswick, Canada

Adrian Wells, PhD, Academic Division of Clinical Psychology,
University of Manchester, Manchester, United Kingdom

Richard M. Wenzlaff, PhD (deceased), Department of Psychology,
University of Texas at San Antonio, San Antonio, Texas

PREFACE

In the last three decades behavioral psychologists have made considerable progress in understanding the role of cognition in the origins, maintenance, and treatment of many psychological disorders. The inclusion of subjective thought as a legitimate focus of empirical investigation reintroduced behavioral researchers and practitioners to the importance of conscious experience in normal and abnormal functioning. Although hidden within the theory and concepts of the information-processing paradigm, conscious thought nevertheless reemerged as a critical factor in the ontogenesis of human experience. In many ways William James's (1890/1950) observations about the stream of consciousness were rediscovered and once again assumed their rightful place within the scientific study of cognition and emotion.

The flow of human thought is exceedingly complex, rich, and ever changing. Social and clinical psychologists have documented through many naturalistic and experimental studies a myriad of thought form and content that constitutes subjective conscious experience. Moreover, what we think and how we construe the world around us profoundly influence our behavior and our emotions. The occurrence of one particular type of conscious thought is the subject of this book. The flow of human thought is frequently punctuated by unintended and unwanted intrusive thoughts, images, or impulses that interrupt our goal-directed pursuits and often seem discordant with our valued ideals and concerns. This unwanted mental activity can redirect attentional resources and interrupt ongoing activity. Depending on the context and their functional significance, many types of intrusive cognition are characterized by heightened subjective distress and are quite impervious to the strongest attempts at suppression or distraction.

Despite the emerging empirical evidence that unwanted intrusive thoughts, images, and impulses are important cognitive features of many clinical disorders, behavioral researchers have only begun to systematically and diligently investigate the role of these cognitive phenomena in the pathogenesis of clinical disorders such as obsessive–compulsive disorder (OCD), posttraumatic stress disorder (PTSD), depression, generalized anxiety disorder, and insomnia. This interest in the role of unwanted conscious thought in normal and abnormal emotional and behavioral states has been fueled by the flurry of research on the deleterious effects of intentional thought suppression that was first documented by another, more recent Harvard psychologist, Daniel Wegner (1994). And yet, the first volume to offer a comprehensive review of the the topic of intrusive thoughts, *Cognitive Interference: Theories, Methods, and Findings* (Sarason, Pierce, & Sarason, 1996), was published only a few years ago. Although the first empirical studies on unwanted intrusive thoughts can be traced back to the early 1970s (Horowitz, 1975; Klinger, 1978; Rachman & de Silva, 1978), a more sustained inquiry into this cognitive phenomenon is relatively recent. This edited book is the first volume devoted exclusively to the role of unwanted intrusive thoughts in clinical disorders.

The topics selected for inclusion in this book focus on clinical disorders in which unwanted intrusive thoughts, images, or impulses are known to play a contributing role in the etiology, persistence, and/or treatment of the disorder. The contributing authors are all leading experts who have researched unwanted intrusive cognition within particular clinical domains. The breadth of coverage was constrained by the limited number of psychological disorders where unwanted intrusive cognition has been investigated. However, the clinical disorders reviewed in these chapters all have an emerging research base that is sufficient to allow a preliminary critical review.

Despite the clinical diversity represented in this book, all the contributors have discussed a number of similar issues. Each has considered (1) the impact of unwanted intrusive cognitive phenomena on salient disorder-specific emotional and behavioral response patterns, (2) the role of higher-order or metacognitive processing and appraisal in the persistence of unwanted cognition, (3) the reciprocal impact of selective attentional processing on intrusive mentation, and (4) the interaction between unwanted mental intrusions and intentional thought suppression. In addition, the contributors discuss various treatment approaches that might be used to ameliorate the negative effect of unwanted distressing intrusive thoughts in the persistence of various psychological

disorders. The book opens with an introductory chapter by Clark and
Rhyno which sets the definitional and conceptual boundaries of unwanted intrusive cognition; the concluding chapter by Purdon highlights
critical issues to be further examined concerning the nature and role of
unwanted intrusive thoughts in psychopathology.

As noted by the contributing authors, many fundamental questions
remain about the origins, function, consequences, and treatment of unwanted intrusive thoughts, images, and impulses.

Why are certain types of unwanted intrusive thoughts so distressing
for some people but not others?

What accounts for the persistence of these intrusions in some clinical
states but their rapid disappearance in most nonclinical contexts?

Are unwanted intrusive thoughts and images a significant contributor to emotional disturbance?

What are the origins and precipitants of this type of unwanted thinking in the stream of consciousness?

Why is control of these thoughts so difficult?

What are the most effective therapeutic strategies for those clients
who are plagued by persistent unwanted distressing cognitive intrusions?

It is hoped that the current volume provides some insight into these
questions and encourages more focused research on the role of unwanted intrusive cognition in psychopathological states.

We were all deeply saddened that one of the contributing authors,
Richard "Rich" Wenzlaff, died suddenly on August 23, 2003, while
playing tennis. Rich was Professor of Psychology and Chair of the
Department of Psychology at the University of Texas at San Antonio. He
is survived by his wife, Ann Eisenberg, a developmental psychologist at
the University of Texas at San Antonio, and his children, Rachel (9) and
Adam (5). Rich's innovative research on the role of thought suppression
in the persistence and recurrence of depression offered refreshing insights into an aspect of cognition that had not been identified by other
cognitive–clinical depression researchers. Rich's piece (Chapter 3) was
written just prior to his death and presents a cogently articulated review
of his theory and research on thought suppression in depression. His
work promised to offer new understanding of depression and had direct
implications for improving our treatment of this serious psychological
disorder and its aftermath. Rich will be greatly missed for his scientific
contributions and for his contributions as a man. It is only fitting that

this volume is dedicated to the great legacy he has left to the profession, his university, his family, and the community.

This book is an outgrowth of a special issue on intrusive thoughts that was published in the July 2002 issue of *Journal of Cognitive Psychotherapy: An International Quarterly*. I am most indebted to the contributing authors who agreed to participate in this volume and who provided such insightful, interesting, and timely reviews of the topic. Their willingness to focus on the key objectives and goals set for the book and to meet deadlines greatly facilitated the editorial process. I also wish to acknowledge financial support for this project from a grant (No. 410-2001-0084) I received from the Social Sciences and Humanities Research Council of Canada. I am grateful for the advice and support received from Jim Nageotte and the staff at The Guilford Press.

DAVID A. CLARK

REFERENCES

Horowitz, M. J. (1975). Intrusive and repetitive thoughts after experimental stress: A summary. *Archives of General Psychiatry, 32*, 1457–1463.

James, W. (1950). *The principles of psychology* (Vol. I). New York: Dover. (Original work published 1890)

Klinger, E. (1978). Modes of normal conscious flow. In K. S. Pope & J. L. Singer (Eds.), *The stream of consciousness*. New York: Plenum Press.

Rachman, S., & de Silva, P. (1978). Abnormal and normal obsessions. *Behaviour Research and Therapy, 16*, 233–248.

Sarason, I. G., Pierce, G. R., & Sarason, B. R. (Eds.). (1996). *Cognitive interference: Theories, methods, and findings*. Mahwah, NJ: Erlbaum.

Wegner, D. M. (1994). Ironic processes of mental control. *Psychological Review, 101*, 34–52.

CONTENTS

1   Unwanted Intrusive Thoughts in Nonclinical Individuals: 1
    Implications for Clinical Disorders
    David A. Clark and Shelley Rhyno

2   Intrusive Thoughts in Posttraumatic Stress Disorder   30
    Sherry A. Falsetti, Jeannine Monnier, and Heidi S. Resnick

3   Seeking Solace but Finding Despair: The Persistence   54
    of Intrusive Thoughts in Depression
    Richard M. Wenzlaff

4   Unwanted Intrusive Thoughts in Insomnia   86
    Allison G. Harvey

5   Worry, Intrusive Thoughts, and Generalized Anxiety Disorder: 119
    The Metacognitive Theory and Treatment
    Adrian Wells

6   Thinking Is Believing: Ego-Dystonic Intrusive Thoughts   145
    in Obsessive–Compulsive Disorder
    David A. Clark and Kieron O'Connor

7   Psychosis and the Phenomenon of Unwanted   175
    Intrusive Thoughts
    Anthony P. Morrison

8 Unwanted Thoughts and Fantasies Experienced   199
   by Sexual Offenders: Their Nature, Persistence,
   and Treatment
   W. L. Marshall and Calvin M. Langton

9 Unwanted Intrusive Thoughts: Present Status   226
   and Future Directions
   Christine Purdon

   Index   245

CHAPTER 1

UNWANTED INTRUSIVE THOUGHTS IN NONCLINICAL INDIVIDUALS

Implications for Clinical Disorders

DAVID A. CLARK
SHELLEY RHYNO

The flow of human thought does not always follow a purposeful, task-oriented, reasoned, or intended path. Instead the natural world of human thought is frequently punctuated with unwanted cognitive activity that interferes with our ability to engage in productive thought and performance (Sarason, Pierce, & Sarason, 1996). Worry, distractions, attentional biases, memory lapses, mindwandering, daydreaming, self-focus, ruminations, and obsessive thought are examples of mental processes that create cognitive interference (Klinger, 1996). These unwanted mental intrusions can interfere in task performance as well as intellectual pursuits and social behavior, and they play a significant role in a number of psychopathological conditions (Sarason et al., 1996).

This volume focuses on a particular type of cognitive interference that is clearly present in a number of psychological disorders. Our subject matter is the unwanted intrusive thoughts, images, or impulses that are primarily self-oriented and emotionally charged and interrupt the

1

flow of thought. They frequently grab attention and may impel one toward some response that is intended to regulate or control the mental intrusion and its associated distress. Thus the occurrence of unwanted intrusive thoughts, their functional role in maladaptive behavioral and emotional states, and deliberate attempts at regulating these thoughts are important topics addressed by the chapter contributors.

In this chapter we examine the nature of clinically relevant unwanted intrusive thoughts, images and impulses in nonclinical samples. After three decades of empirical research, it is abundantly clear that nonclinical individuals experience unwanted mental intrusions that are similar in form and content to the cognitive intrusions that are so problematic in clinical states (for reviews, see Clark, 2004; Papageorgiou & Wells, 2004; Pope & Singer, 1978; Rachman & Hodgson, 1980; Sarason et al., 1996; Wegner & Pennebaker, 1993). The occurrence of clinically relevant cognitive intrusions in nonclinical individuals is clearly illustrated in the following example of an obsession-relevant intrusive impulse recently experienced by one of us (DAC).

It is customary for me to begin the day with an early morning run with a group of fellow runners. Our run takes place in the early morning hours before sunrise and the route involves crossing a couple of bridges over a river that divides our city. On this particular dark, cold late-autumn Canadian morning, I crossed a very busy, two-lane highway bridge with a narrow sidewalk and low guardrails. Suddenly and unexpectedly I felt an intense urge to leap over the bridge railing and imagined myself plunging head first into the frigid water far below. The impulse was so intense that my knees actually felt weak. I mentioned the experience to my co-runner, a sergeant in the Canadian army, who expressed complete bewilderment about my internal mental state.

Upon reflection I was able to identify a number of characteristics of this unwanted intrusive impulse that are typical of this type of cognitive interference. First, the impulse was unwanted and entirely discordant with my current flow of thought and mood. Prior to stepping onto the bridge, I was having a particularly good run and an enjoyable conversation. Second, the impulse was externally cued by the unusually low guardrail and narrow sidewalk. As soon as I left the bridge, the impulse left and did not return despite later running across a second bridge but with a much higher guardrail. Finally, the more I attended to the intrusive impulse, the more intense the sensation. By thinking intently on whether I really could "lose control" and act on the impulse, I was able to intensify the experience but only as long as I was physically on the bridge.

If unwanted intrusive thoughts, images, and impulses are a universal experience, why do some people become so distressed by these cognitive intrusions? How common are unwanted intrusive thoughts in nonclinical persons? What are the similarities and differences between the unwanted mental intrusions in clinical disorders and the same unwelcomed intrusions found in nonclinical samples? How do sudden and unwanted intrusive thoughts differ from other types of cognitive interference such as worry, ruminations, and negative automatic thoughts? What are the origin and function of unwanted cognitive intrusions in the nonclinical state? These are a few of the questions addressed in this chapter. We begin by offering a definition of the phenomena of interest: unwanted intrusive thoughts, images, and impulses.

UNWANTED INTRUSIVE THOUGHTS: DEFINITIONS, INCIDENCE, AND CONSEQUENCE

Definitions

The human mind is a rich tapestry of constantly shifting thoughts, images, feelings, sensations, and impulses. Based on his thought-sampling studies with university students, Klinger (1978, 1996) determined that the median duration for specific thought content was 5 seconds, which means that individuals may experience approximately 4,000 distinct thoughts in a 16-hour day. It is reasonable to expect that some proportion of these thoughts will be unwanted mental intrusions that disrupt current on-task performance and attention. We are reminded of the complexity of the human psyche by the number of different types of cognitive events that psychologists have identified as part of the flow of thought, that is, what William James (1890/1950) referred to as the continuous, but ever-changing personal consciousness, or "stream of thought, of consciousness or of subjective life" (p. 239). As a result of this cognitive diversity, it is important to clearly define one's subject matter. This is also necessitated by the fact that the unwanted intrusive thoughts involved in clinical disorders cannot be restricted to any particular theme, or content. As evident in subsequent chapters, clinically relevant intrusive thoughts can encompass any topic, theme or content that is pertinent to the individual or situation at hand. Our definitions of unwanted intrusive thoughts, then, must specify the process characteristics, dimensions, or properties that enable clear identification of this cognitive phenomena and its differentiation from other types of clinical cognition (Clark & Purdon, 1995; Klinger, 1978; Parkinson & Rachman, 1981a).

For the purposes of this chapter, we define unwanted clinically relevant intrusive thoughts, images or impulses as

> *any distinct, identifiable cognitive event that is unwanted, unintended, and recurrent. It interrupts the flow of thought, interferes in task performance, is associated with negative affect, and is difficult to control.*

This definition is consistent with conceptualizations offered by other researchers interested in this phenomenon. Rachman (1981), for example, defined unwanted intrusive thoughts "as repetitive thoughts, images or impulses that are unacceptable and/or unwanted . . . are accompanied by subjective discomfort" (p. 89). According to Rachman, the necessary and sufficient conditions for a thought to be considered intrusive are that it interrupts an ongoing activity, is attributed to an internal origin, and is difficult to control.

The cognitive phenomena we labeled *clinically relevant unwanted intrusive thoughts* would also be consistent with Klinger's (1978, 1978–1979, 1996) description of a type of thought that is respondent (i.e., spontaneous, unintended thoughts that occur in response to a cue), undirected, and frequently stimulus independent. These thoughts interrupt ongoing activity and may, on occasion, involve content that the individual considers quite usual or strange. Singer (1998) noted that respondent processes include daydreams, fantasies, and nighttime dreams.

Horowitz (1975), in his research on cognitive and affective responses to traumatic stress, defined intrusive thoughts as "any thought that implies nonvolitional entry into awareness, requires suppressive effort or is hard to dispel, occurs perseveratively, or is experienced as something to be avoided" (p. 1458). Although these definitions are fairly precise, some researchers have assumed a broader definition of the phenomena, defining intrusive thoughts as any conscious thought that is internally generated and that distracts (interferes) from on-task activity (Yee & Vaughan, 1996).

Table 1.1 lists the key properties of unwanted intrusive thoughts that are based on our previous definition of the phenomena. The unwanted mental intrusions that are the focus of this inquiry are subjectively experienced as distinct or separate, identifiable thoughts, images,

TABLE 1.1. The Primary Properties or Dimensions of Clinically Relevant Unwanted Intrusive Thoughts, Images, or Impulses

- A distinct thought, image, or impulse that enters conscious awareness
- Attributed to an internal origin
- Considered unacceptable or unwanted
- Interferes in ongoing cognitive and/or behavioral activity
- Is unintended and nonvolitional or has willful independence
- Tends to be recurrent or repetitive
- Easily captures attentional resources; is highly distractible
- Is associated with negative affect (e.g, anxiety, dysphoria, and guilt)
- Difficult to control (dispel)

or impulses that quite suddenly enter conscious awareness. Thus our subject matter concerns conscious thought that is amenable to self-report. Unwanted intrusive thoughts, then, are not chains of mentation or more general patterns of sustained thought but rather discrete "cognitive bytes." Because any thought, image, or impulse could be experienced as a mental intrusion, it is important to consider both the properties or process characteristics of the thought as well as its content when identifying unwanted intrusive thoughts for particular clinical disorders (Clark & Purdon, 1995).

Beck's content-specificity hypothesis (Beck, 1967, 1987; Clark & Beck, 1999), which states that psychological disorders are characterized by a distinct cognitive content, might be helpful in distinguishing the type of unwanted intrusive thought content associated with different emotional states. The unwanted intrusions evident in depressive states would primarily involve thoughts of personal loss or failure, the mental intrusions relevant in anxiety would deal with threat and vulnerability, and the unwanted cognitions related to anger would involve themes of personal injustice and unfairness. As discussed later, researchers have been particularly interested in the role of unwanted intrusive thoughts in obsessive–compulsive disorder (OCD), where the theme involves ego-dystonic concerns (i.e., content that is inconsistent or contrary to a person's sense of self or identity). When investigating unwanted intrusive thoughts, then, it is important to take into consideration whether one is dealing with, for example, depressive, anxious, obsessive, intrusive cognitions.

The person experiencing an unwanted intrusive thought readily acknowledges that the phenomenon is his or her own thought; that is, it has an internal origin. Although this internal attribution would be applicable to all nonpsychotic intrusive thinking, Morrison (Chapter 7, this volume) makes a convincing argument that in psychotic states unwanted intrusive thoughts occur in which the person attributes his or her thoughts to an external source. Whether attributed to an internal or external source, we agree with Rachman (1981) that a critical feature of these mental intrusions is that the individual perceives them as unwanted or unacceptable in order to distinguish this phenomenon from a host of welcomed cognitive intrusions such as inspiration, pleasant daydreams, or fantasy.

One of the most important characteristics of unwanted intrusive thoughts is that they interfere in ongoing task performance (Sarason et al., 1996). Because of this interference, task-irrelevant intrusions have been most often studied within the context of test anxiety and, more recently athletic performance and social interaction (Pierce, Henderson, Yost, & Loffredo, 1996). Not only will unwanted intrusive thoughts interfere in current behavioral performance, but we can expect the intrusions to break into the flow of thought, thereby diverting attention away from some existing cognitive activity. One of the problems with unwanted intrusive thoughts is their capacity to interrupt concentration and impede cognitive and behavioral performance. As noted in Table 1.1, unwanted mentation is not easily ignored when it breaks into conscious awareness. Yee and Vaughan (1996) emphasized that cognitive interference must be understood in terms of impairment in the functioning of attention with interference indicated by the degree to which individuals are distracted from task performance by the imposition of a stimulus. In this sense, unwanted intrusive thoughts, images, and impulses would be an internal stimulus that is highly distracting because it captures attentional resources. Experimental research on control of unwanted intrusive thoughts indicates that individuals have a particularly hard time disattending to these mental intrusions (Edwards & Dickerson, 1987a; Sutherland, Newman, & Rachman, 1982).

Clinically relevant unwanted intrusive thoughts, images, and impulses are unintended or nonvolitional, are associated with negative affect, and are difficult to control. The nonvolitional, undirected or "spontaneous" (i.e., respondent orientation according to Klinger, 1996) quality of unwanted intrusive thoughts is the key property of this cognitive phenomenon. Klinger (1996) noted that intrusive thoughts occur without intended purpose, and Rachman (1981) speaks of the "wilful independence" of intrusive cognitions. Moreover, the unwanted intrusive thoughts relevant to clinical states also possess emotion-arousing properties. These are not benign or fairly neutral spontaneous mentation but, rather, cognition with an "emotional bite." Based on the content-specificity hypothesis, we expect that the type of emotional response associated with the intrusion will depend on its thought content. Given these characteristics, it is not surprising that unwanted intrusive thoughts are more difficult to suppress or ignore. As a result, they often reoccur despite the person's attempt to exert increased mental control.

Incidence

As documented throughout this volume, unwanted intrusive thoughts play an important role in the psychopathology of clinical disorders (see also Sarason et al., 1996). There is increasing evidence that effective treatment of anxiety, depression, insomnia, and other conditions will re-quire clinicians to target relevant distressing intrusive cognitions and the patient's reaction to these thoughts. On the other hand, what evidence do we have that nonclinical individuals experience the same type of un-wanted mental intrusions that we find in clinical disorders? If so, what are the differences between clinical and nonclinical samples? What im-plication does research on nonclinical samples have for our understand-ing of unwanted cognitive intrusions in clinical disorders?

Given the obvious relevance of unwanted intrusive thoughts for OCD, a number of studies have investigated whether nonclinical individ-uals experience unwanted intrusive thoughts, images, or impulses that have a similar content to clinical obsessions. Rachman and de Silva (1978) were the first to report that obsessions do occur in nonclinical individuals. They found that 84% of their nonclinical sample reported unwanted intrusive thoughts, images, or impulses that involved content very similar to clinical obsessions (repugnant themes of dirt, contamina-tion, accidents, injury, aggression, blasphemy, sex, etc.). Subsequent studies confirmed that 80–90% of the nonclinical population experience obsession-relevant unwanted mental intrusions (e.g., Freeston, Ladou-ceur, Thibodeau, & Gagnon, 1991; Niler & Beck, 1989; Parkinson & Rachman, 1981a; Purdon & Clark, 1993; Rachman & de Silva, 1978; Salkovskis & Harrison, 1984). Evidence that most nonclinical individu-als have occasional obsessive-like unwanted intrusive thoughts has played an important role in the development of new cognitive-behavioral for-mulations for OCD (Clark, 2004; Rachman, 1997, 1998, 2003; Sal-kovskis, 1985, 1989, 1999).

Klinger (1978–1979; Klinger & Cox, 1987–1988) conducted two thought-sampling studies in which students recorded their immediate thoughts whenever a timing device they carried with them throughout the day emitted a tone. In addition, participants rated each thought occurrence on 23 different dimensions. In the first study (Klinger, 1978–1979), 12 students produced 285 thought samples over a 24-day sampling period, whereas in the second study (Klinger 1987–1988), 29 undergraduates produced 1,425 thought samples over a 7-day period. Given that Klinger's concept of respondent thoughts is most closely related to our definition of unwanted intrusive thoughts, it is interesting that in the first study 27% of thoughts outside the laboratory were respondent, whereas in the second study 31% of the thoughts were rated as mainly or entirely undirected. Moreover, Klinger (1978–1979) found that 22% of the thoughts were rated by participants as very or somewhat strange or distorted, and later Klinger and Cox (1987–1988) found that 13% of the thoughts were self-rated as " 'out of character,' in gross disregard of others' expectations, or downright shocking" (p. 124). These unwanted intrusive thoughts sound very similar to the obsession-relevant cognitions that Rachman and colleagues identified in nonclinical samples. Klinger (1999) quotes from a thought-sampling dissertation study by Kroll-Mensing in which 33% of thought samples were nondirected and 18% were experienced as unacceptable and uncomfortable.

Although the presence of "normal" obsessions is clearly evident in the thought flow of nonclinical individuals, it is important not to overstate the frequency of this type of cognition in the general population. When assessment of unwanted intrusive thoughts was restricted to obsessional content (e.g., unwanted injury or violence against others, unacceptable sexual acts, dirt, or contamination), nonclinical individuals indicated that even their most common unwanted intrusion only occurred a few times a year (Purdon & Clark, 1994a, 1994b). This low frequency of ego-dystonic intrusive thoughts was replicated in a Korean student sample (Lee & Kwon, 2003). Furthermore, we recently conducted a structured interview on mental control with 100 university students (Wang, Clark, & Purdon, 2003). When asked to report two unwanted thoughts that they found difficult to control in the past week, the most frequently cited thoughts involved ego-syntonic anxious (i.e., worry-relevent) content, followed by thoughts with an obsessive content, then depressive-like thoughts, and finally angry cognitions. Moreover, students reported that these worry-related unwanted intrusive thoughts occurred several times a week but were quite successfully controlled with a moderate degree of effort.

There is other research supporting the view that the unwanted intrusive thoughts of nonclinical individuals are more likely to reflect ego-syntonic worry-related concerns than obsession-relevant ego-dystonic issues. For example, unwanted intrusive thoughts of insecurity, self-doubt, and failure have been shown to be a frequent and important factor in the heightened anxiety that many individuals experience in evaluative settings (i.e., test anxiety; Sarason et al., 1996). Horowitz (1975) has shown that individuals drawn from the general population experience a significant increase in the frequency and repetitiveness of stressful intrusive thoughts after watching distressing films involving accident and injury (see also Tata, 1989). Klinger (1977–1978; Klinger & Cox, 1987–1988) found that 96% of his participants' thoughts concerned their everyday experience, and that thoughts dealt with present life concerns 67% of the time. Likewise, students kept in a dark, sound-attenuated chamber for 24 hours reported thought content that primarily focused on real events occurring in the present and involving friends (Suedfeld, Ballard, Baker-Brown, & Borrie, 1985–1986).

Brewin, Christodoulides, and Hutchinson (1996) also found that nonclinical individuals reported a fairly high frequency of negative intrusive thoughts and memories over a 2-week period. However, in an earlier study by Clark and de Silva (1985), students estimated that negative depressive and anxious entered their mind fairly infrequently (i.e., between biweekly and monthly). Nevertheless, particular circumstances, life situations, or contexts may increase the frequency of unwanted intrusive thoughts. Parkinson and Rachman (1981b) reported that mothers whose children were admitted to hospital for tonsillectomy reported significantly more stress-related intrusive thoughts during a 20-minute period of listening to music than did control mothers. A high percentage of parents of newborns (65%) report that they experience unwanted intrusive thoughts of harm, injury, or illness occurring to their infant (Abramowitz, Schwartz, & Moore, 2004), and 41% of mothers with clinical depression have intrusive thoughts of harming their child (Jennings, Ross, Popper, & Elmore, 1999).

At this point a number of conclusions can be drawn about the clinically relevant unwanted intrusive thoughts in nonclinical individuals. Most nonclinical individuals experience unwanted intrusive thoughts, images, or impulses. A variety of thought content can take the form of an unwanted mental intrusion, including more bizarre ego-dystonic obsession-relevant intrusions. However ego-syntonic anxious or depressive thoughts are likely more common, and it is quite clear that external provocation, such as a stressful stimulus or life circumstance, can trigger a resurgence of unwanted cognitions (Horowitz, 1975; Parkinson & Rachman, 1981b). Information on the exact frequency of various types of unwanted intrusive thoughts in nonclinical populations remains unclear, and it is still not known whether some individuals are more vulnerable to the experience of unwanted cognitive intrusions than other individuals.

Correlates of Unwanted Intrusive Thoughts

A fairly consistent picture is emerging from research on the experience of obsessive, anxious, or depressive unwanted intrusive thoughts in nonclinical samples. The more frequent the unwanted intrusion, the more emotionally arousing or distressing the thought. Frequent and emotionally distressing intrusions are more difficult to control and are more likely to be associated with a negative mood state (Clark & de Silva, 1985; Freeston, Ladouceur, Thibodeau, & Gagnon,1992; Niler & Beck, 1989; Parkinson & Rachman, 1981a; Purdon & Clark, 1994a; Reynolds & Salkovskis, 1991; Salkovskis & Harrison, 1984). Reynolds and Salkovskis (1992) demonstrated a reciprocal relationship between mood and frequency of negative intrusive thoughts. In an initial experimental session, more frequent negative intrusions were associated with a deterioration in mood, whereas in a subsequent experimental session induction of a sad mood led to an increase in negative intrusions and a reduction in positive thoughts. Klinger (1978–1979) reported that participants rated respondent (i.e., intrusive, undirected, spontaneous, and nonvolitional) thoughts as less controllable than operant (more volition, purposeful goal-directed) thoughts.

Faulty Appraisals

There is also evidence that the meaning, significance, or importance attached to the unwanted intrusive thought can have a major impact on its frequency and controllability. Freeston et al. (1991), for example, found that unwanted intrusive thoughts that participants rated as highly disapproving were also considered the most difficult to control. In our own studies on unwanted intrusions in nonclinical individuals, concern that one might act on the intrusive thought was related to greater perceived difficulty controlling the unwanted thought (Clark, Purdon, & Byers, 2000; Purdon & Clark, 1994a, 1994b). In a more recent study, maladaptive beliefs that negative consequences are more likely if intrusive thoughts are not controlled were associated with increased frequency of unwanted intrusions (Clark, Purdon, & Wang, 2003). Lee and Kwon (2003) found that autogenous intrusive thoughts (i.e., ego-dystonic intrusions without an identifiable external trigger) were more difficult to control and tended to be appraised as more unacceptable, immoral, personally significant, and important to control. As well, a number of studies found a positive relationship between questionnaire and rating scale measures of the occurrence and perceived uncontrollability of unwanted negative intrusive or obsessional thoughts on the one hand and higher perceived responsibility for the thought and its anticipated consequences on the other hand (Forrester, Wilson & Salkovskis, 2002; Salkovskis et al., 2000; Wilson & Chambless, 1999; for contrary results, see Foa, Amir, Bogert, Molnar, & Przeworski, 2001).

Attention and Control

There is also evidence that heightened attentiveness to unwanted intrusions and increased effort to control these thoughts may actually result in greater difficulty with the unwanted cognitions. Evidence from a study by Janeck, Calameri, Riemann, and Heffelfinger (2003) indicates that a tendency to be especially attentive toward one's thoughts (i.e., cognitive self-consciousness) may be a factor in negative appraisal of unwanted intrusive thoughts, especially for individuals with OCD. In a thought suppression experiment, Purdon and Clark (2001) found that intentional suppression of obsession-relevant intrusive thoughts heightened the discomfort and unacceptability of the intrusions, with more frequent target thought intrusions associated with a more negative mood state. In a subsequent thought suppression study, Purdon (2001) found that the greater the number of unwanted thoughts during a suppression period, the greater the suppression effort. In an interview study, students who rated themselves as having less control over their unwanted intrusive thoughts were more likely to blame themselves for not trying hard enough to control the thought (Wang et al., 2003). It is apparent from these studies that greater attention and effort to control unwanted thoughts have a negative impact on individuals' experience of the cognition.

We can now construct a profile of unwanted intrusive thoughts in nonclinical individuals. Greater attention and effort to control unwanted thoughts, as well as a tendency to misconstrue these thoughts as highly significant because of anticipated negative consequences or threat to self or others, may actually lead to greater difficulty with the very thoughts one desires to avoid. If this process continues, one could envision the development of a significant clinical problem with unwanted intrusive thoughts.

Clinical versus Nonclinical

In support of this formulation, it is now clear that the primary difference between the unwanted intrusive thoughts in clinical and nonclinical samples is one of degree rather than kind. Studies that have directly compared the characteristics, responses, and appraisals of unwanted intrusive thoughts in clinical and nonclinical individuals generally find quantitative rather than qualitative between-group differences. For example, research comparing the obsession-relevant intrusions of nonclinical individuals with the obsessions of OCD patients found that the primary difference between the two groups is that individuals with OCD experience more frequent, distressing, uncontrollable, and unacceptable intrusions and perceive these thoughts to be less controllable (Calamari & Janeck, 1997; Janeck & Calamari, 1999; Rachman & de Silva, 1978). In addition, OCD patients more strongly resist their obsessions than do nonclinical comparison groups, are more likely to engage in neutralization, have a greater tendency to use maladaptive thought control strategies, and perceive these control efforts to be less successful (Amir, Cashman, & Foa, 1997; Ladouceur et al., 2000).

In a recent study on ego-syntonic or worry-related negative intrusive thoughts, Ruscio and Borkovec (in press) found that both nonclinical high worriers and individuals with diagnosable generalized anxiety disorder (GAD) experienced a brief "burst" of negative intrusive thoughts during a 5-minute focused attention task after they spent 5 minutes concentrating on their primary worry. In terms of subjective ratings, the GAD and non-GAD worriers produced similar ratings on the frequency, distress, and intensity of worry-intrusive thoughts during the postworry induction focused attention task. However, differences were apparent with a higher proportion of the clinical worry group reporting negative intrusions during the postinduction attentional task than did the nonclinical worry group. In addition, the GAD worriers reported less perceived control over their worry intrusions during the experiment, and they showed a tendency to subjectively appraise the thoughts as more dangerous and uncontrollable than did the nonclinical worry group. Together these findings indicate that clinical individuals experience a higher frequency of unwanted intrusive thoughts that may be more easily cued by contextual factors, and they are more likely to appraise these thoughts in a maladaptive and uncontrollable fashion. Again, though, these differences are a matter of degree rather than kind.

UNWANTED INTRUSIVE THOUGHTS
AND OTHER TYPES OF NEGATIVE COGNITION

The stream of consciousness is a busy highway clogged with a variety of thoughts, images, memories, sensations, and feelings. In the last two decades, cognitive–clinical psychologists have identified a number of different types of thought form and content that appear to play an important role in the pathogenesis of clinical disorders. It is important, then, to clarify whether unwanted intrusive thoughts can be distinguished from other types of negative cognition. Is there something unique about mental intrusions that differentiate them from other types of negative cognition, or, in the end, are we merely describing the same mental phenomena from different theoretical perspectives or research traditions?

Obsessions and Unwanted Intrusive Thoughts

Much of the interest in unwanted intrusive thoughts in nonclinical samples came from research into the etiology of obsessions. Clinical obsessions, in many respects, represent the extreme clinical variant of unwanted intrusive thoughts. The conceptualization of intrusive cognition offered in this chapter could be used to characterize more severe clinical obsessions. Thus unwanted intrusive thoughts and obsessions can be placed on a severity continuum, with their distinction being one of degree rather than kind. Table 1.2 summarizes a number of dimensions along which unwanted intrusive thoughts and obsessions can be distinguished. Various cognitive appraisal models have been proposed to explain how a relatively infrequent, ego-dystonic intrusive thought can escalate in frequency and intensity to become a clinical obsession (Clark, 2004; Rachman, 1997, 1998, 2003; Salkovskis, 1985, 1989, 1999). Whether an unwanted ego-dystonic intrusive thought can be considered an obsession or an unwanted mental intrusion will depend on whether the subjective experience of the thought falls toward the more extreme end of the dimensions listed in Table 1.2.

Worry versus Unwanted Intrusive Thoughts

Worry is ubiquitous to the human experience. No doubt everyone has experienced worry at some time in their life. Moreover, worry is a central feature of anxiety states, especially GAD. Worrisome thinking can dominant human thought flow and cause considerable interference in task performance. The most widely accepted definition of worry was formulated by Borkovec, Robinson, Pruzinsky, and DePree (1983):

> Worry is a chain of thoughts and images, negatively affect-laden and relatively uncontrollable. The worry process represents an attempt to engage in mental problem-solving on an issue whose outcome is uncer-

TABLE 1.2. Dimensions That Distinguish Nonclinical Unwanted Intrusive
Thoughts and Clinical Obsessions

Unwanted mental intrusions	Clinical obsessions
Less frequent	More frequent
Less unacceptable/distressing	More unacceptable/distressing
Little associated guilt	Significant feelings of guilt
Less resistance to the intrusion	Strong resistance to the intrusion
Some perceived control	Diminished perceived control over the obsession
Considered meaningless, irrelevant to the self	Considered highly meaningful, threatening important core values of the self (ego-dystonic)
Brief intrusions that fail to dominate conscious awareness	Time-consuming intrusions that dominate conscious awareness
Less concern with thought control	Heightened concern with thought control
Less emphasis on neutralizing distress	Strong focus on neutralizing distress associated with the obsession
Less interference in daily living	Significant interference in daily living

Note. From Clark (2004). Copyright 2004 by The Guilford Press. Reprinted by permission.

tain but contains the possibility of one or more negative outcomes. Consequently, worry relates closely to fear process. (p. 10)

There is considerable evidence that nonclinical individuals engage in worry, although not to the same frequency, intensity, and uncontrollability as patients with GAD (Craske, Rapee, Jackel, & Barlow, 1989; Dupuy, Beaudoin, Rhéaume, Ladouceur, & Dugas, 2001). Like other clinical phenomena, a recent taxometric analysis of selected worry questionnaire items suggests that worry is a dimensional rather than categorical construct (Ruscio, Borkovec & Ruscio, 2001). Based on a 2-week self-monitoring study, Dupuy et al. (2001) found that nonclinical individuals worried 55 minutes per day. Tallis, Eysenck, and Mathews (1992) reported that 50–75% of their nonclinical sample endorsed most of the worry statement items that were selected for the Worry Domains Questionnaire. The types of worry concerns expressed by nonclinical individuals include work/school (19–30%), family/home/interpersonal (26–44%), finances (13–26%), illness/health/injury (2–25%), or miscellaneous (0–15%) (Borkovec, Shadick, & Hopkins, 1991).

A number of researchers have compared worry and unwanted intrusive thoughts (for further discussion, see Wells, Chapter 5, this volume).

Unwanted intrusive thoughts and worry share certain characteristics that can make discrimination difficult. Both types of cognition easily capture attentional resources, interfere in ongoing activities, are difficult to control, and are subjectively unpleasant or distressing (Borkovec et al., 1991). However, a number of key differences have emerged from studies that compared individuals' subjective experience of worry and unwanted intrusive thoughts (Clark & Claybourn, 1997; Langlois, Freeston, & Ladouceur, 2000a, 2000b; Lee, Lee, Kim, Kwon, & Telch, 2003; Wells & Morrison, 1994). Worry predominantly takes a verbal or linguistic form and is more distressing or unpleasant, more realistic but tends to cause greater interference in functioning, is more voluntary but intrusive, is more persistent and of longer duration, and possibly is more difficult to dismiss, although the research is mixed on this last point. In addition, the faulty appraisals that characterize worry tend to focus on whether the dreaded consequences of the worry-related negative events might come true. On the other hand, unwanted intrusions consist of both thoughts and images and are less voluntary, of shorter duration, and more ego-dystonic. The faulty appraisals associated with unwanted intrusions more likely involve concerns about personal responsibility and whether the intrusion reflects negatively on one's personality. Intrusive thoughts and worry may differ less in degree of controllability, their intrusiveness, the extent to which they are resisted, and the types of control strategies used to deal with the unwanted thoughts. Contrary to expectation, there may be a greater compulsion to act on worries than unwanted ego-dysontic intrusive thoughts.

In summary, the distinguishing characteristics of clinically relevant unwanted intrusive thoughts vis-à-vis worry may be that it is experienced as a brief, nonvolitional, undirected, and stimulus-independent "mental flash" that is quite different from one's present train of thought. Worry, on the other hand, appears as a more sustained and persistent pattern of thought that is closely linked in a negative fashion to the individual's current concerns. For this reason, worry is consistently rated as a more problematic cognitive state for nonclinical individuals than are unwanted intrusive thoughts. However, evidence that brief periods of worry can lead to a subsequent increase in negative intrusive thoughts indicates a strong functional relationship exists between the two types of cognitions (Borkovec et al., 1983; York, Borkovec, Vasey, & Stern, 1987; Wells & Papageorgiou, 1995). As well, Langlois, Ladouceur, Patrick, and Freeston (2004) reported that illness intrusions share many important characteristics with other types of ego-syntonic worry. These findings remind us that unwanted mental intrusions and worry are closely related phenomena, and together they can have a significant emotional impact on the individual.

Rumination and Unwanted Intrusions

Persistent and repetitive, or ruminative, negative thinking is another type of cognition that has been linked to adverse emotional states, especially depression. Beck (1967) observed that the moderately or severely depressed person has a tendency to brood or ruminate over negative aspects of the self or external situations. However, it was Nolen-Hoeksema's (1991) conceptualization of rumination that sparked research on its role and function in depression. She defined rumination "as repetitive and passive thinking about one's symptoms of depression and the possible causes and consequences of these symptoms" (Nolen-Hoeksema, 2004, p. 107). Borkovec, Ray, and Stober (1998) commented that depressive rumination appears to have a similar process and content to worry phenomena in GAD. Certainly repetitive thought, a cardinal feature of rumination and worry, is a significant predictor of both anxious and depressive symptoms in nonclinical samples (Segerstrom, Tsao, Alden, & Craske, 2000).

Given that depressive rumination and worry have many similarities, it is important that unwanted intrusive thoughts be distinguishable from ruminative thinking, especially given the heightened incidence of intrusions in depressed states (Brewin et al., 1996; Brewin, Reynolds, & Tata, 1999; Jennings et al., 1999). However, there are no published empirical studies that directly compared unwanted intrusions and rumination in clinical or nonclinical samples. Papageorgiou and Wells (2004) recently provided an informative discussion of the nature of depressive rumination that suggests some key differences between rumination and intrusions. They state that ruminative thinking involves chains of repetitive, recyclic, negative, and self-focused thinking that can be cued by an external event but more often is triggered by a prior thought. The focus of the rumination is often some aspect of the self or one's emotional state, or it could involve negative inferences about a stressful life event. In a series of studies that compared rumination and worry, Papageorgiou and Wells (2004) were able to flesh out a number of key characteristics of rumination such as past orientation, reduced confidence and problem-solving effort, and longer duration.

Although direct comparison studies are needed, it is likely that unwanted intrusive thoughts can be quite easily distinguished from rumination. Rumination represents a much longer train of thought that is recurrent, repetitive, cyclical, highly ego-syntonic, past oriented, and directed. Unwanted intrusions, on the other hand, are brief, sudden, and somewhat unexpected thoughts or images, of relatively short duration, often ego-dystonic, and undirected by the individual. It may be that the repeated occurrence of a similar type of unwanted intrusive thought or image could trigger an episode of depressive rumination.

Negative Automatic Thoughts and Unwanted Intrusions

Beck (1967, 1976) first observed that clinically depressed patients experience a train of negative thought that is not reported but that runs concurrent with more conscious focused thought. Labeled *negative automatic thoughts*, these thoughts appeared to intrude rapidly and with little effort. They were highly self-focused and dealt with negative views about the self, personal world, or future. From his clinical observations, Beck deduced that negative automatic thoughts tended to (1) be very fleeting, (2) be highly specific or discrete, (3) be spontaneous, (4) be plausible to the individual, (5) be idiosyncratic to the individual's personal concerns, (6) precede emotional arousal, and (7) involve a bias or distortion of reality (see Clark & Beck, 1999).

Beck's concept of negative automatic thoughts shares a number of characteristics with unwanted intrusive thoughts, especially within the context of depressed states. In the intervening years, numerous studies using questionnaire, interview, and self-monitoring methods have demonstrated that nonclinical individuals experience negative automatic depressive and anxious thoughts, although they are less frequent, intense, and plausible (i.e., believed) than the negative automatic thoughts that characterize clinical states (for reviews, see Clark & Beck, 1999). This raises the possibility that the same cognitive phenomena could be labeled *unwanted intrusions* in one study and *negative automatic thoughts* in another study, depending on ones theoretical perspective and research tradition.

Salkovskis (1985) argued that negative automatic thoughts as defined by Beck (1976) and unwanted intrusive thoughts (or obsessions) as described by Rachman (1981) can be clearly differentiated in terms of content and process characteristics. The content of unwanted intrusions is more likely perceived as irrational and ego-dystonic, whereas negative automatic thoughts are considered more rational and ego-syntonic. In addition, unwanted intrusive thoughts, images, and impulses are more intrusive, more disruptive of ongoing activity, and more easily accessed, whereas negative automatic thoughts tend to run parallel to conscious awareness, are harder to access, and may cause less momentary interference in task performance.

There are a number of other characteristics that may distinguish unwanted intrusive cognition from negative automatic thoughts. Because negative automatic thoughts are an inherent quality of the depressed or anxious state, they are more plausible, directed, and volitional. Though unwanted intrusive thoughts are influenced by mood state, nevertheless they show less mood contiguity and are less plausible, more nonvolitional, and more spontaneous. A much higher proportion of unwanted mental intrusions occur as images, whereas negative automatic thoughts predominantly occur in the linguistic, verbal mode. Negative automatic thoughts also tend to be longer, more elaborative chains of evaluative thoughts, whereas unwanted mental intrusions are sudden bursts of discrete, highly distracting, and attention-grabbing thoughts, images, or impulses. Until the necessary comparison studies are published, the distinction between clinically relevant unwanted intrusive thoughts and negative automatic thoughts remains based on clinical observation.

ORIGINS OF UNWANTED INTRUSIVE THOUGHTS

Given the ubiquitous nature of unwanted intrusive thoughts, images, and impulses and their significant role in many psychological disorders, why do we have these sudden, inexplicable mental intrusions? What are the origins of these unwanted intrusions given their apparent discordance with self-interests, their disrupting influence on task performance, and their minimal relevance to goal-directed pursuits? Are they an inconsequential by-product of our problem-solving capability, or an inherent part of human imagination or curiosity seeking? (L. Ford, October 22, 2003, personal communication)

Unfortunately, empirical research into unwanted intrusive thoughts has not devoted much attention to the origin and role of this cognitive phenomenon in normal functioning. Salkovskis (1988), for example, suggests that unwanted intrusive thoughts are an inherent aspect of generating ideas for problem solving. He notes that "brainstorming" is a critical element in human problem solving. To consider all possible solutions to a current concern or problem, it is important that novel ideas are generated without prior censorship in a manner that maintains attentional priority. Unwanted mental intrusions, then, are considered a product of human problem-solving capacity where the generation and conscious awareness of ideas must occur prior to any evaluative process. Salkovskis contends that even our normally unacceptable intrusive thoughts may be useful under changed circumstances. The intrusive and compelling nature of these thoughts or ideas ensures that they are noticed and evaluated for possible relevance to current concerns, goals, and problems. Intrusive thoughts produced by an "idea generator" with little relevance to our immediate goals or concerns will not persist because of limited attentional resources. However, intrusions which are evaluated as relevant to immediate concerns will persist and attain salience regardless of their acceptability. In support of this perspective, Salkovskis cites research showing that nonclinical individuals have both positive (pleasant) and negative (unpleasant) intrusions that are experienced in a similar manner (Edwards & Dickerson, 1987b; England & Dickerson, 1988).

Although Salkovskis's view on the origins of unwanted intrusive thoughts has not been elaborated in subsequent years, it is broadly consistent with formulations proposed by Rachman (1981, 2003) and Klinger (1978, 1996). Next we consider three explanations of the etiology of unwanted mental intrusions proposed by Rachman (1981, 2003), Klinger (1978, 1996), and Horowitz (1975).

Rachman's Account

Rachman's view on the origins of unwanted intrusive thoughts primarily concerns the etiology of obsessions. Rachman (1981) commented that external cues are important in the provocation of unwanted intrusive impulses (i.e., sudden urge to jump in front of an oncoming subway train), but the role of the environmental context in triggering unwanted intrusive thoughts or images is much less clear. In fact, he noted that intrusive thoughts are often more frequent and intense during periods of solitude.

Rachman contends that setting conditions and internal origins may be more critical in the genesis of unwanted intrusive thoughts and images (Rachman, 1978, 1981, 2003; Rachman & Hodgson, 1980). Two conditions that may be particularly important in the provocation of unwanted intrusive thoughts and images are stress and a dysphoric mood state. Research reviewed by Rachman indicates that individuals have more frequent and distressing mental intrusions when exposed to stressful conditions and they have greater difficulty ignoring or suppressing unwanted thoughts during a sad mood state (see Wenzlaff, Chapter 3, this volume). As well, Rachman (2003) raised the possibility that dysphoria may result in a greater tendency to misinterpret the significance and feared consequences of the intrusion.

Rachman (1978) suggests that certain personality characteristics, such as heightened sensitivity to threat or danger, neuroticism (high negative emotionality), conscientiousness, and timidity, may also increase sensitivity or responsiveness to unwanted intrusive thoughts and images. Individuals high in these personality traits may be more inclined to interpret their thoughts as highly significant and unacceptable events that challenge their basic values and concerns. As well, a person with heightened sensitivity to external danger or threat cues will be provoked by a wider range of stimuli. As a result, he or she will experience more unwanted distressing intrusive thoughts, images, and impulses.

In summary, Rachman suggests a number of possible precipitants of unwanted mental intrusions, including external cues, stress, dyphoric mood, and certain predisposing personality characteristics. Although Rachman's ideas are useful in understanding the provocation of unwanted intrusions, especially those with obsessive content, they do not really address the more fundamental question of the origins and function of this cognitive phenomenon in nonclinical individuals.

Klinger's Thought-Shifting Theory

The intrusion of unwanted thoughts, images, or impulses into the flow of thought can be viewed as a sudden shift in thought content. From this perspective, an explication of the variables responsible for shifts in thought content would indicate how unwanted intrusive thoughts are generated. The main tenet of Klinger's (1996) model is that "thought content shifts when an individual encounters a cue that arouses emotion because of its association with one of the individual's current concerns" (p. 4). The concept of *current concern*, then, plays a central role in understanding the frequent, rapid shifts in thought content.

Current concerns is a motivational construct that refers to "the latent state of an organism between the two time points of commitment to striving for a particular goal and either goal attainment or disengagement from that goal" (Klinger, 1996, p. 4). Current concerns are presumed to underlie various cognitive processes including the formation of thought content. Moreover, an individual's current concerns will make him or her particularly sensitive or emotionally reactive to cues associated with valued goals or the means for attaining these goals (Klinger, 1996). These concern-related cues may be external stimuli, nonverbal events, or even other events within the stream of consciousness (Klinger, 1999). If some goal-directed response cannot be initiated by the cued concern-related thought, then the thought will remain a spontaneous, idle cognitive response. Klinger (1996) states that cues leading to shifts in thought content will be evaluated at various levels of information processing. At a central, preconscious level, gross features of a cue are evaluated and a *protoemotional response* is generated. This leads to further higher-level processing that confirms or disconfirms the cue's relevance to current concerns. If the relevance of the cue is disconfirmed, then processing ends, whereas confirmation of the cue's relevance to current concerns will lead to further processing and/or some response or action (Klinger, 1999).

There are two important qualifications about the processing of emotional cues associated with current concerns (Klinger, 1996, 1998, 1999). First, the processing of concern-related emotional cues will conflict with ongoing activity for attention and other processing resources. If attention to the emotional cue can be inhibited so that attentional resources can remain focused on the ongoing activity, then the concern-related emotional cues may be processed without entering conscious awareness. However, the concern-related emotional cues will enter consciousness if they exceed a certain threshold for interrupting the ongoing stream of thought. In other words, a certain amount of preconscious processing occurs with concern-related emotional cues. A second qualification is that cues that elicit hard-wired emotional responses or a conditioned emotional response may produce conscious thought content in the absence of a current concern, although in most instances emotional responses reflect current concerns.

Research support can be found for Klinger's view of a close relation between current concerns and greater responsive to emotional cues. In an early study involving a dichotic listening task, Klinger (1978) found that participants attended more closely to concern-related passages, recalled more words from these passages, and generated more thoughts in response to the concern-related passage than to the non-concern-related passage. Other studies have shown that individuals exhibit enhanced processing of concern-related material (for review, see Klinger, 1996). These findings suggest that the ability of intrusive thoughts to gain attentional priority might stem from their connection to the individual's current concerns.

Thus what can be concluded from this model about the origins of unwanted intrusive thoughts? First, motivation (i.e., an individual's primary goals or current concerns) will have a powerful impact on the types of thoughts, images, or impulses that intrude into conscious awareness. Second, any internal or external cue relevant to a person's current concerns (i.e., goal pursuits) can elicit an emotional response, and this emotional response may precede extensive cognitive processing. Third, some degree of preconscious emotional and cognitive processing will occur in response to concern-related emotional cues. Thus the intrusion of an unwanted thought, image, or impulse is the result of an emotionally arousing concern-related cue that triggers a shift in thought content. To understand why an individual has certain unwanted intrusive thoughts, it is necessary to determine his or her current concerns, including any dormant or latent concerns, as well as the cues that are capable of eliciting an emotional response.

Horowitz's Formulation

Horowitz (1975) proposed a cognitive reformulation derived from the prevailing psychoanalytic explanation at that time for the repeated intrusion of thoughts and feelings following termination of a stressful event or stimulus. The account is based on three propositions about active memory: (1) active memory storage is characterized by an intrinsic tendency to repeat its represented contents, (2) this will continue until storage of contents in active memory is terminated, and (3) termination of active memory contents will occur only when cognitive processing is complete. According to Horowitz, the contents of active memory follow an automatic "completion tendency." The complete cognitive processing of stressful or traumatic events occurs with the assimilation and accommodation of information dealing with the meaning, interpretation, and implication of the event with the planning and assessment of one's coping resources.

Horowitz (1975) states that external stressful events will stimulate in active memory an internalized representation of the experience, which itself is influenced by internal factors such as the motivational state of the person, defensive and coping strategies, and the personal meaning of the event. There is a tendency for the internal representation of the event in active memory to reemerge repeatedly into consciousness when control capacity is low and concentration on external demands can not be maintained. As well, internal or external cues may trigger recollections. Thus intrusive and repetitive thoughts of the stressful event will continue until there is an integration of new and old information. Representations (memories) of the stressful event may conflict with a person's inner model of the world and thus remain in active memory until these inner models are modified to accord with the new stressful experience (Horowitz, 2003). That is, schemas of the self, world, and others must be revised so that new memories of the traumatic or stressful event are created that adequately fit with existing memory representations. When this occurs, the stress-relevant representations in active memory are erased and, as a consequence, stress-related intrusive thoughts cease. The stressful event now becomes coded with other relevant associations in inactive memory.

Horowitz's formulation is particularly helpful in understanding unwanted cognition that is provoked by highly stressful or traumatic events. It provides less insight into the apparently irrelevant, uncharacteristic intrusive thoughts that often interrupt the normal flow of thought. Nevertheless, Horowitz reminds us that certain aspects of memory storage may be inclined toward the conscious intrusion and repetition of unwanted material. In addition, his formulation emphasizes that unwanted intrusive thoughts may represent a failure to integrate new information of external events with existing internal working models of the self and world.

CONCLUSION

In this chapter we have discussed the existence of unwanted intrusive thoughts, images, and impulses in nonclinical populations. Although three decades have passed since the first empirical studies on unwanted cognitions in nonclinical individuals, a convergence of thought on the nature, role, and function of this phenomenon in normal functioning is lacking. Theory and research on unwanted intrusive thoughts have proceeded quite separately within different research streams. The social psychologists interested in consciousness and thought flow have pursued their research agenda on thought content quite independent of the clinical research on the same phenomenon. Even within the clinical domain, there has been little cross-fertilization in research on unwanted intrusive thoughts in the context of OCD and the work on cognitive intrusions in other anxiety states such as performance evaluation or test anxiety. It is hoped that the definitional issues addressed in this chapter, the differentiation of unwanted intrusive thoughts from other types of negative cognition, and a consideration of the origins of intrusive thoughts in nonclinical states will help advance our research into this phenomena. The chapters that follow provide a more focused discussion of the processes involved in the transition from nonclinical unwanted intrusive thoughts to the more frequent, distressing, and uncontrollable mental intrusions so prominent in a variety of clinical states.

ACKNOWLEDGMENT

Work on this chapter was supported by a grant (No. 410-2001-0084) from the Social Sciences and Humanities Research Council of Canada awarded to David A. Clark.

REFERENCES

Abramowitz, J. S., Schwartz, S. A., & Moore, K. M. (2004). *Obsessional thoughts in postpartum females and their partners: Content, severity, and relationship with depression*. Manuscript submitted for publication.

Amir, N., Cashman, L., & Foa, E. B. (1997). Strategies of thought control in obsessive–compulsive disorder. *Behaviour Research and Therapy, 35*, 775–777.

Beck, A. T. (1967). *Depression: Clinical, experimental, and theoretical aspects.* New York: Harper & Row.

Beck, A. T. (1976). *Cognitive therapy and the emotional disorders.* New York: New American Library.

Beck, A. T. (1987). Cognitive models of depression. *Journal of Cognitive Pyschotherapy: An International Quarterly, 1*, 5–37.

Borkovec, T. D., Ray, W. J., & Stober, J. (1998). Worry: A cognitive phenomenon intimately linked to affective, physiological, and interpersonal behavioral processes. *Cognitive Therapy and Research, 22*, 561–576.

Borkovec, T. D., Robinson, E., Prudinsky, T., & DePree, J. A. (1983). Preliminary investigation of worry: Some characteristics and processes. *Behaviour Research and Therapy, 21*, 9–16.

Borkovec, T. D., Shadick, R. N., & Hopkins, M. (1991). The nature of normal and pathological worry. In R. M. Rapee & D. H. Barlow (Eds.), *Chronic anxiety: Generalized anxiety disorder and mixed anxiety–depression* (pp. 29–51). New York: Guilford Press.

Brewin, C. R., Christodoulides, J., & Hutchinson, G. (1996). Intrusive thoughts and intrusive memories in a nonclinical sample. *Cognition and Emotion, 10*, 107–112.

Brewin, C. R., Reynolds, M., & Tata, P. (1999). Autobiographical memory processes and the course of depression. *Journal of Abnormal Psychology, 108*, 511–517.

Calamari, J. E., & Janeck, A. S. (1997). *Negative intrusive thoughts in obsessive–compulsive disorder: Appraisal and response differences.* Poster presented at the National Convention of the Anxiety Disorders Association of America, New Orleans.

Clark, D. A. (2004). *Cognitive-behavioral therapy for OCD*. New York: Guilford Press.

Clark, D. A., & Beck, A. T. (with Alford, B.) (1999). *Scientific foundations of cognitive theory and therapy of depression*. New York: Wiley.

Clark, D. A., & Claybourn, M. (1997). Process characteristics of worry and obsessive intrusive thoughts. *Behaviour Research and Therapy, 35*, 1139–1141.

Clark, D. A., & de Silva, P. (1985). The nature of depressive and anxious, intrusive thoughts: Distinct or uniform phenomena? *Behaviour Research and Therapy, 23*, 383–393.

Clark, D. A., & Purdon, C. L. (1995). The assessment of unwanted intrusive thoughts: A review and critique of the literature. *Behaviour Research and Therapy, 33*, 967–976.

Clark, D. A., Purdon, C., & Byers, E. S. (2000). Appraisal and control of sexual and non-sexual intrusive thoughts in university students. *Behaviour Research and Therapy, 38*, 439–455.

Clark, D. A., Purdon, C., & Wang, A. (2003). The Meta-Cognitive Beliefs Questionnaire: Development of a measure of obsessional beliefs. *Behaviour Research and Therapy, 41*, 655–669.

Craske, M. G., Rapee, R. M., Jackel, L., & Barlow, D. H. (1989). Qualitative dimensions of worry in DSM-III-R generalized anxiety disorder subjects and nonanxious controls. *Behaviour Research and Therapy, 27*, 397–402.

Dupuy, J.-B., Beaudoin, S., Rhéaume, J., Ladouceur, R., & Dugas, M. J. (2001). Worry: Daily self-report in clinical and non-clinical populations. *Behaviour Research and Therapy, 39*, 1249–1255.

Edwards, S., & Dickerson, M. (1987a). Intrusive unwanted thoughts: A two-stage model of control. *British Journal of Medical Psychology, 60*, 317–328.

Edwards, S., & Dickerson, M. (1987b). On the similarity of positive and negative intrusions. *Behaviour Research and Therapy, 25*, 207–211.

England, S. L., & Dickerson, M. (1988). Intrusive thoughts: unpleasantness not the major cause of uncontrollability. *Behaviour Research and Therapy, 26*, 279–282.

Foa, E. B., Amir, N., Bogert, K. V. A., Molnar, C., & Przeworski, A. (2001). Inflated perception of responsibility for harm in obsessive-compulsive disorder. *Journal of Anxiety Disorders, 15*, 259–275.

Forrester, E., Wilson, C., & Salkovskis, P. M. (2002). The occurrence of intrusive thoughts transforms meaning in ambiguous situations: An experimental study. *Behavioural and Cognitive Psychotherapy, 30*, 143–152.

Freeston, M. H., Ladouceur, R., Thibodeau, N., & Gagnon, F. (1991). Cognitive intrusions in a non-clinical population: I. Response style, subjective experience, and appraisal. *Behaviour Research and Therapy, 29*, 585–597.

Freeston, M. H., Ladouceur, R., Thibodeau, N., & Gagnon, F. (1992). Cognitive intrusions in a non-clinical population: II. Associations with depressive, anxious, and compulsive symptoms. *Behaviour Research and Therapy, 30*, 263–271.

Horowitz, M. J. (1975). Intrusive and repetitive thoughts after experimental stress: A summary. *Archives of General Psychiatry, 32,* 1457–1463.

Horowitz, M. J. (2003). *Treatment of stress response syndromes.* Washington, DC: American Psychiatric Association Press.

James, W. (1950). *The principles of psychology* (Vol. 1). New York: Dover. (Original work published 1890)

Janeck, A. S., & Calamari, J. E. (1999). Thought suppression in obsessive–compulsive disorder. *Cognitive Therapy and Research, 23,* 497–509.

Janeck, A. S., Calamari, J. E., Riemann, B. C., & Heffelfinger, S. K. (2003). Too much thinking about thinking?: Metacognitive differences in obsessive–compulsive disorder. *Journal of Anxiety Disorders, 17,* 181–195.

Jennings, K. D., Ross, S., Popper, S., & Elmore, M. (1999). Thoughts of harming infants in depressed and nondepressed mothers. *Journal of Affective Disorders, 54,* 21–28.

Klinger, E. (1978). Modes of normal conscious flow. In K. S. Pope & J. L. Singer (Eds.), *The stream of consciousness.* New York: Plenum Press.

Klinger, E. (1978–1979). Dimensions of thought and imagery in normal waking states. *Journal of Altered States of Consciousness, 4,* 97–113.

Klinger, E. (1996). The contents of thoughts: Interference as the downside of adaptive normal mechanisms in thought flow. In I. G. Sarason, G. R. Pierce, & B. R. Sarason (Eds.), *Cognitive interference: Theories, methods, and findings* (pp. 3–23). Mahwah, NJ: Erlbaum.

Klinger, E. (1998). The search for meaning in evolutionary perspective and its clinical implications. In P. T. Wong & J. A. Fry (Eds.), *The human quest for meaning: The handbook of psychological research.* Mahwah, NJ: Erlbaum.

Klinger, E. (1999). Thought flow: Properties and mechanisms underlying shifts in content. In J. Singer & P. Salovey (Eds.), *At play in the fields of consciousness: Essays in honor of Jerome Singer* (pp. 29–50). Mahwah, NJ: Erlbaum.

Klinger, E., & Cox, W. M. (1987–1988). Dimensions of thought flow in everyday life. *Imagination, Cognition and Personality, 7,* 105–128.

Ladouceur, R., Freeston, M. H., Rhéaume, J., Dugas, M. J., Gagnon, F., Thibodeau, N., & Fournier, S. (2000). Strategies used with intrusive thoughts: A comparison of OCD patients with anxious and community controls. *Journal of Abnormal Psychology, 109,* 179–187.

Langlois, F., Freeston, M. H., & Ladouceur, R. (2000a). Differences and similarities between obsessive intrusive thoughts and worry in a non-clinical population: Study 1. *Behaviour Research and Therapy, 38,* 157–173.

Langlois, F., Freeston, M. H., & Ladouceur, R. (2000b). Differences and similarities between obsessive intrusive thoughts and worry in a non-clinical population: Study 2. *Behaviour Research and Therapy, 38,* 175–189.

Langlois, F., Ladouceur, R., Patrick, G., & Freeston, M. H. (2004). Characteristics of illness intrusions in a non-clinical sample. *Behaviour Research and Therapy, 42,* 683–696.

Lee, H.-J., & Kwon, S.-M. (2003). Two different types of obsession: Autogenous obsessions and reactive obsessions. *Behaviour Research and Therapy*, *41*, 11–29.

Lee, H.-J., Lee, S.-H., Kim, H.-S., Kwon, S.-M., & Telch, M. J. (2003). *A comparison of autogenous/reactive obsessions and worry in a nonclinical population.* Poster presented at the annual meeting of the Association for the Advancement of Behavior Therapy, Boston.

Niler, E. R., & Beck, S. J. (1989). The relationship among guilt, dysphoria, anxiety and obsessions in a normal population. *Behaviour Research and Therapy*, *27*, 213–220.

Nolen-Hoeksoma, S. (1991). Response to depression and their effects on the duration of depressive episodes. *Journal of Abnormal Psychology*, *100*, 569–582.

Nolen-Hoeksoma, S. (2004). The response styles theory. In C. Papageorgiou & A. Wells (Eds.), *Depressive rumination: Nature, theory and treatment* (pp. 107–123). Chichester, UK: Wiley.

Papageorgiou, C., & Wells, A. (2004). Nature, functions, and beliefs about depressive rumination. In C. Papageorgiou & A. Wells (Eds.), *Depressive rumination: Nature, theory and treatment* (pp. 3–20). Chichester, UK: Wiley.

Parkinson, L., & Rachman, S. (1981a). Part II. The nature of intrusive thoughts. *Advances in Behaviour Research and Therapy*, *3*, 101–110.

Parkinson, L., & Rachman, S. J. (1981b). Part III. Intrusive thoughts: The effects of an uncontrived stress. *Advances in Behaviour Research and Therapy*, *3*, 111–118.

Pierce, G. R., Henderson, C. A., Yost J. H., & Loffredo, C. M. (1996). Cognitive interference and personality: Theoretical and methodological issues. In I. G. Sarason, G. R. Pierce, & B. R. Sarason (Eds.), *Cognitive interference: Theories, methods and findings* (pp. 285–296). Mahwah, NJ: Erlbaum.

Pope, K. S., & Singer, J. L. (Eds.). (1978). *The stream of consciousness: Scientific investigations into the flow of human experience.* New York: Plenum Press.

Purdon, C. (2001). Appraisal of obsessional thought recurrences: impact on anxiety and mood state. *Behavior Therapy*, *32*, 47–64.

Purdon, C., & Clark D. A. (1993). Obsessive intrusive thoughts in nonclinical subjects. Part I. Content and relation with depressive, anxious and obsessional symptoms. *Behaviour Research and Therapy*, *31*, 713–720.

Purdon, C. L., & Clark, D. A. (1994a). Obsessive intrusive thoughts in nonclinical subjects. Part II. Cognitive appraisal, emotional response and thought control strategies. *Behaviour Research and Therapy*, *32*, 403–410.

Purdon, C., & Clark, D. A. (1994b). Perceived control and appraisal of obsessional intrusive thoughts: A replication and extension. *Behavioural and Cognitive Psychotherapy*, *22*, 269–285.

Purdon, C., & Clark, D. A. (2001). Suppression of obsession-like thoughts in nonclinical individuals: Impact on thought frequency, appraisal and mood state. *Behaviour Research and Therapy*, *39*, 1163–1181.

Rachman, S. (1978). An anatomy of obsessions. *Behavioural Analysis and Modification, 2,* 235–278.

Rachman, S. (1981). Part 1. Unwanted intrusive cognitions. *Advances in Behaviour Research and Therapy, 3,* 89–99.

Rachman, S. J. (1997). A cognitive theory of obsessions. *Behaviour Research and Therapy, 35,* 793–802.

Rachman, S. J. (1998). A cognitive theory of obsessions: Elaborations. *Behaviour Research and Therapy, 36,* 385–401.

Rachman, S. (2003). *The treatment of obsessions.* Oxford, UK: Oxford University Press.

Rachman, S., & de Silva, P. (1978). Abnormal and normal obsessions. *Behaviour Research and Therapy, 16,* 233–248.

Rachman, S., & Hodgson, R. J. (1980). *Obsessions and compulsions.* Englewood Cliffs, NJ: Prentice Hall.

Reynolds, M., & Salkovskis, P. M. (1991). The relationship among guilt, dysphoria, anxiety and obsessions in a normal population—An attempted replication. *Behaviour Research and Therapy, 29,* 259–265.

Reynolds, M., & Salkovskis, P. M. (1992). Comparison of positive and negative intrusive thoughts and experimental investigation of the differential effects of mood. *Behaviour Research and Therapy, 30,* 273–281.

Ruscio, A. M., & Borkovec, T. D. (in press). Experience and appraisal of worry among high worriers with and without generalized anxiety disorder. *Behaviour Research and Therapy.*

Ruscio, A. M., Borkovec, T. D., & Ruscio, J. (2001). A taxometric investigation of the latent structure of worry. *Journal of Abnormal Psychology, 110,* 413–422.

Salkovskis, P. M. (1985). Obsessional–compulsive problems: A cognitive-behavioural analysis. *Behaviour Research and Therapy, 23,* 571–584.

Salkovskis, P. M. (1988). Intrusive thoughts and obsessional disorders. In D. Glasgow & N. Eisenberg (Eds.), *Current issues in clinical psychology* (Vol. 4). London: Gower.

Salkovskis, P. M. (1989). Cognitive-behavioural factors and the persistence of intrusive thoughts in obsessional problems. *Behaviour Research and Therapy, 27,* 677–682.

Salkovskis, P. M. (1999). Understanding and treating obsessive–compulsive disorder. *Behaviour Research and Therapy, 37,* S29–S52.

Salkovskis, P. M., & Harrison, J. (1984). Abnormal and normal obsessions—A replication. *Behaviour Research and Therapy, 23,* 571–584.

Salkovskis, P. M., Wroe, A. L., Gledhill, A., Morrison, N., Forrester, E., Richards, C., et al. (2000). Responsibility attitudes and interpretations are characteristic of obsessive compulsive disorder. *Behaviour Research and Therapy, 38,* 347–372.

Sarason, I. G., Pierce, G. R., & Sarason, B. R. (1996). Domains of cognitive interference. In I. G. Sarason, G. R. Pierce, & B. R. Sarason (Eds.), *Cognitive interference: Theories, methods and findings* (pp. 139–152). Mahwah, NJ: Erlbaum.

Segerstrom, S. C., Tsao, J. C. I., Alden, L. E., & Craske, M. G. (2000). Worry and rumination: Repetitive thought as a concomitant and predictor of negative mood. *Cognitive Therapy and Research, 24,* 671–688.

Singer, J. (1998). Daydreams, the stream of consciousness, and self-representations. In R. Bornstein & L. Masling (Eds.), *Empirical perspectives on the psychoanalytic unconscious. Empirical studies of psychoanalytic theories* (Vol. 7, pp. 141–186). Washington, DC: American Psychological Association.

Suedfeld, P., Ballard, E. J., Baker-Brown, G., & Borrie, R. A. (1985–1986). Flow of consciousness in restricted environmental stimulation. *Imagination, Cognition and Personality, 5,* 219–230.

Sutherland, G., Newman, B., & Rachman, S. (1982). Experimental investigations of the relations between mood and intrusive unwanted cognitions. *British Journal of Medical Psychology, 55,* 127–138.

Tallis, F., Eysenck, M., & Mathews, A. (1992). A questionnaire for the measurement of nonpathological worry. *Personality and Individual Differences, 13,* 161–168.

Tata, P. (1989). *Stress-induced intrusive thoughts and cognitive bias.* Paper presented at the World Congress of Cognitive Therapy, Oxford, UK.

Wang, A., Clark, D. A., & Purdon, C. (2003). *Frequency and effort of mental control over unwanted cognitions.* Poster presented at the annual conference of the Association for Advancement of Behavior Therapy, Boston.

Wegner, D. M., & Pennebaker, J. W. (Eds.). (1993). *Handbook of mental control.* Englewood Cliffs, NJ: Prentice Hall.

Wells, A., & Morrison, A. P. (1994). Qualitative dimensions of normal worry and normal obsessions: A comparative study. *Behaviour Research and Therapy, 32,* 867–870.

Wells, A., & Papageorgiou, C. (1995). Worry and the incubation of intrusive images following stress. *Behaviour Research and Therapy, 33,* 579–583.

Wilson, K. A., & Chambless, D. L. (1999). Inflated perceptions of responsibility and obsessive–compulsive symptoms. *Behaviour Research and Therapy, 37,* 325–335.

Yee, P. L., & Vaughan, J. (1996). Integratinig cognitive, personality, and social approaches to cognitive interference and distractibility. In I. G. Sarason, G. R. Pierce, & B. R. Sarason (Eds.), *Cognitive interference: Theories, methods and findings* (pp. 77–97). Mahwah, NJ: Erlbaum.

York, D., Borkovec, T. D., Vasey, M., & Stern, R. (1987). Effects of worry and somatic anxiety induction on thoughts, emotion and physiological activity. *Behaviour Research and Therapy, 25,* 523–526.

CHAPTER 2

INTRUSIVE THOUGHTS
IN POSTTRAUMATIC
STRESS DISORDER

SHERRY A. FALSETTI
JEANNINE MONNIER
HEIDI S. RESNICK

Posttraumatic stress disorder (PTSD) as defined by the text revision of the fourth edition of the *Diagnostic and Statistical Manual of Mental Disorders* (DSM-IV-TR; American Psychiatric Association, 2000) involves the development of reexperiencing symptoms, avoidance behavior, and increased physiological arousal following exposure to a traumatic event. Intrusive symptoms, such as repetitive thoughts, images, memories, or impulses related to the trauma, that are usually uncontrollable and unwanted are included in the symptom category of reexperiencing.

We use the term *trauma-related intrusions* to refer to a broad range of cognitive phenomena that includes images, memories, and impulses as well as lexical cognitions. Images and memories may include but are not limited to visualizing the perpetrator's face in cases of interpersonal violence, seeing the trauma reoccur, or visualizing what occurred immediately before or after the traumatic event. Victims who are injured may also have intrusions of being at the hospital and obtaining treatment. Intrusive cognitions may include thoughts that occurred at the time of the traumatic event, such as thoughts of fear of injury or death, thoughts of disgust, and thoughts of escape. Impulses often focus on the urge to survive the situation by fighting and/or fleeing. In this chapter, the term *trauma-related intrusions* is used to refer to all these phenomena.

Trauma-related intrusions have been linked with a variety of subjective and psychophysiological disturbances (Horowitz, 1969; Rachman, 1981) and are predictive of the development and maintenance of PTSD (Davidson & Baum, 1993; Halligan, Michael, Clark, & Ehlers, 2003). This chapter reviews current theory on PTSD, studies related to the psychopathology of intrusive thoughts in PTSD, the assessment of this cognitive phenomenon, mental control of trauma-related intrusions, and the nature and impact of PTSD treatment on trauma-related intrusions. Finally, this chapter discusses future directions for research in the area of trauma related intrusions in PTSD.

THEORIES OF PTSD

Several cognitive-behavioral and cognitive theories have been adopted to explain trauma reactions, including learning theories, information processing theories, and, more recently, cognitive constructivist theories. These formulations have many similarities in their explanation of the role of trauma-related intrusions in the development and maintenance of PTSD.

Learning theory (Axelrod, & Cichon, 1984; Holmes & St. Lawrence, 1983; Kilpatrick, Veronen, & Best, 1985; Kilpatrick, Veronen, & Resick, 1982), for example, proposes that during a stressful event, previously neutral stimuli become associated with the event. Thus, when presented with the associated stimuli following the event, fear and anxiety may be evoked. Furthermore, negative reinforcement, or the withdrawal of negative stimuli, helps to promote behavioral avoidance of the conditioned fear and anxiety cues because of the reinforcing properties of anxiety reduction due to an avoidance response. Fear and anxiety responses can also generalize to stimuli that are similar to the conditioned stimuli. Although not stated explicitly, it is suggested that the avoidance behaviors would maintain trauma-related intrusions, as no new learning could take place to break the pairing of the trauma and conditioned cues. A weakness of learning theory is the failure to explain the development of uncued intrusive thoughts, or how individuals not present during a trauma—for instance, the murder of a loved one—may also develop trauma-related intrusions.

Similarly, information-processing theories (Chemtob, Roitblat, Hamada, Carlson, & Twentyman, 1988; Foa, Steketee, & Olasov-Rothbaum, 1989) suggest that those suffering from PTSD develop fear structures or networks as a result of trauma exposure. These structures hold images and memories of threatening events as well as information regarding emotions and plans for action. These fear structures comprise threat schemas that are weakly activated at all times in people with PTSD. Thus, for someone with PTSD, the activated threat schema or network can cause many events to be interpreted as potentially danger-ous and can also bring forth reexperiencing emotions (e.g., trauma-related intrusions) and physiological reactions associated with traumatic events. Trauma-related intrusions are part of the fear network that can be triggered by other parts of the network. For example, seeing someone who looks similar to the perpetrator may trigger intrusive images or thoughts of the traumatic event. Conversely, physiological sensations may serve as cue that can trigger intrusive thoughts. This model is broader than learning theory in that it also takes into account cognitive processes that may lead to the development and maintenance of PTSD.

More recently, constructivist theory has been applied to understand reactions to trauma exposure. In general, constructivist theorists pro-pose that individuals actively construct their own mental representations of the world (Meichenbaum, 1993). These representations, sometimes referred to as schemas, have personal meaning and are based on each in-dividual's unique life experiences. PTSD researchers (McCann & Pearl-man, 1990; Resick & Schnicke, 1993) have proposed that these schemas can be disrupted by trauma. Specifically, McCann and Pearlman (1990) proposed that individuals have specific schemas about safety, trust, inde-pendence, power, esteem, and intimacy about themselves and about other people. Depending on the individual's previous life experiences, trauma exposure may either serve to disrupt or confirm these schemas. Resick and Schnicke (1993) offered a more integrative view by combin-ing ideas from learning, information processing, and constructivist theo-ries to explain trauma reactions. This integrative perspective has been specifically tailored to explain the reactions of rape victims. In their conceptualization of PTSD, they proposed that rape is a traumatic expe-rience that victims are often unable to integrate successfully with prior beliefs and experiences. Instead, the event is either changed to fit prior beliefs (assimilation) or their prior beliefs are altered (accommodation). They further hypothesize that symptoms of intrusion and avoidance occur because the event has not been assimilated or accommodated suc-cessfully.

Ehlers and Clark (2000) proposed a more cognitive integrative model of PTSD that drew on prior PTSD theories and their own cognitive–clinical perspective. This model proposes that persistent PTSD occurs only in those who process a traumatic event in a manner that leads them to perceive this event as a serious, current threat. It is the perception of current threat that is related to trauma-related intrusions and other PTSD symptoms.

Two processes are thought to lead to a sense of current threat: individual differences in the appraisal of the trauma and/or its sequelae and individual differences in the nature of the memory for the event and its link to other autobiographical memories. Excessively negative appraisals of the trauma and/or its sequelae result in an increased sense of current threat. Also, a disturbance of autobiographical memory, which may be characterized by poor elaboration as well as other factors, such as data-driven processing (i.e., processing sensory impressions and perceptual characteristics rather than the meaning of the event), results in an increased sense of current threat. The model proposed that eliminating such negative appraisals and autobiographical memory disturbances can reduce the experience of PTSD.

Ehlers et al. (2002) proposed the warning signal hypothesis to explain the occurrence of intrusive memories. They first examined the nature of intrusive memories across several studies and found that visual trauma-related intrusions were much more common than intrusive thoughts. Interestingly, the images were usually of stimuli present moments before the part of the trauma that had the most emotional impact. Ehlers et al. (2002) suggest that these intrusive memories may function as a warning signal, and thus are accompanied by a sense of serious current threat.

Halligan, Clark, and Ehlers (2002; Halligan et al., 2003) hypothesized that intrusions develop from the way in which information is processed. Specifically, intrusions are more likely to occur when information is processed in a data-driven manner, such as processing the sensory impressions and perceptual characteristics rather than processing conceptually. Conceptual processing focuses on the context and meaning of an event.

Cognitive-behavioral theories of PTSD and trauma-related intrusions specifically have evolved from a relatively simple conditioning paradigm to a more complex cognitive perspective, as research in this field has advanced our understanding of the development and maintenance of PTSD. Cognitive models have received some empirical support that certain modes of information processing do indeed seem to be associated with PTSD. These models do not address why one individual may be more inclined to process information in a data-driven way compared to another person, however. To fully understand individual differences in vulnerability to the development of PTSD, future models would do well to also include event characteristics as well as characteristics of the individual. For example, certain events may be so life threatening, or so threatening to the integrity of the individual (combat, sexual assault), that the brain cannot process its meaning at the same time that it is focused on survival. Certain individuals may also be more prone to avoiding anxiety-provoking situations and thus are less likely to engage in natural exposure or more adaptive thinking about the trauma in a way that would derive meaning. Individuals who have been victimized more than once are more likely to develop PTSD and perhaps are also more likely to engage in cognitive processes that maintain a sense of current threat, or to avoid in hopes of escaping future victimization.

THE PSYCHOPATHOLOGY OF TRAUMA-RELATED INTRUSIONS IN PTSD

A recent body of research has focused specifically on the psychopathology of trauma-related intrusions. Evidence suggests that images are more common in PTSD than thoughts or purely lexical cognitions (Ehlers & Steil, 1995; Ehlers et al., 2002). Reynolds and Brewin (1999) found that PTSD intrusive thoughts typically contain content of personal illness or injury or personal assault. de Silva and Marks (1998) proposed that individuals also experience intrusive thoughts that are not memories of the traumatic event but, rather, questions about the event. These thoughts fall into three broad categories: (1) threat and danger (e.g., Am I safe?), (2) negative thoughts about the self (e.g., Am I a bad person?), and (3) thoughts about the meaning of the event (e.g., Why did this happen to me?). The frequency and distressing nature of these non-recollection-based intrusions are similar to recollection-based intrusions (de Silva & Marks, 1998).

It is also evident that intrusive thoughts may not necessarily reflect traumatic incidents in an accurate way. For example, Merckelbach, Muris, Horselenberg, and Rassin (1998) found that 22% of those in a nonclinical sample reported that their intrusive thoughts were exaggerated versions of what actually happened. They suggested that such intrusions might represent "worse-case scenarios" of what could have happened. Exaggerated intrusions appeared to be more similar to flashbacks than nonexaggerated intrusions and occurred at a higher frequency than realistic intrusions.

It is clear that intrusive cognitions are a common reaction to trauma exposure. Durham, McCammon, and Allison (1985) found that in a sample of disaster workers (e.g., rescue, fire, and medical personnel and police officers), this was the most frequently reported symptom, with 74% of their sample reporting intrusive thoughts. Intrusive thoughts in PTSD can be triggered by numerous cues (de Silva & Marks, 1998). For example, stressful stimuli can trigger intrusive thoughts (e.g., a violent movie can trigger intrusive thoughts about a rape). In addition, an internal event, such as a related memory, can trigger unwanted intrusive cognitions. Physiological arousal may also precipitate intrusive thoughts or images. Sodium lactate infusion has been observed to precipitate flashbacks among PTSD-positive combat veterans (Jensen et al., 1997; Rainey et al., 1987). A study of yohimbine-induced panic attacks noted that 40% of participants who had PTSD experienced flashbacks following administration of yohimbine (Southwick et al., 1993). However, intrusive thoughts may also spontaneously occur with no apparent cue or stimulus. Schreuder, Kleijn, & Rooijamns (2000) reported that 56% of veterans in their sample reported trauma-related nightmares or anxiety dreams more than 40 years after war trauma. Presumably this is an example of an uncued intrusive memory.

Trauma-related intrusions appear to have a strong relationship to the experience of distress following a traumatic event. Davidson and Baum (1993) found that intrusiveness of recalled imagery associated with stressful combat events was an important predictor of long-term symptoms of stress irrespective of intensity of exposure. In addition, the interaction of combat exposure and trauma-related intrusions was significantly related to symptoms of chronic stress. Rothbaum, Foa, Riggs, Murdock, and Walsh (1992) reported similar findings in rape victims. Specifically, they found that PTSD status at 3 months postassault could be predicted by self-report of early trauma-related intrusions. These data suggest that trauma-related intrusions may reflect an important individual difference variable that could help predict long-term response to stress.

In an effort to increase understanding of the association of intrusive thoughts and distress, investigators have identified key qualities of intrusions that relate to distress. For example, Dougall, Craig, and Baum (1999) found that characteristics of intrusive memories reflecting the extent to which they were unwanted or uncontrollable were key determinants of distress. Frequency was not found to be a major factor in distress (Dougall et al., 1999). Schooler, Liegey Dougall, and Baum (1999) found that early uncued thoughts and the severity of distress caused by trauma-related intrusions in the month after a trauma were associated with higher frequencies of trauma-related intrusions and avoidance at 6-, 9-, and 12-month follow-up. Similar to other investigators, Schooler et al. (1999) found that those who experienced uncued trauma-related intrusions were more likely to experience later distress.

Steil and Ehlers (2000) found in a sample of motor vehicle accident victims that whether or not trauma-related intrusions are experienced as distressing depended on their idiosyncratic meaning. Idiosyncratic meanings are found in both the occurrence of the intrusion ("having this thought means I am crazy") and the content of the intrusion, which usually relates to the traumatic event and its sequelae. Negative idiosyncratic meanings were related to the distress caused by the trauma-related intrusion, such that intrusive thoughts to which dysfunctional meanings were assigned were related to high levels of trauma-related intrusion distress. When victims assigned meanings such as, "I am going crazy," "I am inferior to other people," "My life is ruined," "It is my fault," or "It will happen again," they were more likely to experience distress than were trauma victims who did not assign such meaning. This relationship remained significant when intrusion frequency, trauma severity, and general anxiety-related catastrophic cognitions were partialed out.

Halligan et al. (2002; 2003) examined disorganized trauma memories in the development of PTSD, peritraumatic cognitive processing in the development of intrusive memories and PTSD, and ongoing dissociation and negative appraisals of memories in maintaining symptomatology. Halligan et al. (2002) reported that data-driven processing (i.e., processing sensory perceptions rather than the meaning of the event) was associated with intrusive symptoms in an analogue study.

A later cross-sectional study (Halligan et al., 2003) compared groups with current, past, or no PTSD. Results of this study suggested that peritraumatic cognitive processing including dissociation, data-driven processing, and lack of self-referent processing is related to the development of disorganized memories and PTSD. Negative appraisals of dissociation served to maintain PTSD symptoms. These results were replicated in another longitudinal study in which cognitive and memory assessments completed within 12 weeks posttrauma predicted symptoms at 6 months. Specifically, negative interpretations of memory disorganization and intrusive thoughts predicted chronic PTSD symptoms. These findings are consistent with the results of Steil and Ehlers (2000).

In other investigations, various correlates of PTSD trauma-related intrusions have been identified. Resnick (1997) found that initial panic symptoms were predictive of PTSD intrusion symptoms at 3-month follow-up in a sample of women seen at the emergency room following a rape. In a comparison of trauma-related intrusions in matched samples of patients with PTSD and major depression, Reynolds and Brewin (1999) demonstrated that fear was characteristic of trauma-related intrusions in both groups but high levels of helplessness were uniquely associated with trauma-related intrusions in those with PTSD. Age at the time of the trauma may also be related to severity of trauma-related intrusions, with those who are older reporting more trauma-related intrusions (Hagström, 1995; Yehuda, Schmeidler, Siever, Binder-Brynes, & Elkin, 1997). Hagström (1995) found that individuals who experienced a threat to their lives during the trauma experienced more intrusive thoughts.

Trauma-related intrusions in PTSD have also been associated with memory deficits (Wessel, Merckelbach, & Dekkers, 2002). Wessel et al. (2002) explored the role of autographical memory specificity, intrusive memory, and general memory ability in Dutch-Indonesian survivors of the World War II era. They found that intrusion and avoidance, as measured by the Impact of Event Scale (Horowitz, Wilner, & Alvarez, 1979), predicted the tendency to produce less specific memories in response to negative but not positive word cues on an autobiographical memory test. The mechanism that underlies this effect is unclear. The authors hypothesized that perhaps either self-focused rumination or the repetitive execution of the retrieval process for intrusive memories hampers the recall of other memory material. This would not explain why the bias is only for negative emotional material, however.

Researchers have also examined the biological impact of traumatic exposure, including its impact on trauma-related intrusions. Intrusions appear to be related to several stress-related biological outcomes, including resting blood pressure and hypothalamic–pituitary–adrenal axis function (Baum, Cohen, & Hall, 1993; Goenjian et al., 1996). MacFarlane (1992) proposed that trauma-related intrusions may constitute continued episodes of distress, thereby over time altering HPA axis function. Others have found that intrusive thoughts are related to immune function. Ironson et al. (1997) found that intrusive thoughts were associated with lower natural killer cell cytotoxicity. While the implication of lower natural killer cell cytotoxicity (NKCC) is not well understood, lower rates of NKCC have been linked to serious diseases such as cancer (Whiteside & Herberman, 1989).

The relationship between trauma exposure/PTSD and brain structure has also been investigated. As with immune function, this relationship is not well understood, but trauma-related intrusions have been found to relate to brain structure. For example, De Bellis et al. (1999) found that trauma-related intrusions were positively correlated with ventricular volume in a sample of children with PTSD. They also found that intrusions were negatively correlated with brain volume, total corpus callosum size, and regional measures of size.

Finally, some investigators have focused on the persistence of trauma-related intrusions. Ehlers and Steil (1995) developed a model to explain the maintenance of intrusive thoughts in which two pathways were proposed: avoidance and distress. Their model suggests that the distress pathway leads to the short-term maintenance of intrusions through arousal and reexperiencing symptoms, and the avoidance pathway leads to the maintenance of intrusions in both the short and long term.

Steil and Ehlers (2000) found that whether or not intrusions are maintained depends, in part, on their idiosyncratic meaning. Negative idiosyncratic meanings, such as "I am going crazy," "I am inferior to other people," "My life is ruined," "It is my fault," or "It will happen again" predicted avoidance coping strategies. In turn, these coping strategies maintained intrusive thoughts by limiting exposure to reminders of the intrusion through a variety of means such as thought suppression, rumination, and distraction.

Building on the work of Steil and Ehlers (2000), Engelhard, van den Hout, Arntz, and McNally (2002) examined intrusion-based reasoning and PTSD in a small sample exposed to a train disaster and compared them to a control group. Intrusions regarding the train disaster were highly associated with predicting danger in other situations for those with PTSD. They concluded that it might not only be the catastrophic interpretations of the intrusions themselves that maintain PTSD but also whether individuals interpret situations as more dangerous because of intrusions.

In sum, the research suggests that intrusions can include actual accounts of a traumatic event, thoughts about the meaning of the event, and thoughts about the meaning of self and also may not always be factually accurate but may be intrusions of a worst-case scenario. Research also indicates that trauma-related intrusions are common and can be induced by physiological arousal. Distress following the trauma appears to be an important predictor of trauma-related intrusions and the idiosyncratic meaning given to the occurrence of intrusions may predict how distressing the intrusions themselves are viewed by an individual. What is yet to be investigated is why some individuals might be more inclined to attribute a negative idiosyncratic meaning or process information in a data-driven manner than other individuals also exposed to a trauma.

ASSESSMENT AND MEASUREMENT OF UNWANTED INTRUSIVE MEMORIES IN PTSD

The assessment of intrusive memories is a key component for understanding their role in PTSD and other trauma reactions, as well as for the treatment of PTSD. Most measures of PTSD assess intrusive thoughts and images as a component of the reexperiencing symptoms. Useful structured interviews for the assessment of PTSD include the Clinician Administered PTSD Scale (CAPS; Blake et al., 1990) and the Structured Clinical Interview for DSM-IV (SCID; First, Spitzer, Gibbon, & Williams, 1995). The CAPS includes separate versions for lifetime and current PTSD. Each version includes measures of frequency and intensity of PTSD symptoms. In addition, the CAPS allows for the assessment of the impact of symptoms on social and occupational functioning. Cutoff scores for the CAPS have been developed and there is high agreement between this measure and the SCID (.89) in diagnosing PTSD (Blake et al., 1990). The SCID has been used in many other studies with victims of crime or those exposed to other types of traumatic events.

There are also a number of self report measures available that assess PTSD. The Impact of Event Scale (IES; Horowitz et al., 1979) has been widely used to assess intrusions and avoidance related to traumatic events. This measure has demonstrated good test–retest reliability and respectable internal reliability for both subscales across samples of motor vehicle accident victims, rape victims, and natural disaster victims (Bryant & Harvey, 1996; Burge, 1988; Steinglass & Gerrity, 1990). Weiss and Marmar (1997) published a revised version of the IES in which they modified the "frequency of symptom" scale into a measure a distress, and added a subscale to assess hyperarousal. Thus, the measure can now assess all components of PTSD in order to determine the level of distress associated with the symptoms.

The Intrusive Thoughts Questionnaire (ITC; Dougall et al., 1999) is a promising new measure of intrusive symptoms in PTSD. The ITC has good reliability and validity for the assessment of PTSD-related intrusive thoughts. In addition, the measure provides more information about intrusive thoughts than other measures currently available. The ITC assesses: (1) the frequency of intrusive thoughts; (2) the predictability or occurrence of these thoughts in the presence or absence of cues; (3)

whether intrusions are negative and/or upsetting; (4) the degree to which these thoughts are unwanted; (5) the extent to which intrusions are controllable once they occur; and (6) the occurrence of trauma-related dreams during sleep. With this in-depth examination of intrusive thoughts, the ITC promises to improve the understanding of the role of intrusive thoughts in reaction to trauma exposure.

Foa and her colleagues developed the Posttraumatic Cognitions Inventory (PTCI) as a measure of the appraisals of trauma and its sequelae that are thought to be involved in the development of PTSD (Foa, Ehlers, Clark, Tolin, & Orsillo, 1999b). Initial evidence supports the validity and reliability of the PTCI in assessing three factors hypothesized to underlie PTSD: (1) negative cognitions about self; (2) negative cognitions about the world; and (3) self-blame. Scores on the PTCI predicted PTSD severity, depression, and general anxiety. They also discriminated between traumatized individuals with and without PTSD. Foa et al. (1999b) suggest that the PTCI may be useful as a clinical assessment tool and may be used to identify erroneous cognitions that can be targeted in cognitive-behavioral treatments for PTSD.

Selection of PTSD measures will largely depend on the purpose of the assessment. For clinical research on PTSD or trauma-related intrusions, the ITC and PTCI will provide detailed information regarding trauma-related intrusions. For therapists who are treating PTSD, the CAPS or IES may be sufficient.

Mental Control and Persistence of Intrusive Thoughts in PTSD

Quasi-experimental studies have demonstrated a relationship between intrusive thoughts and intentional control responses such that suppression increases the frequency of unwanted intrusive thoughts. These results suggest that suppression of intrusive thoughts may be important in the development and maintenance of PTSD. For example, Trinder and Salkovskis (1994) found that nonclinical participants who were instructed to suppress their thoughts experienced more thoughts and found these thoughts more uncomfortable than those who were asked to think about the thoughts and those who were asked to write them down. Shipherd and Beck (1998) also found that the deliberate suppression of intrusive thoughts resulted in a rebound in frequency of such thoughts in those with PTSD. Lawrence, Fauerbach, and Munster (1996) also demonstrated such a relationship. Avoidance behaviors and intrusive thoughts near the time of a trauma were significantly related to experiencing intrusive thoughts 4 months following the event. After controlling for intrusive thoughts at the first assessment, avoidance behavior continued to predict intrusive thoughts at 4 months posttrauma.

TREATMENT OF UNWANTED INTRUSIONS IN PTSD

At present no PTSD treatment packages have specific intervention strategies for trauma-related intrusions, nor is the treatment outcome research at the stage of conducting dismantling studies aimed at answering questions about which components of treatment are most effective for disorder-specific symptoms. What we can conclude from the PTSD treatment outcome literature is that there are currently several effective cognitive-behavioral treatments and these interventions do appear to decrease intrusive memories. Solomon and Johnson (2002), in a review of the PTSD outcome literature, concluded that imaginal exposure and hypnosis were most likely to affect the intrusive symptoms of PTSD. We refer the reader to other sources for detailed descriptions of cognitive-behavioral treatment options and provide information specific to each treatment's effect on intrusions if available. In this chapter we provide a more detailed discussion of a treatment approach we developed, multiple channel exposure therapy (M-CET),with particular attention to its impact on trauma-related intrusive thoughts.

Full descriptions of stress inoculation therapy (SIT), prolonged exposure (PE), cognitive processing therapy (CPT), and M-CET can be found in the following resources: (1) SIT (Kilpatrick et al., 1982; Foa, Rothbaum, & Steketee, 1993; Resnick & Newton, 1992; Resick & Jordan, 1988; Veronen & Kilpatrick, 1983); (2) PE (Foa, Rothbaum, Riggs, & Murdock, 1991); (3) CPT (Resick, 1992; Resick & Schnicke, 1990, 1992, 1993; Calhoun & Resick, 1993); and (4) M-CET (Falsetti & Resnick, 1997, 2000a, 2000b; Falsetti, Resnick, & Gibbs, 2001; Falsetti, Erwin, Resnick, & Davis, 2003).

Studies investigating SIT, PE, CPT, and M-CET have tended to support the efficacy of these treatments for PTSD. Foa et al. (1991) found that both SIT and PE significantly reduced intrusions at posttreatment. Foa, Dancu, et al. (1999a) again reported significant posttreatment reductions in PTSD symptoms, although no specific results pertaining to intrusions were reported. It can be inferred from the results of these studies that intrusions likely decreased in the active treatment conditions.

In a more direct investigation of cognitive change, Foa, Molnar, and

Cashman (1995) reported on differences in rape trauma narratives in a sample of 14 sexual assault victims who completed two information sessions and seven sessions of repeated imaginal exposure. They found that narrative content changes derived from exposure sessions over the course of treatment were consistent with successful processing of traumatic memories. Specifically, narratives were found to increase in length over time and to contain greater percentages of words reflecting thoughts and feelings and a decrease in the percentage of words denoting actions and dialogue. Results also indicated that a reduction in fragmented memories was associated with lower trauma-related PTSD symptoms. These findings are intriguing in that they indicate the occurrence of cognitive processing during exposure treatment which is suggestive that trauma-related intrusive thoughts may also have declined as a result of treatment.

In addition to the Foa et al. (1991; 1995; 1999a) studies, other researchers have also supported the efficacy of exposure therapy. Marks, Lovell, Noshirvani, Livanou, and Thrasher (1998) found that exposure alone, cognitive restructuring alone, and exposure plus cognitive restructuring all produced marked improvement and were generally superior to relaxation training alone. However, no data were presented specific to intrusive symptoms.

Cognitive processing treatment has emerged as another, more cognitive approach, that is showing promise as a treatment for PTSD. Resick and Schnicke (1992) reported significant improvements with CPT on depression and PTSD measures pretreatment to 6 months posttreatment. At pretreatment 90% of the sample met criteria for PTSD, whereas at posttreatment none of the women met diagnostic criteria for the disorder. Similarly, major depression decreased from 62% of the women meeting criteria depression prior to treatment to only 42% continuing to meet criteria at posttreatment. This study reported specifically on intrusion scores as measured by the IES Intrusion subscale (Horowitz et al., 1979) and the Reexperiencing subscale of the PTSD Symptom Scale (Foa, Riggs, Dancu, & Rothbaum, 1993). Results on both of these subscales indicated significant pre- to posttreatment differences. A more recent study by Resick and colleagues (2002) compared CPT with PE and a wait-list condition. Both treatments were found to be efficacious and superior to the wait-list condition. No results were reported that were specific to intrusive memories.

M-CET (Falsetti & Resnick, 2000a, 2000b) is a more eclectic approach that borrows intervention strategies from CPT (Resick & Schnicke, 1993), SIT (Kilpatrick et al., 1982), and panic control treatment (Barlow

& Craske, 1988). The rationale for this treatment approach is that panic attacks are highly prevalent in PTSD, and learning contingencies and faulty information processing appear critical to symptom formation in the disorder. Thus cognitive-behavioral treatments for PTSD based on learning and information-processing theories are hypothesized to be effective by exposing patients to an activated fear memory of the traumatic event or by exposure to event-related cues (i.e., places, situations, smell, and sounds) that are not in and of themselves dangerous but which became associated with fear at the time of a traumatic event. During the course of successful treatment the patient initially experiences high levels of physiological arousal that decrease over time with repeated exposure sessions until extinction of fear responses occurs. However, for patients who have panic attacks and who are fearful of the attacks, fear exposure may be overwhelming and thus unacceptable to the patient. M-CET is unique in that it provides exposure to physiological arousal symptoms prior to cognitive and behavioral exposure to trauma-related symptoms.

M-CET is a 12-week treatment that can be offered either individually and in a group format. It is relevant to individuals who have experienced many types of traumatic events and are suffering from PTSD and panic attacks as a result of their traumatic experience(s). M-CET provides exposure through directly accessing the three channels that have been hypothesized to comprise the fear response system: physiological, cognitive, and behavioral (Lang, 1977). Exposure to the physiological channel is conducted through interoceptive exposure to physiological reactions, a method developed by Barlow and Craske (1988) in their treatment of panic disorder.

Exposure to the cognitive channel is conducted through writing assignments about the traumatic event. This method of exposure has been used effectively with rape victims by Resick and Schnicke (1992) as a component of CPT. Finally, exposure to the behavioral channel is achieved through *in vivo* exposure to conditioned cues to the traumatic event. This type of exposure has been used in SIT (Kilpatrick et al., 1982; Resick & Jordan, 1988) for rape victims.

In addition to the exposure components, M-CET also provides education about PTSD and panic symptoms and includes several cognitive components to address faulty cognitions about trauma. Cognitive interventions are employed to assist participants in challenging faulty thinking and to fully process traumatic memories. Psychoeducation, breathing retraining, and cognitive restructuring have also been adapted from current treatments for panic disorder (Mastery of your Anxiety and Panic

[MAP]; Barlow & Craske, 1988) and PTSD (CPT; Resick & Schnicke, 1993).

Falsetti, Resnick, and colleagues (Falsetti et al., 2001, 2003) (2001; 2002) completed a 4-year controlled study of M-CET for PTSD with comorbid panic attacks. Here we include data specific to the evaluation of M-CET for reducing the frequency and severity of intrusive thoughts. The treatment conditions (initial and delayed) and control conditions (control only and control then treatment) were combined and comparisons made between the participants who completed the treatment (n = 24) and control (n = 23) conditions. All treatment participants attended 12, once-weekly sessions.

Intrusive thoughts were assessed using four separate measures. Two structured interviews were used to assess symptoms of PTSD, including intrusive memories. The CAPS (Blake et al., 1990) included a question assessing the frequency of unwanted memories (i.e., "In the past week, have you experienced unwanted memories of the event(s) without being exposed to something that reminded you of the event?" "How often?") and the severity of this experience (i.e., "At their worst, how much distress or discomfort did these memories cause you?"). The SCID (First et al., 1995) included a question about lifetime and current intrusive thoughts (i.e., "Did you think about [this event/any of these events] when you didn't want to or did [it/they] come to you suddenly and vividly when you didn't want [it/them] to, perhaps even when there was nothing there to remind you of it/them?"). Two self-report measures, the Modified PTSD Symptom Scale (MPSS; Resick, Falsetti, Resnick, & Kilpatrick, 1991) and the IES (Horowitz et al., 1979), were also used. The MPSS included an assessment of the frequency and severity of intrusive thoughts (i.e., "Have you had recurrent or intrusive distressing thoughts or recollections about the event(s)?"). The IES also included an assessment of the frequency of intrusive thoughts (i.e., "Other things kept making me think about it; I thought about it when I didn't mean to").

The overall rates of intrusive thoughts were relatively high for the participants prior to the beginning of treatment. At the initial assessment, 85% of participants reported lifetime intrusive thoughts and 96% reported current trauma-related intrusive thoughts on the SCID. The mean frequency score for the CAPS question regarding unwanted memories was 2.68 (possible range 0–5) and the mean intensity score was 2.81 (possible range 0–5). Similar results were found for the self-report measures. On the MPSS, participants averaged 1.96 (possible range 0–3) for frequency of intrusive thoughts and 2.28 (possible range 0–4) for severity of distress associated with the intrusive thoughts. The two questions on the IES assessing intrusive thoughts had mean scores of 3.29 and 3.53 (possible range 0–5). These scores suggest that participants experienced frequent and severe intrusive thoughts prior to becoming involved in any intervention.

The wait-list control and treatment groups were compared on the above items at pre- and postassessment. At the pre-assessment, one between-group difference was found. The treatment group reported less distress related to the intrusive thoughts than did the control group, $F (1, 47) = 3.99$, $p = .052$, as measured by the CAPS. At the immediate postassessment, significant between-group differences were found for intrusive thoughts as assessed by the SCID. Specifically, fewer participants in the treatment group (37.5%) than the control group (91.3%) reported experiencing intrusive thoughts, $\chi^2(1, n = 47) = 14.73$, $p < .001$. Between-group differences were also found for the CAPS questions regarding the frequency and severity of intrusive thoughts. The treatment group reported significantly less frequent unwanted intrusive memories, $F (1, 47) = 13.64$, $p < .001$, and less distress associated with the trauma-related memories, $F (1, 47) = 12.75$, $p < .001$ at posttreatment compared to the control group. Similar results were found on the IES with the treatment group reporting less frequent intrusive thoughts, $F (1, 47) = 10.85$, $p < .002$ and unwanted intrusive images, $F (1, 47) = 8.25$, $p < .006$ at posttreatment compared to the control group. Finally, results revealed a trend for the treatment group to report reduced frequency of intrusive thoughts, $F (1, 47) = 3.27$, $p < .077$, and significantly less intensity of intrusive thoughts, $F (1, 47) = 12.00$, $p < .001$, as measured by the MPSS.

Ehlers and Clark (2000) hypothesized that in order for PTSD treatment to be effective, putting the trauma into the past requires that the traumatic memory be elaborated and integrated into the context of the individual's experience to reduce intrusive reexperiencing. They suggest that the mechanism for this elaboration is the promoting of a better discrimination between stimuli that occurred at the time of the trauma and stimuli that occur in the person's immediate context.

Cognitive-behavioral treatments do appear to increase stimulus discrimination through the use of cognitive restructuring, as well as through behavioral exposure, which decreases the fear response to nondangerous stimuli. Cognitive restructuring can be used to directly challenge negative interpretations of intrusive thoughts, as well as self-blame. In addition, narratives of traumatic events appear to become more cohesive following cognitive-behavioral treatment, suggesting that deeper conceptual processing has taken place. In our clinical work

(Falsetti et al., 2001; Falsetti & Resnick, 2000a, 2000b) and that of Foa et al. (1999a) and Resick and Schnicke (1992), there are also decreases in self-blame and in the negative idiosyncratic meaning found in narratives of those who respond to treatment. These factors may explain the effectiveness of cognitive-behavioral treatments in reducing intrusions.

FUTURE DIRECTIONS

Although it has long been accepted that intrusive memories are a symptom criteria of PTSD, only recently have intrusions come under more in-depth study regarding their origins, nature, frequency, severity, correlates with long-term outcome, and treatment. Because of the relative infancy of this research, much further work is needed. A review of the literature highlights some important gaps in our knowledge. First we need a better understanding of the nature and characteristics of intrusive thoughts. As noted by de Silva and Marks (1999), current diagnostic criteria for PTSD include both images and perceptions as well as thoughts as potential examples of intrusive and distressing recollections. In addition, flashbacks are described in DSM-IV-TR (American Psychiatric Association, 2000) as a type of reexperiencing symptom that includes "acting or feeling as if the traumatic event were recurring" (p. 428). As suggested by de Silva and Marks (1999), further data are needed to more carefully distinguish between cognitions that are predominantly lexical versus recollections that involve predominantly imagery or combinations of the two. Similarly, we suggest that the element of subjective sense of "reliving" be assessed in research to further clarify differences between flashbacks and mental imagery. As noted by de Silva and Marks (1999), additional research also needs to focus on memories that occur in other sensory modalities, including auditory, olfactory, and tactile.

Also of particular interest is the paucity of research on intrusive images and thoughts of family members of homicide or other traumatic events in which the person was not present but develops intrusive symptoms. Our clinical experience suggests that secondary victims report intrusive images of their loved one's death, despite the fact that they were not present at the scene. It appears common that the mind creates images of what the traumatic event may have looked like and intrusive images and thoughts are then experienced. A systematic investigation into the prevalence of this phenomena as well as theory aimed at explaining the potential purpose of such images could greatly increase our understanding of intrusions and assist in developing treatment for this population.

Further research is also needed on understanding the relationship of cognitive avoidance and thought suppression in the maintenance of intrusive thoughts in PTSD. Currently, we know that greater initial distress is associated with intrusive thoughts and also with PTSD in general. Perhaps if thought avoidance and suppression can be prevented early on, the development of PTSD and intrusive thoughts can be reduced. Resnick, Acierno, Holmes, Kilpatrick, and Jager, (1999) conducted a preliminary intervention with rape victims that suggests encouraging rape victims to refrain from avoidance behaviors reduces the onset of later PTSD.

As treatment outcome research on PTSD progresses, it will also be important to look at what components of treatment are most effective for the main symptom clusters of PTSD as well as individual symptoms, including trauma-related intrusions. The current treatment outcome literature indicates that cognitive-behavioral treatments such as PE therapy, SIT, CPT, and M-CET may all be effective in significantly decreasing intrusions. However, we know little about which components of treatment are most effective in reducing trauma-related intrusions. Future dismantling studies will assist in testing theories such as Ehlers and Clark's (2000) to determine if indeed it is the elaboration of the trauma that reduces intrusive thoughts and what strategies (writing, PE) are best at producing that elaboration.

A number of implications can be drawn from Halligan et al.'s (2002, 2003) finding that data-driven processing is associated with intrusions. They do not hypothesize, however, why traumatic events would be more likely to be processed in this manner. Could it be that traumatic events are more likely to be processed in this manner because there are no well-elaborated schema to conceptually process the event? In other words, in the midst of a traumatic event, it is difficult to understand what is happening and to find meaning because the event is not one that is normally experienced. A related possibility is that the life-threatening nature of trauma activates more primordial brain systems that focus on physical safety and survival, thereby circumventing higher-level conceptual processing. This might explain why those who survive repeated trauma, such as childhood sexual assault survivors and victims of repeated domestic violence, still have difficulty processing these experiences conceptually at the time they are happening even though they may have well-elaborated fear schemas. Together these speculations suggest that treatment should focus on the meaning of the trauma so that schemas become more organized and coherent, thereby leading to a reduction in intrusive memories.

Although much more needs to be learned about the nature of trauma-related intrusive thoughts in PTSD, a few preliminary conclusions can be drawn. Intrusive thoughts and memories of the trauma and related sequelae are a fundamental symptom feature of PTSD. Reductions in trauma-related intrusions appear to be an important aspect of improvement in PTSD. Failure to achieve reduction in trauma-related intrusions is indicative of poor treatment response. However, two critical issues remain for further research. What are the key cognitive mechanisms that underlie the persistence of trauma-related intrusions and what are the most effective intervention strategies for achieving symptomatic improvement in intrusive reexperiencing symptoms?

ACKNOWLEDGMENT

This work was supported in part by NIMH Grant No. 5R21MH053381-03.

REFERENCES

American Psychiatric Association. (2000). *Diagnostic and statistical manual of mental disorders* (4th ed., text rev.). Washington, DC: Author.

Barlow, D. H., & Craske, M. G. (1988). *Mastery of your anxiety and panic manual*. Albany, NY: Center for Stress and Anxiety Disorders.

Baum, A., Cohen, L., & Hall, M. (1993). Control and intrusive memories as possible determinants of chronic stress. *Psychosomatic Medicine, 55*, 274–286.

Blake, D. D., Weathers, F. W., Nagy, L. M., Kaloupek, D. G., Klaumizer, G., Charney, D., et al. (1990). A clinician rating scale for assessing current and lifetime PTSD: The CAPS-1. *The Behavior Therapist, 13*, 187–188.

Bryant, R. A., & Harvey, A. G. (1996). Initial posttraumatic strss response following motor vehicle accidents. *Journal of Traumatic Stress, 9*, 223–234.

Burge, S. K. (1988). Post-traumatic stress disorder in victims of rape. *Journal of Traumatic Stress, 1*, 193–210.

Chemtob, C., Roitblat, H. L., Hamada, R. S., Carlson, J. G., & Twentyman, C. T. (1988). A cognitive action theory of post-traumatic stress disorder. *Journal of Anxiety Disorders, 2*, 253–275.

Davidson, L., & Baum, A. (1993). Predictors of chronic stress among Vietnam veterans: Stressor exposure and intrusive recall. *Journal of Traumatic Stress, 6*, 195–212.

De Bellis, M. D., Keshavan, M. S., Clark, D. B., Casey, C. B. J., Giedd, J. N., Boring,

A. M., et al. (1999). Developmental traumatology Part II: Brain development. *Biological Psychiatry, 45,* 1271–1284.

de Silva, P., & Marks, M. (1998). Intrusive thinking in posttraumatic stress disorder. In W. Yule (Ed.), *Post-traumatic stress disorder: Concepts and therapy* (pp. 161–175). New York: Wiley.

de Silva, P., & Marks, M. (1999). The role of traumatic experiences in the genesis of obsessive–compulsive disorder. *Behaviour Research and Therapy, 37,* 941–951.

Dougall, A. L., Craig, K. J., & Baum, A. (1999). Assessment of characteristics of intrusive thoughts and their impact on distress among victims of traumatic events. *Psychosomatic Medicine, 61,* 38–48.

Durham, T. W., McCammon, S. L., & Allison, E. J. (1985). The psychological impact of disaster on rescue personnel. *Annals of Emergency Medicine, 14,* 664–668.

Ehlers, A., & Clark, D. M. (2000). A cognitive model of posttraumatic stress disorder. *Behaviour Research and Therapy, 38,* 319–345.

Ehlers, A., Hackman, A., Steil, R., Clohessy, S.. Wenninger, K., & Winter, H. (2002). The nature of intrusive memories after trauma: The warning signal hypothesis. *Behaviour Research and Therapy, 40,* 995–1002.

Ehlers, A., & Steil, R. (1995). Maintenance of intrusive memories in posttraumatic stress disorder: A cognitive approach. *Behavioural and Cognitive Psychotherapy, 23,* 217–249.

Engelhard, I. M., van den Hout, M. A., Arntz, A., & McNally, R. J. (2002). A longitudinal study of "intrusion-based reasoning" and posttraumatic stress disorder after exposure to a train disaster. *Behavior Research and Therapy, 40,* 1415–1424.

Falsetti, S. A., Erwin, B. A., Resnick, H. S., & Davis, J. L. (2003). Multiple channel exposure therapy of PTSD: Impact of treatment on functioning and resources. *Journal of Cognitive Psychotherapy, 17,* 133–147.

Falsetti, S. A., Resnick, H. S., & Gibbs, N. A. (2001). Treatment of PTSD with panic attacks combining cognitive processing therapy with panic control treatment techniques. *Group Dynamics: Theory, Research and Practice, 5,* 252–260.

Falsetti, S. A., & Resnick, H. S. (1997). Treatment of PTSD with comorbid panic attacks. *Clinical Quarterly, 7,*(3), 46–48.

Falsetti, S. A., & Resnick, H. S. (2000a). Cognitive-behavioral treatment of PTSD with comorbid panic attacks. *Journal of Contemporary Psychology, 30,* 163–179.

Falsetti, S. A., & Resnick, H. S. (2000b). Treatment of PTSD using cognitive and cognitive behavioral therapies. *Journal of Cognitive Psychotherapy, 14,* 97–122.

First, M. B., Spitzer, R. L., Gibbon, M., & Williams, J. B. (1995). *Structured clinical interview for DSM-IV Axis I Disorders—Patient edition (SCID-I/P, Ver-*

sion 2). New York: Biometrics Research Department, New York State Psychiatric Institute.

Foa, E. B., Dancu, C. V., Hembree, E. A., Jaycox, L. H., Meadows, E. A., & Street, G. P. (1999a). A comparison of exposure therapy, stress inoculation training, and their combination for reducing posttraumatic stress disorder in female assault victims. *Journal of Consulting and Clinical Psychology, 67*, 194–200.

Foa, E. B., Ehlers, A., Clark, D. M., Tolin, D. F., & Orsillo, S. M. (1999b). The posttraumatic cognitions inventory (PTCI): Development and validation. *Psychological Assessment, 11*, 303–314.

Foa, E. B., Molnar, C., & Cashman, L. (1995). Change in rape narratives during exposure therapy for posttraumatic stress disorder. *Journal of Traumatic Stress, 8*, 675–690.

Foa, E. B., Riggs, D. S., Dancu, C. V., & Rothbaum, B. O. (1993). Reliability and validity of a brief instrument for assessing posttraumatic stress disorder. *Journal of Traumatic Stress, 6*, 459–473.

Foa E. B., & Rothbaum, B. O. (1998). *Treating the trauma of rape.* New York: Guilford Press.

Foa, E. B., Rothbaum, B. O., Riggs, D. S., & Murdock, T. B. (1991). Treatment of posttraumatic stress disorder in rape victims: A comparison between cognitive-behavioral procedures and counseling. *Journal of Consulting and Clinical Psychology, 59*, 715–723.

Foa, E. B., Rothbaum, B. O., & Steketee, G. S. (1993). Treatment of rape victims. *Journal of Interpersonal Violence, 8*, 256–276.

Foa, E. B., Steketee, G., & Olasov-Rothbaum, B. (1989). Behavioral/cognitive conceptualizations of posttraumatic stress disorder. *Behavior Therapy, 20*, 155–176.

Goenjian, A. K., Yehuda, R., Pynoos, R. S., Steinberg, A. M., Tashjian, M., Yang, R. K., et al. (1996). Basal cortisol, dexamethasone suppression of cortisol, and MHPG in adolescents after the 1988 earthquake in Armenia. *American Journal of Psychiatry, 153*, 929–934.

Hagström, R. (1995). The acute psychological impact on survivors following a train accident. *Journal of Traumatic Stress, 8*, 391–402.

Halligan, S. L., Clark, D. M., & Ehlers, A. (2002). Cognitive processing, memory, and the development of PTSD symptoms: Two experimental analogue studies. *Journal of Behavior and Experimental Psychiatry, 33*, 73–89.

Halligan, S. L., Michael, T., Clark, D. M., & Ehlers, A. (2003). Posttraumatic stress disorder following assault: Trauma, memory, and appraisals. *Journal of Consulting and Clinical Psychology, 71*, 419–431.

Holmes, M. R., & St. Lawrence, J. S. (1983). Treatment of rape-induced trauma: Proposed behavioral conceptualization and review of the literature. *Clinical Psychology Review, 3*, 417–433.

Horowitz, M. (1969). Psychic trauma: Return of images after a stress film. *Archives of General Psychiatry, 20*, 552–559.

Horowitz, M. J., Wilner, N., & Alvarez, W. (1979). Impact of Event Scale: A measure of subjective stress. *Psychosomatic Medicine, 41*, 209–218.

Ironson, G., Wynings, C., Schneiderman, N., Baum, A., Rodriguez, M., Green-wood, D., et al. (1997). Posttraumatic stress symptoms, intrusive thoughts, loss, and immune function after Hurricane Andrew. *Psychsomatic Medicine, 59,* 128–141.

Jensen, C. F., Keller, T. W., Peskind, E. R., McFall, M. M., Veith, R. C., Martin, D., et al. (1997). Behavioral and neuroendocrine responses to sodium lactate infusion in subjects with posttraumatic stress disorder. *American Journal of Psychiatry, 154,* 266–268.

Kilpatrick, D. G., Veronen, L. J., & Best, C. L. (1985). Factors predicting psychological distress among rape victims. In C. R. Figley (Ed.), *Trauma and its wake: Vol. 1 The study and treatment of posttraumatic stress disorder* (pp. 113–141). New York: Brunner/Mazel.

Kilpatrick, D. G., Veronen, L. J., & Resick, P. A. (1982). Psychological sequelae to rape: Assessment and treatment strategies. In D. M. Dolays & R. L. Meredith (Eds.), *Behavioral medicine: Assessment and treatment strategies* (pp. 473–497). New York: Plenum Press.

Lawrence, J. W., Fauerbach, J. F., & Munster, A. (1996). Early avoidance of traumatic stimuli predicts chronicity of intrusive thoughts following burn injury. *Behavior Research Therapy, 34,* 643–646.

MacFarlane, A. C. (1992). Stress and disaster. In S. E. Hobful & M. de Vries (Eds.), *Extreme stress and communities: Impact and intervention* (pp. 247–265). Dordrecht, The Netherlands: Kluwer Academic.

Marks, I., Lovell, K., Noshirvani, H., Livanou, M., & Thrasher, S. (1998). Treatment of posttraumatic stress disorder by exposure and/or cognitive restructuring. *Archives of General Psychiatry, 55,* 317–325.

McCann. L., & Pearlman, L. A. (1990). *Psychological trauma and the adult survivor: Theory, therapy & transformation.* New York: Brunner/Mazel.

Merckelbach, H., Muris, P., Horselenberg, R., & Rassin, E. (1998). Traumatic intrusions as "worse case scenarios." *Behaviour Research and Therapy, 36,* 1075–1079.

Rachman, S. (1981). Unwanted intrusive cognitions. *Advances in Behaviour Research and Therapy, 13,* 89–99.

Rainey, J. M., Aleem, A., Ortiz, A., Yerigani, V., Pohl, R., & Berchou, R. (1987). A laboratory procedure for the induction of flashbacks. *American Journal of Psychiatry, 144,* 1317–1319.

Resick, P. A. (1992). Cognitive treatment of crime-related post-traumatic stress disorder. In R. D. Peters, R. J. McMahon, & V. L. Quinsey (Eds.), *Aggression and violence throughout the life span* (pp.171–191). Newbury Park, CA: Sage Publication.

Resick, P. A., Falsetti, S. A., Resnick, H. S., & Kilpatrick, D. G. (1991). *The Modified PTSD Symptom Scale—Self report.* St. Louis, MO: University of Missouri and Crime Victims Treatment and Research Center, Medical University of South Carolina.

Resick, P. A., & Jordan, C. G. (1988). Group stress inoculation training for victims of sexual assault: A therapist manual. In P. A. Keller & S. R. Heyman (Eds.),

Innovations in clinical practice: A source book (Vol. 7, pp. 99–111). Sarasota, FL: Professional Resource Exchange.

Resick, P. A., & Schnicke, M. K. (1990). Treating symptoms in adult victims of sexual assault. *Journal of Interpersonal Violence, 5,* 488–506.

Resick, P. A., & Schnicke, M. K. (1992). Cognitive processing therapy for sexual assault victims. *Journal of Consulting and Clinical Psychology, 60,* 748–756.

Resick, P. A., & Schnicke, M. K. (1993). *Cognitive processing therapy for rape victims: A treatment manual.* Newbury Park, CA: Sage.

Resnick, H. S. (1997). Acute panic reactions among rape victims: Implications for prevention of postrape psychopathology. *National Center for PTSD Clinical Quarterly, 7,* 41–45.

Resnick, H., Acierno, R., Holmes, M., Kilpatrick, D. G., & Jager, N. (1999). Prevention of post-rape psychopathology: Preliminary findings of a controlled acute rape treatment study. *Journal of Anxiety Disorders, 13,* 359–370.

Resnick, H. S., & Newton, T. (1992). Assessment and treatment of post-traumatic stress disorder in adult survivors of sexual assault. In D. Foy (Ed.), *Treating PTSD* (pp. 99–126). New York: Guilford Press.

Reynolds, M., & Brewin, C. R. (1999). Intrusive memories in depression and posttraumatic stress disorder. *Behaviour Research & Therapy, 37,* 201–215.

Rothbaum, B. O., Foa, E. B., Riggs, D. S., Murdock, T., & Walsh, W. (1992). A prospective examination of post-traumatic stress disorder in rape victims. *Journal of Traumatic Stress, 5,* 455–475.

Schooler, T. Y., Liegey Dougall, A., & Baum, A. (1999). Cues, frequency, and the disturbing nature of intrusive thoughts: Patterns seen in rescue workers after the crash of flight 427. *Journal of Traumatic Stress, 12,* 571–585.

Schreuder, B. J. N., Kleijn, W. C., Rooijamns, H. G. M. (2000). Nocturnal re-experiencing more than forty years after war trauma. *Journal of Traumatic Stress, 13,* 453–463.

Shipherd, J. C., & Beck, J. G. (1998). The effects of suppressing trauma-related thoughts on women with rape-related posttraumatic stress disorder. *Behaviour Research and Therapy, 37,* 99–12.

Southwick, S. M., Krystal, J. H., Morgan, C. A., Johnson, D., Nagy, L. M., Nicolaou, A., et al. (1993). Abnormal noradrenergic function in posttraumatic stress disorder. *Archives of General Psychiatry, 50,* 266–274.

Steil, R., & Ehlers, A. (2000). Dysfunctional meaning of posttraumatic intrusions in chronic PTSD. *Behaviour Research and Therapy, 38,* 537–558.

Steinglass, P., & Gerrity, E. (1990). Natural disasters and post-traumatic stress disorder: Short-term versus long-term recovery in two disaster affected communities. *Journal of Applied Social Psychology, 20,* 1746–1765.

Veronen, L. J., & Kilpatrick, D. G. (1983). Stress management for rape victims. In D. Meichenbaum & M. E. Jaremko (Eds.), *Stress reduction and prevention* (pp. 341–374). New York: Plenum Press.

Weiss, D. S., & Marmar, C. R. (1997). The Impact of Event Scale—Revised. In J. P. Wilson & T. M. Keane (Eds.), *Assessing psychological trauma and PTSD* (pp. 399–411). New York: Guilford Press.

Whiteside, T. L., & Herberman, R. B. (1989). The role of natural killer cells in human disease. *Clinical Immunology and Immunopathology, 53*, 1–23.

Wessel, I., Merckelbach, H., & Dekkers, T. (2002). Autobiographical memory specificity, intrusive memory, and general memory skills in Dutch-Indonesian Survivors of World War II era. *Journal of Traumatic Stress, 15*, 227–234.

Yehuda, R., Schmeidler, J., Siever, L. J., Binder-Brynes, K., & Elkin, A. (1997). Individual differences in posttraumatic stress disorder symptom profiles in holocaust survivors in concentration camps or in hiding. *Journal of Traumatic Stress, 10*, 453–463.

CHAPTER 3

SEEKING SOLACE BUT FINDING DESPAIR

The Persistence of Intrusive Thoughts in Depression

RICHARD M. WENZLAFF

In the normal course of mental life, unwanted, negative thoughts occasionally arise, prompting critical self-reflection and a downturn in mood. These intrusive thoughts may be unpleasant, but they are typically infrequent and manageable and may even be helpful by alerting us to potential problems that signal the need for a different course of action (Neese, 2000). In some cases, however, unwanted, negative thoughts can persist and escalate in frequency and intensity, creating a mental state that is ripe for the development and maintenance of depression. This emotionally precarious situation can be exacerbated by misguided attempts to suppress the offending thoughts that can ironically create a state of mind that is more vigilant for the unwanted material.

Over the past two decades, research showing an intimate association between dysfunctional patterns of thinking and depressive moods has enhanced our understanding of the role of cognition in depression and informed the techniques and goals of cognitive therapy. This research has focused primarily on two areas: (1) cognitive biases, as reflected in attention and memory, and (2) dysfunctional attitudes, including unrealistic expectations and hopelessness. Until recently, investigators have not specifically examined the origins and impact of intrusive, depressive thoughts—perhaps because these intrusions were considered to be secondary to cognitive biases and dysfunctional attitudes. However, recent research suggests that intrusive depressive thoughts are worth examining in their own right because they may hold important clues concerning the role of cognition in depression and the mental control processes that help maintain the disorder.

This chapter examines the common characteristics of intrusive, depressive thoughts, their origins, and their role in the development and maintenance of depression. Topics of measurement, theory, and research are explored to illuminate the role of misguided mental control in the development and perpetuation of intrusive, depressive thoughts. The chapter concludes with a consideration of the kinds of treatment that this analysis suggests are most likely to be effective.

THE NATURE OF INTRUSIVE THOUGHTS IN DEPRESSION

Unwanted, intrusive thoughts are undesirable cognitions that are difficult to control and have the potential to undermine mood. Investigators have found that such intrusive thoughts are relatively common, with approximately 80–90% of the general population experiencing them on occasion (Clark & de Silva, 1985; Purdon & Clark, 1999; Rachman & de Silva, 1978; Salkovskis & Harrison, 1984). Typically, these normal intrusions are infrequent, mild, or moderate in intensity and somewhat controllable. In contrast, clinically significant intrusions are much more frequent, intense, and uncontrollable (Wang & Clark, 2002). Most of the research in this area has focused on obsessive–compulsive disorder because intrusive thoughts are among the defining features of the disorder and constitute a primary target of treatment. Although research on intrusive thoughts in depression is relatively new, the existing evidence suggests that depressive intrusions are clinically significant and play an important role in the course of the disorder.

Intrusive thoughts in depression should be distinguished from the automatic negative thoughts in depression identified by Beck (1967). One key difference is that the intrusive thoughts that are experienced by depressed individuals could be negative—and might be largely expected to take this form—but could also be neutral or even positive in affective tone. Intrusive thoughts in normal individuals and across several forms of psychopathology share the special quality of being inconsistent with ongoing prior thought—and consequently seeming to "pop out" in consciousness. The depressed person may be involved in thinking on some topic that is far from depressive, for instance, only to have a depressive thought come to mind that is seemingly irrelevant and uninvited in the current context. The depressed person could also have an intrusive thought that is anxiety-laden, however, or perhaps one that is simply jarring or irrelevant to the person's present purposes. Although the intrusive thoughts experienced in depression might be expected to be predominantly negative, their intrusiveness is the unique quality that distinguishes them from more intentional or expected thoughts.

A second and more subtle distinction between the automatic negative thoughts described by Beck and the intrusive thoughts emphasized here is the degree to which the thoughts redirect the person's thinking. Intrusive thoughts may often have the property of redirecting thinking toward depressive topics when it was previously aimed elsewhere (cf. Salkovskis, 1985; Wenzlaff, Wegner, & Roper, 1988). Automatic negative thoughts, in turn, could simply follow in a chain of negative thinking and be quite thematic and predictable—even though they are experienced as uncontrollable. The sudden reorienting of attention to the intrusive thought makes such thought often more noticeable and disturbing than sequences of negative thoughts that occur in rumination or continued worry (Gold & Wegner, 1995).

Levels of Intrusiveness

One of the first steps in assessing the significance of depressive thought intrusions is to determine whether they exceed normal levels of intrusive thought found in the general population. To gauge the relative intensity, frequency, and uncontrollability of intrusive thoughts in depression for this chapter, analyses were carried out on the combined results of several studies that involved depressed and nondepressed participants and included a common measure of unwanted, intrusive thoughts (Wenzlaff & Eisenberg, 2001; Wenzlaff & Luxton, 2003; Wenzlaff, Rude, Taylor, Stultz, & Sweatt, 2001; Wenzlaff, Rude, & West, 2002b). Each of these studies used the White Bear Suppression Inventory (WBSI; Wegner & Zanakos, 1994). As shown in Table 3.1, the WBSI consists of three subscales: Thought Suppression, Unwanted Intrusive Thoughts, and Self-Distraction (Blumberg, 2000; Wenzlaff & Luxton, 2003). The reliability of the WBSI is good and there is strong evidence for its validity (Muris, Merckelbach, & Horselenberg, 1996;

Spinhoven & van der Does, 1999; van den Hout, Merckelbach, & Pool, 1996; Wegner & Zanakos, 1994).

Using responses to the 13-item Beck Depression Inventory—Short Form (BDI-SF; Beck & Beck, 1972), and following guidelines suggested by Beck and Beamesderfer (1974), the nondepressed group was defined as having scores of 3 or less and the depressed group as having scores of 13 or more.[1] A one-way analysis of variance indicated that the depressed group had significantly higher intrusive thought scores ($M = 32.60$) than did the nondepressed group ($M = 25.00$), $F(1, 419) = 186.04$, $p < .001$, $\eta^2 = .31$. An inspection of the items comprising the intrusive thought subscale (see Table 3.1) indicates that high scores are indicative of high intensity, frequency, and uncontrollability of unwanted thoughts.

Additional evidence for the intrusiveness of negative thoughts in depression comes from studies involving instructed thought suppression (e.g., Wenzlaff et al., 1988). Such studies show that whereas nondepressed individuals are largely successful in keeping negative thoughts out of mind, depressed individuals experience frequent, negative intrusions while trying to exert mental control. For example, Wenzlaff and Bates (1998) presented participants with a series of scrambled sentences (e.g., "future dismal the positive very looks") that could each be unscrambled by reordering five of the six words. Each scrambled sentence could form either a positive statement (e.g., "the future looks very positive") or a negative one ("the future looks very dismal"). When participants were instructed to form only positive statements, the nondepressed group formed negative sentences only 2% of the time, whereas the depressed group inadvertently produced negative solutions 14% of the time.

The Self-Relevance of Depressive Intrusions

Having established that depression involves abnormal levels of intrusive thoughts, it becomes important to determine whether depressive intrusions differ from the intrusive thoughts associated with the anxiety dis-

---

[1]In this research and elsewhere in this chapter, depression is defined in terms of high scores on questionnaires—specifically, the BDI (Beck & Beck, 1972; Beck & Beamesderfer, 1974). As critics of questionnaires have noted, this convention does not allow comparisons of such individuals with those who meet diagnostic criteria for syndrome depression. The approach in this chapter is consistent with evidence indicating no clear discontinuity in depressive symptoms between the distributions of individuals identified in these two ways (Lewinsohn, Solomon, Seeley, & Zeiss, 2000).

TABLE 3.1. White Bear Suppression Inventory

Factor 1: Thought Suppression

1. There are things I prefer not to think about.
8. I always try to put problems out of mind.
11. There are things that I try not to think about.
14. I have thoughts that I try to avoid.

Factor 2: Unwanted Intrusive Thoughts

2. Sometimes I wonder why I have the thoughts I do.
3. I have thoughts that I cannot stop.
4. There are images that come to mind that I cannot erase.
5. My thoughts frequently return to one idea.
6. I wish I could stop thinking of certain things.
7. Sometimes my mind races so fast I wish I could stop it.
9. There are thoughts that keep jumping into my head.
15. There are many thoughts I have that I don't tell anyone.

Factor 3: Self-Distraction

10. Sometimes I stay busy just to keep thoughts from intruding on my mind.
12. Sometimes I really wish I could stop thinking.
13. I often do things to distract myself from my thoughts.

orders. This is an important consideration because of the high rate of comorbidity of depression and anxiety (Brady & Kendall, 1992; Clark & Beck, 1989). The absence of distinguishing characteristics between depression- and anxiety-related intrusions would limit our ability to draw conclusions about the unique role that thought intrusions might play in depression. A review of the relevant research suggests that one of the features that distinguishes depressive intrusions involves the self-relevance of the thoughts.

According to cognitive theories, negative self-views and unrealistic self-standards are among the primary predisposing factors for depression (e.g., Beck, 1967; Ingram, 1984; Teasdale & Barnard, 1993). An array of research supports this assumption by showing a strong association between low self-esteem and depression and by demonstrating that self-relevant, negative material is more frequently endorsed by depressed individuals than by other groups (e.g., Pyszczynski & Greenberg, 1987). Perhaps most central to the issue of intrusive thoughts is the finding that depressed individuals are more likely than other groups spontaneously to report pejorative thoughts about themselves (Hollon & Kendall, 1980; Hollon, Kendall, & Lumry, 1986). These findings are consistent with research showing that depression is associated with heightened levels of self-focused attention (Pennebaker, Mehl, & Niederhoffer, 2003), which can make unfavorable, self-relevant information more accessible (Pyszczynski & Greenberg, 1987).

Presumably depressed individuals' self-critical thoughts stem from, and are congruent with, their low sense of self-worth. In contrast, the thoughts that characterize obsessive–compulsive disorder tend to be "ego-dystonic" in the sense that they are inconsistent with self-perceptions (Clark & Purdon, 1993, 1995; Purdon, 2001; Purdon & Clark, 1999; Wang & Clark, 2002). For example, intrusive thoughts of harming a loved one are ego-dystonic if they are inconsistent with the person's actual feelings and moral standards (Wang & Clark, 2002; Wells & Papageorgiou, 1998). In the case of generalized anxiety disorder, the intrusive thoughts take the form of exaggerated worries about real-life events and circumstances (Wang & Clark, 2002). Thus, self-critical, ego-syntonic content appears to be one of the important features that distinguishes depressive thought intrusions from the intrusive thoughts associated with anxiety disorders. This distinction is supported by research showing that a negative view of the self distinguishes individuals with major depression from those with anxiety disorders (Di Nardo & Barlow, 1990; Watson & Kendall, 1989). Further support for the distinction between depressive and anxious thought intrusions comes from a study by Clark (1992). Using a revised form of the Distressing Thoughts Questionnaire, Clark found that the thoughts associated with depression involved themes of personal loss and failure, whereas the thoughts associated with anxiety concerned possible harm and danger.

ORIGINS OF DEPRESSIVE INTRUSIONS

A variety of factors contribute to the development and maintenance of intrusive thoughts in depression, including cognitive biases, mood-relevant associations, and misguided mental control. These factors can interact in ways that help ensure that attention is automatically directed toward negative self-relevant material, thereby creating a mental environment that is conducive to intrusive negative thoughts.

Cognitive Biases

Depressed individuals seem to view their worlds through a mental prism that highlights negative aspects of their experiences while minimizing the positive facets of their lives. According to cognitive theory, this type of negative bias arises from learned patterns of thinking or "schemas" that guide perceptions and judgments and organize new information and experiences (Beck, 1967; Clark, Beck, & Alford, 1999). There is growing evidence that a depressive perspective develops early in life and can be fostered by a variety of factors, including dysfunctional parenting (Blatt & Homann, 1992), social skills deficits (Cole, Jacquez, & Maschman, 2001), maltreatment (Cutler & Nolen-Hoeksema, 1991; Gibb, Alloy, & Tierney, 2001), and stressful life events (Compas, 1987; Compas, Grant, & Ey, 1994). The common outcome of these unfortunate experiences is a depressive mind-set and a fragile sense of self-worth, which contribute to an automatic tendency to construe the world—especially the self—in negative ways.

Research supports the idea of a depressive schema by showing that depression is associated with a tendency to selectively focus on negative information. For example, in a study by Wenzlaff et al. (2001), dysphoric and nondysphoric participants identified words that were hidden in a letter grid containing equal numbers of positive, negative, and neutral words. The task involved finding words by selecting adjacent letters running sequentially forward, backward, up, or down. Dysphoric participants identified more negative than positive words, whereas the nondysphoric group found more positive than negative items.

Research using a modified version of the Stroop color-naming task has also provided evidence of an attentional bias among depressed individuals (for a review, see Ingram, Miranda, & Segal, 1998). The emotional Stroop task requires participants to name the colors of presented words that have depressive, neutral, or manic connotations. If depressed individuals possess a cognitive bias for depressive material, their attention should be drawn to depressed-content words, thereby interfering with their ability to name the color of the words. Indeed, unlike nondepressed individuals, depressed participants were slower in naming the colors of depressed-content words, compared to neutral or manic-content words (Gotlib & McCann, 1984; Williams & Nulty, 1986).

In their review of the research on attentional biases in depression Clark et al. (1999) suggest a number of refinements in our understanding of depressive biases. For example, negative attentional biases among depressed individuals have been found most consistently in studies involving conceptually based cognitive tasks (e.g., expectancies and self-evaluations) as opposed to perceptual types of information. In addition, nondepressed individuals often display a self-enhancing bias that depressed individuals apparently lack. When this positivity bias is taken into account, the judgments of depressed individuals may be more evenhanded (but not necessarily more accurate) than those of nondepressed people. Questions also remain concerning whether depressive biases are more apt to occur during the encoding or output phases of information processing.

Cognitive biases among depressed individuals have also been documented with respect to judgments and attributions. For example, compared to nondepressed people, dysphoric and depressed individuals are more likely to magnify the importance of failures (Wenzlaff & Grozier, 1988) and discount achievements (Sweeney, Anderson, & Bailey, 1986). Research on memory biases has produced differential results, depending on whether the task involves implicit or explicit memory. Explicit memory tasks make explicit reference to a specific learning experience and prompt participants to recall the information, whereas implicit memory tasks make no reference to the learning experience but infer implicit memory from facilitation of performance as a function of exposure to prior information. For example, one type of implicit memory task involves first exposing participants to a word list and then providing them with word stems (e.g., fea_____). Participants display implicit memory to the extent that they complete stems to form words from the earlier list.

In general, depressed individuals display a relatively robust negativity bias on explicit memory tasks (Blaney, 1986), whereas their performance on implicit memory tasks is more mixed (Clark et al., 1999). The mixed results for implicit memory may reflect the fact that most implicit memory tests are data-driven and therefore rely on perceptual processing which, as noted earlier, is less likely than conceptual tasks to be affected by cognitive biases (Clark et al., 1999; Roediger, 1990).

On balance, then, the evidence indicates that depressed individuals' cognitions are tainted by negativity in a variety of domains including attentional processes, judgments, and memory. Although the precise nature and function of the mechanisms underlying depressive biases are not well established (Mathews & Wells, 2000), it is clear that they represent a state of mind that is conducive to the development of intrusive negative thoughts. Moreover, the depressive mood state itself can increase the likelihood of depressive intrusions by facilitating associations to negative material.

Mood-Congruent Thought

The idea that thoughts are associated with each other in meaningful ways in memory is one of the fundamental assumptions of cognitive psychology. Theorists have incorporated this notion in an associative network model of cognition (e.g., Anderson & Bower, 1973; Collins & Quillian, 1969). The network analogy holds that thoughts are interconnected and that some thoughts are more closely linked than others. This metaphor is used to explain why when a particular thought is activated by perception or by memory retrieval, it leads through a process of spreading activation to an increased likelihood of retrieval of semantically related thoughts.

According to associative network theories, thoughts can be linked by both meaning and emotion (Bower, 1981; Isen, 1984). For instance, the concept *bird* may activate associations to *sparrow* before it would to *penguin* because *sparrow* is more closely associated to the semantic properties of the target concept. Mood states can also prompt related thoughts through associative links. For example, sadness may trigger the thought "Life is unfair," which in turn may lead to the thought "The future is dismal," and so on. Indeed, a variety of studies have shown that depressive moods—both natural and experimentally induced—cue related, negative thoughts and memories (Bargh & Tota, 1988; Blaney, 1986; Bower, 1981).

The enhanced accessibility of negative thoughts during depression increases the likelihood that the depressed person will be confronted with unwanted intrusive thoughts. Unfortunately, this situation can lead to a downward spiral where the depressive mood state cues unwanted thoughts, which in turn trigger associations to other negative thoughts, causing a further deterioration of mood that prompts more negative associations, and so on. Recent research suggests that when confronted with this situation, depressed individuals often engage in thought suppression in an attempt to control the intrusive thoughts that are undermining their well-being. However, thought suppression is a precarious enterprise that can ultimately backfire by ironically fostering a wariness of unwanted thoughts that helps ensure their return.

Thought Suppression

Numerous studies (Spinhoven & van der Does, 1999; Wegner & Zanakos, 1994; Wenzlaff, Meier, & Salas, 2002a; Wenzlaff et al., 2001; Wenzlaff et al., 2002b) have found a strong, positive correlation between depression and chronic thought suppression as measured by the WBSI (Wegner & Zanakos, 1994; see Table 3.1). The high correlation between depression and chronic suppression suggests that many depressed individuals are engaged in an ongoing struggle to inhibit the intrusive thoughts that plague them. Unfortunately, depressed individuals' suppression efforts can ultimately have the unintended effect of intensifying unwanted thoughts. To understand the dilemma posed by thought suppression it is necessary to consider the processes involved in this type of mental control.

Instructing people not to think about a particular thought can ironically make the thought more accessible and intrusive. This observation was made initially for the thought of a white bear by Wegner, Schneider, Carter, and White (1987) and now has been replicated in a substantial array of studies (see Wegner, 1989; Wegner & Smart, 1997; Wenzlaff & Wegner, 2000). This finding has led to the development of *ironic process theory* (Wegner, 1994), which suggests that thought suppression involves two mechanisms: an intentional distraction process that diverts attention away from unwanted thoughts and a monitoring system that remains vigilant for intrusions that call for renewed distraction. Although the distraction process is effortful and consciously guided, the monitoring system is usually unconscious and less demanding of mental effort. Under normal circumstances, these two processes work in concert so that distraction diverts awareness from unwanted thoughts while the monitoring system subtly prompts it to further action at the first sign of failure.

At one level, then, the distraction and monitoring processes are complementary, helping ensure that unwanted thoughts are relegated to the fringes of consciousness. At another level, however, the monitoring system can undermine the goal of suppression by maintaining vigilance for the very thoughts that have been targeted for elimination. Indeed, a variety of studies show that when distraction is disrupted by competing cognitive demands, unwanted thoughts become more pervasive than they would have been if suppression had not been attempted (for a review, see Wenzlaff & Wegner, 2000). For example, studies have found that the imposition of cognitive demands (e.g., time pressures or concurrent memory tasks) during suppression has the effect of not merely diminishing control but of making the target material more accessible and influential than it would have been without suppression. For example, Wegner and Erber (1992, Expt. 1) instructed participants to think or not to think about a target word (e.g., "house"), and then assessed their tendency to respond with the target word to related prompts (e.g., "home") and unrelated cues (e.g., "adult"). With the imposition of time pressure, participants who were engaged in suppression responded to the related prompts with the target word more often than did either suppressing participants not under time constraint or nonsuppressing participants.

In a second experiment, Wegner and Erber (1992) measured the accessibility of target words using a Stroop-type color-naming interference task in which the participants' latency to name the color in which the word was printed was taken as a measure of the accessibility of the word. Participants attempting to suppress a target word showed greater accessibility of the word than did participants trying to think of the target word, but only when they were given a mental load in the form of a 9-digit number to rehearse during the Stroop task (see also Wegner, Erber, & Zanakos, 1993).

DEPRESSION AND SUPPRESSION

There are at least three reasons that depressed individuals are especially likely to suffer the ironic consequences of thought suppression. First, depressed individuals are likely to choose distracters that have an emotional association to the material they are trying to suppress. Second, the depressive mood can drain cognitive resources, thereby undermining the effortful process of distraction. Third, depressed individuals often experience high levels of subjective stress that can tax their ability to employ effective distraction.

Suppression-Related Distracters

When depressed individuals target unwanted thoughts for suppression, they must divert their attention to other—preferably more desirable—thoughts. In depression, however, the types of distracters that are most accessible are often tainted by the same negativity that characterizes the thoughts the person is trying to suppress. Several factors can enhance the accessibility of negative distracters in depression, including cognitive biases, negative life experiences, and the depressive mood itself. Network models of memory indicate that thoughts and moods are associated in meaningful and reciprocal ways (Bower, 1981). Thus, negative thoughts are likely to elicit negative moods and negative moods are apt to make negative thoughts more accessible (Blaney, 1986; Bower, 1981). This state of affairs suggests that depressed individuals' mental control efforts are hindered by the selection of distracters that are emotionally related to the suppression target. In this regard, Wenzlaff et al. (1988) found that in a college student sample, compared to nondepressed individuals, depressed participants chose more negative distracters while trying to suppress negative information. The negative distracters served as reminders of the unwanted material, eventually leading to an increase in thoughts about the suppression target (also see Renaud & McConnell, 2002). A similar pattern of results was obtained by Conway, Howell, and Giannopoulos (1991) who found that dysphoric participants had more difficulty initially suppressing negative thoughts than positive cognitions. Howell and Conway (1992) replicated those results and also showed the converse effect by finding that nondysphoric individuals had more difficulty suppressing positive thoughts.

In a related vein, Wenzlaff, Wegner, and Klein (1991) tested the idea that mood-related distracters create an association between the mood state and the suppression target. The investigators found that reinstating the original mood (using a mood manipulation) that existed during suppression facilitated the return of the suppressed thought. Conversely, participants who were induced to think about a previously suppressed topic experienced a reinstatement of the mood state that existed when they had originally engaged in suppression. Thus, thoughts that are targeted for suppression can become associated with the mood state that is present during suppression. Subsequently the suppression target and the mood state become linked, such that the reinstatement of one prompts the reoccurrence of the other.

Mood-Related Depletion of Cognitive Resources

The distraction component of thought suppression involves an effortful process that can be disrupted when cognitive resources are depleted, thereby enabling unwanted thoughts to exert greater influence. There is a great deal of research showing that during instructed suppression, the imposition of a cognitive load (e.g., rehearsing a series of numbers) leads to a surge in unwanted thoughts (for reviews, see Wegner, 1989, 1994; Wegner & Wenzlaff, 1996; Wenzlaff & Wegner, 2000). Recent research has examined this effect with respect to the naturally occurring suppression associated with depression.

In a study by Wenzlaff and Bates (1998), participants engaged in a task that involved unscrambling words that could form either positive or negative sentences. The results indicated that under normal circumstances, depressed individuals formed more negative statements than did nondepressed participants. However, this negative bias became especially pronounced with the introduction of a cognitive load. This load-related surge in negative thinking was positively correlated with a measure of chronic thought suppression.

Although externally imposed cognitive demands may undermine depressed individuals' suppression efforts, it is also clear that these individuals are plagued by negative thoughts even when external circumstances are conducive to thought suppression (Wenzlaff & Bates, 1998). This observation suggests that there are internal factors that undermine depressed individuals' thought suppression efforts. Indeed, the depressed mood itself may drain cognitive resources that are needed for effortful distraction. Considerable research indicates that depression absorbs cognitive capacity, thereby interfering with the ability to engage in effortful processing (Hartlage, Alloy, Vazquez, & Dykman, 1993).

Stress-Related Depletion of Cognitive Resources

Although the relationship between stress and cognitive performance can be complex (Klein, 1996), a variety of studies have indicated that high levels of stress can disrupt cognitive ability, resulting in reduced memory capacity (Bacon, 1974; Hamilton, 1982), a narrowing of perceptual focus (Combs & Taylor, 1952; Easterbrook, 1959), and attentional deficits (Sanders, 1981). To the extent that life stress depletes cognitive resources, it should undermine the effortful distraction process of thought suppression, thereby allowing the monitoring process to usher unwanted thoughts into consciousness. Depressed individuals may be especially likely to suffer these stress-related consequences because not only are they apt to engage in suppression, but they also appear to be especially likely to experience life stress.

Research indicates that a surge in life stress precedes the onset of depression (Monroe & Hadjiyannakis, 2002). Although there are outstanding questions about the nature of the relationship between stress and depression (Kessler, 1997) and whether the stressors are externally imposed or internally generated (Hammen, 1991), investigators agree that there is a significant temporal link between the stress and depression. From the current perspective, the subjective experience of stress would further undermine depressed individuals' ability to suppress intrusive thoughts. This possibility was supported by a recent longitudinal study examining the relationship between suppression, life stress, and depressive thoughts.

Wenzlaff and Luxton (2003) recruited 103 college students that consisted of high suppressors and low suppressors. Pre- and posttest measures over a 10-week period assessed depression, depressive rumination, and stressful events that arose during the assessment interval. After controlling for initial levels of depression and rumination, the investigators found that high suppressors at the initial assessment who subsequently experienced high levels of stress, experienced a greater increase in depressive thoughts and depressive symptoms after 10 weeks than did any other group. The findings are consistent with the idea that stress undermines thought suppression, thereby allowing negative thoughts to emerge and undermine mood. The results are also consistent with ironic processes theory, although the correlational nature of the study precludes definitive conclusions in that regard.

The Futile Persistence of Suppression

As we have seen, the evidence indicates that depressed individuals are particularly ill equipped to benefit from thought suppression. In addition to having inadequate cognitive resources to maintain effortful distraction, depressed individuals are apt to choose distracters that are affectively related to the suppression target, thus ensuring that awareness will eventually be redirected to the unwanted material. Despite these problems, depressed individuals persist in their efforts to suppress negative thoughts (Wenzlaff & Bates, 1998). This persistence is not only futile; it is also likely to be counterproductive. In the absence of effective distraction, the vigilance supplied by the automatic monitoring process would usher more unwanted thoughts into awareness than would have occurred if suppression had never been attempted. This possibility is supported by recent longitudinal studies showing that thought suppression is associated with a worsening of intrusive thoughts (Wenzlaff & Bates, 1998) and depressive symptoms (Rude, Wenzlaff, Gibbs, Vane, & Whitney, 2002) and with the subsequent occurrence of depression as assessed by diagnostic interview (Rude, Valdez, Odom, & Ebrahimi, 2003).

Given the counterproductive nature of thought suppression, it may—on first consideration—be difficult to understand why depressed individuals continue to use this form of mental control. However, the problems associated with thought suppression are probably not obvious to the depressed person who is seeking relief from negative thoughts. After all, conventional wisdom suggests that a positive frame of mind is important for emotional well-being (Wenzlaff, 1993), thereby encouraging depressed individuals to seek remedy for their emotional plight through mental control. When this approach fails, the depressed person may misattribute the escalation of negative thinking to personal inadequacies or life events. These misattributions could lead the individual to renew mental control efforts, thus perpetuating a process that helps ensure the persistence of unwanted thoughts. Over time, however, it is possible that the problems of thought suppression may cause depressed individuals to despair of ever gaining control over their mental lives. Thus, in the advanced stages of depression, they may forsake control and resign themselves to negative thinking and rumination.

THE ROLE OF INTRUSIVE NEGATIVE THOUGHTS IN DEPRESSION

The research considered thus far provides compelling evidence that a variety of factors contribute to the intrusive thoughts that plague depressed individuals. However, questions remain concerning the role that these unwanted thoughts play in the emotional disturbance. Cognitive theory suggests that negative thoughts are not only symptoms of depression but also precede the mood disturbance and contribute to its development. Another possibility, however, is that intrusive depressive thoughts are simply by-products of depression and do not play a direct role in the etiology of the disorder. This issue—which is central to both cognitive theory and the treatments approaches it has spawned—has been the focus of considerable debate and empirical study. In this section, we examine the evidence that bears on this issue.

Treatment Effects

The results of psychotherapy research support the possibility that negative thoughts contribute to the development and maintenance of depression. Cognitive therapy typically leads to substantial improvement in approximately 50–60% of the cases, equaling the results of drug interventions (Elkin, 1994; Hollon, 1996; Sacco & Beck, 1995). Moreover, recovery is usually accompanied by a significant reduction in dysfunctional thinking (Hamilton & Abramson, 1983; Simons, Garfield, & Murphy, 1984). The relative success of cognitive treatment, however, does not necessarily demonstrate that negative thinking causes depression. One complicating factor is that approximately the same percentage of depressed patients who respond favorably to cognitive therapy also benefit from drug treatment alone (Oei & Free, 1995). Moreover, it is possible that interventions that are unrelated to a disorder's etiology may, nevertheless, be therapeutic. For example, the sexual performance of a patient with erectile dysfunction may be restored by medication, even though the treatment may not address the psychological cause of the problem.

Cognitive Vulnerability

If dysfunctional thoughts promote depression, they should precede the mood disturbance. In an attempt to identify cognitive antecedents to depression, investigators have typically studied the cognitions of formerly depressed individuals who have relapse rates as high as 80% (Judd, 1997). This research generally shows that, under normal circumstances, formerly depressed individuals do not show elevated levels of negative thinking relative to nondepressed people. In a comprehensive review of this research, Ingram et al. (1998) state that "an inescapable conclusion from the majority of these studies is that depressive cognition is largely [mood] state dependent" (p. 157).

The Mood-State Hypothesis

In an effort to detect a cognitive vulnerability to depression, some investigators have tested the idea that a relatively minor downturn in mood can reactivate depressive biases by triggering relevant associations (Miranda & Persons, 1988). Partial support for this idea comes from correlational studies that find that formerly depressed individuals display more dysfunctional attitudes during naturally occurring negative mood shifts (Miranda & Persons, 1988; Miranda, Persons, & Byers, 1990; Roberts & Kassel, 1996). To provide a more precise test of the mood–state hypothesis, several studies have used mood induction procedures with formerly depressed and never-depressed individuals. With some notable exceptions (e.g., Dykman, 1997), most of these studies have shown that during induced negative mood shifts, formerly depressed individuals are more likely than never-depressed people to endorse dysfunctional attitudes (for a review, see Ingram et al., 1998).

Although the mood-priming studies suggest that formerly depressed individuals possess latent dysfunctional cognitions, recent evidence indicates that these negative patterns of thinking may be more virulent than previously suspected. Compared to people who have never had an episode of depression, formerly depressed individuals report higher levels of chronic thought suppression (Wenzlaff & Bates, 1998; Wenzlaff & Eisenberg, 2001; Wenzlaff et al., 2002b) and expend more effort trying to maintain a positive frame of mind (Coyne & Calarco, 1995). These findings suggest that despite the absence of a depressive mood, formerly depressed individuals continue to struggle with intrusive thoughts. Thus, when mental control is disrupted, these suppressed thoughts should have a more pronounced effect on perceptions and judgments.

Suppressed Biases

In the first study to test the possibility that suppression can mask depressive biases, Wenzlaff and Bates (1998) found that the addition of a cognitive load caused a depressive shift in formerly depressed individuals' performance on an experimental task. The task involved unscrambling sentences that could form either a depressive theme or a positive theme. Under no-load conditions, the formerly depressed and never depressed groups equally favored positive sentences. However, the imposition of a cognitive load caused formerly depressed individuals to shift toward negative statements, making their responses resemble those of a depressed group. This load-induced shift in negative thinking was significantly related to high levels of chronic thought suppression.

In a follow-up study, Wenzlaff et al. (2001) assessed formerly depressed individuals' performance on a novel measure of thought accessibility that involved detecting emotionally relevant words in a letter grid. The results indicated that under normal circumstances, both the formerly depressed and never depressed groups identified mostly positive words. However, under cognitive load, the formerly depressed group identified more negative words, reaching levels equivalent to an actively depressed group. A similar pattern of findings was obtained in a study where participants interpreted homophones under varying time constraints (Wenzlaff & Eisenberg, 2001). Unlike never depressed participants, formerly depressed individuals interpreted recorded homophones (e.g., dye/die) in a more negative fashion when they were under time pressure. In each of these studies, the load-related surge in negative thinking was significantly correlated with chronic thought suppression as measured by the WBSI (Wegner & Zanakos, 1994). Because cognitive demands are more apt to interfere with controlled processes rather than automatic ones (Posner & Snyder, 1975; Shiffrin & Schneider, 1977), the load-induced shift suggests that, despite their desire to maintain a positive frame of mind, formerly depressed individuals are predisposed to construe information in a negative manner.

The evidence suggests, then, that suppression—and the negative thoughts that prompt it—often persist following a depressive episode. In the absence of added cognitive demands, formerly depressed individuals' mental control efforts can mask negative thoughts, helping preserve a fragile sense of well-being. However, an increase in life stress can undermine suppression, leading to a surge in negative thinking that could foster a relapse. This situation may help explain why stress often precipitates a depressive episode (Brown & Harris, 1989). Once the depressive mood takes hold, negative thoughts become more accessible and further undermine mental control, thereby increasing that risk of ironic effects. Under these circumstances, the depressive mood is likely to persist until life circumstances improve or the individual adopts more effective coping strategies.

TREATMENT IMPLICATIONS

The research considered thus far highlights the pernicious nature of intrusive thoughts in depression. Included among the array of factors that promote and maintain depressive intrusions are cognitive biases, mood-congruent associations, thought suppression, mood-related depletion of cognitive resources, and life stress. The challenge for therapists is to find ways to diffuse these factors while supplying the cognitive and behavioral tools to help the depressed person gain peace of mind. The remainder of this chapter considers therapeutic considerations and techniques that may help alleviate the depressed patient's mental and emotional turmoil.

Goal Framing

Cognitive therapy offers a variety of techniques to help depressed patients recognize the irrationality of their intrusive thoughts and supplant them with more adaptive cognitions, including reality testing, reattribution, and recording techniques (Beck et al., 1979). Similarly, cognitive therapists have developed useful methods for helping patients identify, scrutinize, and dispute the dysfunctional attitudes and beliefs that often underlie the depressive intrusions (Ellis, 1962; Hollon & Beck, 1986). Once patients are aware of the irrational and dysfunctional nature of their intrusive thoughts and dysfunctional beliefs, they are in a position to adopt more positive ways of thinking. This is a critical stage of the therapeutic process where it is important that the client not fall back on familiar but counterproductive (e.g., thought suppression) coping strategies. From this perspective, goal framing becomes an important consideration.

Recent research suggests that a simple change in the goal of mental control may reduce or eliminate the ironic effects of thought suppression. According to ironic processes theory (Wegner, 1994), there is an important difference between trying *to* think positive thoughts (an approach-oriented goal) and trying *not* to think negative thoughts (an avoidance-oriented goal). When the goal of mental control is to think positive thoughts, the automatic monitoring process is alert for either neutral or negative thoughts that would signal failure. In contrast, the avoidance goal of suppressing negative thoughts invokes a monitoring process that is exclusively vigilant for negative thoughts. Thus, although both goals involve the effortful redirection of attention to positive material, the monitoring process associated with suppression is more likely to produce negative thoughts as its ironic effect.

Support for the superiority of approach-oriented strategies comes from recent personality research exploring the implications of individual differences in the conceptualization of personal goals. This work compares two types of people: those who emphasize moving toward desirable outcomes and those who focus on trying to avert unwanted outcomes. This research indicates that, compared to an approach orientation, an emphasis on avoidance has more deleterious consequences for a host of achievement-relevant and general well-being outcomes (Elliot & Sheldon, 1997; Elliot, Sheldon, & Church, 1997). These results are consistent with research that has experimentally manipulated the emphasis on approach or avoidance goals (Elliot & Harackiewicz, 1996; Roney & Sorrentino, 1995). Recent research has specifically examined the consequences of approach and avoidance forms of mental control. In a series of studies, Wenzlaff and Bates (2000) instructed participants to either try to think positive thoughts or try not to think negative thoughts. The investigators examined the efficacy of these approaches when mental control was disabled (e.g., under cognitive load). The results indicated that whereas avoidance led to an ironic rebound of negative thoughts, the approach orientation did not. However, this research employed a normal sample of participants, leaving it unclear whether an approach orientation is useful for depressed individuals.

As we have already seen, depressed individuals have difficulty directing their attention to positive material. Approach-oriented mental control requires both the sufficient availability and accessibility of goal-relevant material for attentional focus. Unfortunately, depressed individuals may lack these prerequisites. For example, depressed individuals may not have a sufficient repertoire of desirable thoughts and memories to tap because they may have had precious few positive experiences (Beevers, Wenzlaff, Hayes, & Scott, 1999). Moreover, it may be especially difficult to access whatever desirable thoughts are available because their associative links to the depressive mood state are weak, whereas links to negative thoughts are especially strong (Bower, 1981). This state of affairs is likely to cause depressed individuals to forsake approach-oriented mental control in favor of suppression, setting the stage for ironic effects. However, therapeutic techniques that engage the depressed individuals in pleasant activities and experiences (Beck et al., 1979; Lewinsohn & Clarke, 1984) may increase the accessibility of positive thoughts, thereby arming patients with the tools needed for approach-oriented mental control.

Opening Up

In virtually all forms of psychotherapy, the client acknowledges the existence of a problem and is encouraged to openly discuss it with the therapist. Recent research suggests the act of disclosure itself has significant psychological and physical benefits (Pennebaker, 1990, 1997; Pennebaker, Colder, & Sharp, 1990). For example, the simple act of writing about upsetting experiences—although painful in the days of writing— produces long-term improvements in mood and indicators of well-being compared with writing about control topics (Pennebaker, 1990; Smyth, 1998). In a study by Lepore (1997), prospective graduate students who wrote about their thoughts and feelings about graduate entrance exams experienced a significant decline in depressive symptoms from 1 month to 3 days before taking the exam. Students in the control group, who wrote about a trivial topic, maintained a relatively high level of depressive symptoms over the same period.

It may be that the beneficial effects of expressive writing and talking arise because expression reduces the person's tendency to pursue thought suppression. There is evidence that secret keeping is often implemented by the suppression of the secret thought, as people find it useful not to think of the secret when they are hoping to keep from expressing it in their verbal communication or nonverbal gestures (Lane & Wegner, 1995). Some of the salutary consequences of disclosure may arise because divulging thoughts that have been kept hidden releases the person from the continued burden of denying those thoughts to consciousness. In the case of depressive thoughts, disclosure may be helpful because it reduces the person's focus on active suppression and so undermines the production of ironic effects of suppression.

It is important to note that adaptive disclosure is different from the counterproductive rumination associated with depression (Nolen-Hoeksema, 1996). In rumination, depressed individuals dwell on negative thoughts in a failed attempt to gain insight about their feelings and state of mind. The inability to resolve these issues may cause depressed individuals to continue to focus on negative thoughts, thereby inviting more unhappiness, despondency, and hopelessness. In contrast, adaptive disclosure begins as a process of expressing thoughts and feelings without the expectation of new insights or resolution.

Adaptive expression may yield emotional and physiological benefits for a variety of reasons. First, it discourages unproductive rumination and avoids the ironic effects of thought suppression. In addition, whereas rumination and suppression may inflate the perceived importance of negative thoughts, adaptive expression is likely to diffuse negative thoughts by desensitizing the person to them. Finally, unlike intentional rumination that imposes undue pressure to find solutions, expression may allow for the gradual realization of new insights and a more integrated perspective of the self (Pennebaker, 1990).

Mindfulness

There is growing scientific interest in an ancient approach to well-being that involves being attentive to and aware of what is taking place in the present—a state that has been called mindfulness. This state has been described as "the clear and single-minded awareness of what actually happens to us and in us at the successive moments of perception" (Thera, 1962, p. 5) and "keeping one's consiousness alive to the present reality" (Hanh, 1976, p. 11). Research shows that mindfulness is associated with a variety of psychological and physical benefits (Kabat-Zinn, Lipworth, & Burney, 1985; Miller, Fletcher, & Kabat-Zinn, 1995). For example, Brown and Ryan (2003) found that both dispositional and state mindfulness predicted self-regulated behavior and positive emotional states. In a separate study, the investigators also found that increases in mindfulness over time related to declines in mood disturbance and stress among patients with cancer.

One way of understanding mindfulness therapies is to suggest that they tend to counteract a distressed person's natural tendency to try to suppress unwanted thoughts. Rather than instituting new or more effective forms of mental control or distraction, the instruction to be mindful instead promotes an abandonment of mental control intentions and a relinquishment of the ineffective thought suppression strategy (Wegner, 1994, 1997). This kind of therapy may have salutary effects because it replaces the use of a self-defeating mental control technique with a simple relaxation of the control motive.

The relevance of mindfulness to depressive thought intrusions has not gone unnoticed by investigators. In one study, for example, the investigators examined the relapse rates of patients who were treated either with standard therapy or with a modified version of cognitive therapy that incorporated techniques designed to promote mindfulness (Teasdale, Segal, & Williams, 1995). The results indicated that mindfulness training significantly reduced the relapse rates for patients with three or more previous episodes of depression (77% of the sample). It appears that mindfulness training reduced relapse rates by helping patients disengage from depressive thoughts.

It is worth emphasizing that in mindfulness or other therapeutic approaches, it is important that the client take ownership of the change process. Experienced therapists recognize the clinical value of carefully facilitating depressed patients' sense of self-determination in finding more adaptive ways of thinking (Teasdale, 1996). A variety of empirical studies echo the importance of self-determination in the therapeutic process. For example, Simons, Lustman, Wetzel, and Murphy (1985) found that depressed patients who benefited most from cognitive therapy were those who at the outset showed a tendency to take responsibility for their thoughts. Another study found that patients with an internal locus of control showed more emotional improvement when they were encouraged to attribute changes to their own efforts instead of to a placebo pill (Liberman, 1978). The provision of choice increases intrinsic motivation as reflected by greater task persistence and more internal causal attributions (Deci & Ryan, 1985; Dember, Galinsky, & Warm, 1992; Swann & Pittman, 1977). Choice can also increase the impact of strategic self-presentation on private self-appraisals (Jones, Rhodewalt, Berglas, & Skelton, 1981; Rhodewalt & Agustsdottir, 1986). Finally, much evidence shows that counterattitudinal behavior is especially likely to produce corresponding attitude change under conditions of high choice (Wicklund & Brehm, 1976).

A series of experiments tested the idea that perceptions of choice can alter the self-relevance and emotional impact of thoughts (Wenzlaff & LePage, 2000). Individuals who were experiencing negative moods engaged in an exercise that involved generating positive thoughts. The critical manipulation involved leading participants to believe that the thought exercise was either required (low-choice condition) or optional (high-choice condition). The results indicated that in the high-choice condition, participants experienced a significant improvement in mood, producing thoughts that were highly self-relevant and especially memorable. Participants in the low-choice condition reported no change in mood and their thoughts were not as self-relevant and memorable as those generated by the high-choice group.

Research, then, supports psychotherapeutic approaches that foster a sense of self-determination and it advises against heavy-handed methods of persuasion that place the person in a passive role. A patient may comply with instructions to entertain more adaptive thoughts, but if the person does not claim ownership of those new thoughts, they are unlikely to resonate at an emotional level. Thus, in facilitating new beliefs and attitudes, therapists may find that a Socratic method (Beck, Rush, Shaw, & Emery, 1979)—that prompts patients to discover for themselves the value and personal meaning of new ways of thinking and knowing—leads to better results than a more didactic and directive style.

Cautionary Note

Some techniques associated with cognitive therapy may have the unintended effect of fostering depressive thoughts by making the patient more vigilant for their occurrence. For example, some therapists recommend thought stopping as a way of reducing the frequency of maladaptive thoughts (Wolpe, 1958, 1973). Specifically, clients are encouraged to emit a subvocal "Stop" whenever they begin to engage in self-defeating ruminations. To the extent that this technique encourages thought suppression, it may ultimately do more harm than good by promoting an ironic vigilance for the very thoughts the person is trying to eliminate. Evidence exists that thought-stopping techniques can often be counterproductive in precisely this way (Wegner, Eich, & Bjork, 1994), suggesting that thought stopping is unlikely to be a useful therapeutic technique.

The client's potential inclinations to suppress thoughts might also be a problem in other applications of cognitive-behavioral therapy, although evidence in these cases is not yet available. A problem may arise, for example, with the use of self-monitoring techniques that sensitize clients to the occurrence of dysfunctional thoughts. Some forms of cognitive therapy encourage clients to be watchful for negative thinking and to document their dysfunctional thoughts (Burns, 1989). Once they become aware of their dysfunctional thinking, clients can learn to dispute the thoughts and entertain more adaptive responses. The benefits of this approach rest on the ability of the client—with the help of the therapist—to reject dysfunctional thoughts and supplant them with adaptive cognitions. If the client is unable to generate compelling alternatives to dysfunctional thoughts, the self-monitoring exercise may backfire by promoting unproductive rumination. Although the effects of such monitoring and replacement strategies are not yet known, it would be useful to examine whether techniques that encourage suppression, even tangentially, might have some unexpected countertherapeutic influences.

SUMMARY

The mental lives of depressed individuals are tainted by cognitive biases that promote intrusive, negative thoughts. These thoughts are evident during depression but can be veiled by thought suppression prior to the onset of the mood disturbance. Although suppression may mask a cognitive vulnerability to depression, it can also ironically enhance it by fostering vigilance for unwanted thoughts. During depression, thought suppression is rendered ineffective by the enhanced accessibility of negative thoughts and a lack of adequate cognitive resources. A variety of techniques may prove useful in helping depressed individuals overcome the problems caused by their intrusive thoughts and misguided attempts to gain mental control. Treatment interventions for depression may be enhanced by devoting special attention to the importance of self-determination in changing dysfunctional patterns of thinking, framing the goals of mental control in positive ways, and encouraging the adaptive disclosure and release of unwanted thoughts.

ACKNOWLEDGMENTS

Research reported here was supported by a National Institutes of Health grant (No. GM 08194). Richard M. Wenzlaff died prior to publication, and his draft of this chapter was revised by Daniel M. Wegner. Thanks are due to Stephanie S. Rude for her comments.

REFERENCES

Anderson, J. R., & Bower, G. H. (1973). *Human associative memory.* New York: Wiley.

Bacon, S. J. (1974). Arousal and the range of cue utilization. *Journal of Experimental Psychology, 102,* 81–87.

Bargh, J. A., & Tota, M. E. (1988). Context-dependent automatic processing in depression: Accessibility of negative constructs with regard to self and not others. *Journal of Personality and Social Psychology, 54,* 925–939.

Beck, A. T. (1967). *Depression: Clinical, experimental, and theoretical aspects.* New York: Harper & Row.

Beck, A. T., & Beamesderfer, A. (1974). Assessment of depression: The depression inventory. In P. Pichot (Ed.), *Psychological measurements in psychopharmacology: Modern problems in pharmacopsychiatry* (Vol. 7, pp. 151–169). Basel, Switzerland: Karger.

Beck, A. T., & Beck, R. (1972). Screening depressed patients in family practice: A rapid technique. *Postgraduate Medicine, 52*, 81–85.

Beck, A. T., Rush, A. J., Shaw, B. F., & Emery, G. (1979). *Cognitive therapy of depression.* New York: Guilford Press.

Beevers, C. G., Wenzlaff, R. M., Hayes, A. M., & Scott, W. D. (1999). Depression and the ironic effects of thought suppression: Therapeutic strategies for improving mental control. *Clinical Psychology: Science and Practice, 6*, 133–148.

Blaney, P. H. (1986). Affect and memory: A review. *Psychological Bulletin, 99*, 229–246.

Blatt, S. H. J., & Homan, E. (1992). Parent-child interaction in the etiology of dependent and self-critical depression. *Clinical Psychology Review, 12*, 47–91.

Blumberg, S. J. (2000). The White Bear Suppression Inventory: Revisiting its factor structure. *Personality and Individual Differences, 29*, 943–950.

Bower, G. H. (1981). Mood and memory. *American Psychologist, 36*, 129–148.

Brady, E. U., & Kendall, P. C. (1992). Comorbidity of anxiety and depression in children and adolescents. *Psychological Bulletin, 111*, 244–255.

Brown, G. W., & Harris, T. O. (1989). Depression. In G. W. Brown & T. O. Harris (Eds.), *Life events and illness* (pp. 49–93). New York: Guilford Press.

Brown, K. W., & Ryan, R. M. (2003). The benefits of being present: The role of mindfulness in psychological well-being. *Journal of Personality and Social Psychology, 84*, 822–848.

Burns, D. D. (1989). *The feeling good handbook.* New York: Penguin Books.

Clark, D. A. (1992). Depressive, anxious and intrusive thoughts in psychiatric inpatients and outpatients. *Behaviour Research and Therapy, 30*, 93–102.

Clark, D. A., & Beck, A. T. (1989). Cognitive and cognitive-behavioral treatments of anxiety and depression. In P. Kendall & D. Watson (Eds.), *Anxiety and depression: Distinctions and overlapping features* (pp. 379–411). Orlando, FL: Academic Press.

Clark, D. A., Beck, A. T., & Alford, B. A. (1999). *Scientific foundations of cognitive theory and therapy of depression.* New York: Wiley.

Clark, D. A., & de Silva, P. (1985). The nature of depressive and anxious, intrusive thoughts: Distinct or uniform phenomena? *Behaviour Research and Therapy, 23*, 383–393.

Clark, D. A., & Purdon, C. (1993). New perspectives for a cognitive theory of obsessions. *Australian Psychologist, 28*, 161–167.

Clark, D. A., & Purdon, C. (1995). The assessment of unwanted intrusive thoughts: A critique of the literature. *Behaviour Research and Therapy, 33*, 967–976.

Cole, D. A., Jacquez, F. M., & Maschman, T. L. (2001). Social origins of depressive cognitions: A longitudinal study of self-perceived competence in children. *Cognitive Therapy and Research, 25*, 377–396.

Collins, A. M., & Quillian, M. R. (1969). Retrieval time from semantic memory. *Journal of Verbal Learning and Verbal Behavior, 8*, 240–248.

Combs, A. W., & Taylor, C. (1952). The effect of the perception of mild degrees of threat on performance. *Journal of Abnormal and Social Psychology, 47*, 420–424.

Compas, B. E. (1987). Stress and life events during childhood and adolescence. *Clinical Psychology Review, 7*, 275–302.

Compas, B. E., Grant, K. E., & Ey, S. (1994). Psychosocial stress and child/adolescent depression: Can we be more specific? In W. M. Reynolds & H. F. Johnson (Eds.), *Handbook of depression in children and adolescents* (pp. 509–523). New York: Plenum Press.

Conway, M., Howell, A., & Giannopoulos, C. (1991). Dysphoria and thought suppression. *Cognitive Therapy and Research, 15*, 153–166.

Coyne, J. C., & Calarco, M. M. (1995). Effects of the experience of depression: Application of focus groups and survey methodologies. *Psychiatry, 58*, 149–163.

Cutler, S. E., & Nolen-Hoeksema, S. (1991). Accounting for sex differences in depression through female victimization: Childhood sexual abuse. *Sex Roles, 24*, 425–438.

Deci, E. L., & Ryan, R. M. (1985) *Intrinsic motivation and self-determination in human behavior.* New York: Plenum Press.

Dember, W. N., Galinsky, T. L., & Warm, J. S. (1992). The role of choice in vigilance performance. *Bulletin of the Psychonomic Society, 30*, 201–204.

Di Nardo, P. A., & Barlow, D. H. (1990). Syndrome and symptom co-occurrence in the anxiety disorders. In J. D. Maser & C. R. Cloninger (Eds.), *Comorbidity of mood and anxiety disorders* (pp. 205–230). Washington, DC: American Psychiatric Press.

Dykman, B. M. (1997). A test of whether negative emotional priming facilitates access to latent dysfunctional attitudes. *Cognition and Emotion, 11*, 197–222.

Easterbrook, J. A. (1959). The effect of emotion on cue utilization and the organization of behavior. *Psychological Review, 56*, 183–201.

Elkin, I. (1994). The NIMH Treatment of Depression Collaborative Research Program: Where we began and where we are. In A. E. Bergin & S. L. Garfield (Eds.), *Handbook of psychotherapy and behavior change* (4th ed., pp. 114–139). New York: Wiley.

Elliot, A. J., & Harackiewicz, J. (1996). Approach and avoidance achievement goals and intrinsic motivation: A mediational analysis. *Journal of Personality and Social Psychology, 70*, 461–475.

Elliot, A. J., & Sheldon, K. M. (1997). Avoidance achievement motivation: A personal goals analysis. *Journal of Personality and Social Psychology, 73*, 171–185.

Elliot, A. J., Sheldon, K. M., & Church, M. A. (1997). Avoidance personal goals and subjective well-being. *Personality and Social Psychology Bulletin, 23*, 915–927.

Ellis, A. (1962). *Reason and emotion in psychotherapy.* New York: Lyle Stuart.

Gibb, B. E., Alloy, L. B., & Tierney, S. (2001). History of childhood maltreatment, negative cognitive styles, and episodes of depression in adulthood. *Cognitive Therapy and Research, 25*, 425–446.

Gold, D. B., & Wegner, D. M. (1995). The origins of ruminative thought: Trauma, incompleteness, nondisclosure, and suppression. *Journal of Applied Social Psychology, 25*, 1245–1261.

Gotlib, I. H., & McCann, C. D. (1984). Construct accessibility and clinical depression: A longitudinal investigation. *Journal of Abnormal Psychology, 96*, 199–204.

Hamilton, E. W., & Abramson, L. Y. (1983). Cognitive patterns and major depressive disorder: A longitudinal study in a hospital setting. *Journal of Abnormal Psychology, 92*, 173–184.

Hamilton, V. (1982). Cognition and stress: An information processing model. In L. Goldberger & S. Bresnitz (Eds.), *Handbook of stress: Theoretical and clinical aspects* (pp. 105–120). New York: Free Press.

Hammen, C. (1991). Generation of stress in the course of unipolar depression. *Journal of Abnormal Psychology, 100*, 555–561.

Hanh, T. N. (1976). *The miracle of mindfulness.* Boston: Beacon Press.

Hartlage, S., Alloy, L. B., Vasquez, C., & Dykman, B. (1993). Automatic and effortful processing in depression. *Psychological Bulletin, 113*, 247–278.

Hollon, S. D. (1996). The efficacy and effectiveness of psychotherapy relative to medications. *American Psychologist, 53*, 1025–1030.

Hollon, S., & Beck, A. T. (1986). Research on cognitive therapies. In S. L. Garfield & A. E. Bergin (Eds.), *Handbook of psychotherapy and behavior change* (4th ed., pp. 443–482). New York: Wiley.

Hollon, S. D., & Kendall, P. C. (1980). Cognitive self-statements in depression: Development of an automatic thoughts questionnaire. *Cognitive Therapy and Research, 4*, 383–395.

Hollon, S. D., Kendall, P. C., & Lumry, A. (1986). Specificity of depressotypic cognitions in clinical depression. *Journal of Abnormal Psychology, 95*, 52–59.

Howell, A., Conway, M. (1992). Mood and the suppression of positive and negative self-referent thoughts. *Cognitive Therapy and Research, 16*, 535–555.

Ingram, R. E. (1984). Toward an information-processing analysis of depression. *Cognitive Therapy and Research, 8*, 443–478.

Ingram, R. E., Miranda, J., & Segal, Z. V. (1998). *Cognitive vulnerability to depression.* New York: Guilford Press.

Isen, A. (1984). Toward understanding the role of affect in cognition. In R. S. Wyer & T. K. Srull (Eds.), *Handbook of social cognition* (Vol. 2, pp. 179–236). Hillsdale, NJ: Erlbaum.

Jones, E. E., Rhodewalt, F., Berglas, S., & Skelton, J. A. (1981). Effects of strategic self-presentation on subsequent self-esteem. *Journal of Personality and Social Psychology, 41*, 407–421.

Judd, L. L. (1997). The clinical course of unipolar major depressive disorders. *Archives of General Psychiatry, 54*, 989–991.

Kabat-Zinn, J., Lipworth, L., & Burney, R. (1985). The clinical use of mindfulness meditation for the self-regulation of chronic pain. *Journal of Behavioral Medicine, 149,* 936–943.

Kessler, R. C. (1997). The effects of stressful life events on depression. *Annual Review of Psychology, 48,* 191–214.

Klein, G. (1996). The effects of acute stressors on decision making. In J. E. Driskell & E. Salas (Eds.), *Stress and human performance* (pp. 49–88). Mahwah, NJ: Erlbaum.

Lane, J. D., & Wegner, D. M. (1995). The cognitive consequences of secrecy. *Journal of Personality and Social Psychology, 69,* 237–253.

Lepore, S. J. (1997). Expressive writing moderates the relation between intrusive thoughts and depressive symptoms. *Journal of Personality and Social Psychology, 73,* 1030–1037.

Lewinsohn, P. M., & Clarke, G. N. (1984). Group treatment of depressed individuals: The "coping with depression" course. *Advances in Behavior Research and Therapy, 6,* 99–114.

Lewinsohn, P. M., Solomon, A., Seeley, J. R., & Zeiss, A. (2000). Clinical implications of "subthreshold" depressive symptoms. *Journal of Abnormal Psychology, 109,* 345–351.

Liberman, B. L. (1978). The role of mastery in psychotherapy: Maintenance of improvement and prescriptive change. In J. D. Frank, R. Hoehn-Saric, S. D. Imber, B. L. Liberman, & A. R. Stone (Eds.), *Effective ingredients of successful psychotherapy* (pp. 35–72). New York: Brunner/Mazel.

Mathews, G., & Wells, A. (2000). Attention, automaticity, and affective disorder. *Behavior Modification, 24,* 69–93.

Miller, J. J., Fletcher, K., & Kabat-Zinn, J. (1995). Three-year follow-up and clinical implications of a mindfulness meditation-based stress reduction intervention in the treatment of anxiety disorders. *General Hospitial Psychiatry, 17,* 192–200.

Miranda, J., & Persons, J. B. (1988). Dysfunctional attitudes are mood-state dependent. *Journal of Abnormal Psychology, 97,* 76–79.

Miranda, J., Persons, J. B., & Byers, C. N. (1990). Endorsement of dysfunctional beliefs depends on current mood state. *Journal of Abnormal Psychology, 99,* 237–241.

Monroe, S. M., & Hadjiyannakis, K. (2002). The social environment and depression: Focusing on severe life stress. In I. H. Gotlib & C. L. Hammen, (Eds.), *Handbook of depression* (pp. 314–340). New York: Guilford Press.

Muris, P., Merckelbach, H., & Horselenberg, R. (1996). Individual differences in thought suppression: The White Bear Suppression Inventory: Factor structure, reliability, validity and correlates. *Behaviour Research and Therapy, 34,* 501–513.

Neese, R. M. (2000). Is depression an adaption? *Archives of General Psychiatry, 57,* 14–20.

Nolen-Hoeksema, S. (1996). Chewing the cud and other ruminations. In R. S.

Wyer (Ed.), *Advances in social cognition* (Vol. 9, pp. 135–144). Mahwah, NJ: Erlbaum.

Oei, T. P. S., & Free, M. L. (1995). Do cognitive behaviour therapies validate cognitive models of mood disorders? A review of the empirical evidence. *International Journal of Psychology, 30,* 145–179.

Pennebaker, J. W. (1990). *Opening up: The healing power of confiding in others.* New York: Morrow.

Pennebaker, J. W. (1997). Writing about emotional experiences as a therapeutic process. *Psychological Science, 8,* 162–166.

Pennebaker, J. W., Colder, M., & Sharp, L. K. (1990). Accelerating the coping process. *Journal of Personality and Social Psychology, 58,* 528–537.

Pennebaker, J. W., Mehl, M. R., & Niederhoffer, K. (2003). Psychological aspects of natural language use: Our words, our selves. *Annual Review of Psychology, 54,* 547–577.

Posner, M. I., & Snyder, C. R. R. (1975). Attention and cognitive control. In R. L. Solso (Ed.), *Information processing and cognition: The Loyola symposium* (pp. 55–85). Hillsdale, NJ: Erlbaum.

Purdon, C. (2001). Appraisal of obsessional thought recurrences: Impact on anxiety and mood state. *Behavior Therapy, 32,* 47–64.

Purdon, C., & Clark, D. A. (1999). Meta-cognition in obsessive compulsive disorders. *Clinical Psychology and Psychotherapy, 6,* 102–110.

Pyszczynski, T., & Greenberg, J. (1987). Self-regulatory perseveration and the depressive self-focusing style: A self-awareness theory of reactive depression. *Psychological Bulletin, 102,* 122–138.

Rachman, S., & de Silva, P. (1978). Abnormal and normal obsessions. *Behaviour Research and Therapy, 16,* 233–248.

Renaud, J. M., & McConnell, A. R. (2002). Organization of the self-concept and the suppression of self-relevant thoughts. *Journal of Experimental Social Psychology, 38,* 79–86.

Rhodewalt, F., & Agustsdottir, S. (1986). Effects of self-presentation on the phenomenal self. *Journal of Personality and Social Psychology, 50,* 47–55.

Roberts, J. E., & Kassel, J. D. (1996). Mood-state dependence in cognitive vulnerability to depression: The roles of positive and negative affect. *Cognitive Therapy and Research, 20,* 1–12.

Roediger, H. L. (1990). Implicit memory: Retention without remembering. *American Psychologist, 45,* 1043–1056.

Roney, C., & Sorrentino, R. (1995). Reducing self-discrepancies or maintaining self-congruence? Uncertainty orientation, self-regulation, and performance. *Journal of Personality and Social Psychology, 68,* 485–497.

Rude, S. S., Valdez, C. R., Odom, S., & Ebrahimi, A. (2003). Negative cognitive biases predict subsequent depression. *Cognitive Therapy and Research, 27,* 415–429.

Rude, S. S., Wenzlaff, R. M., Gibbs, B., Vane, J., Whitney, T. (2002). Negative interpretive biases predict subsequent depressive symptoms. *Cognition and Emotion, 16,* 423–440.

Sacco, W. P., & Beck, A. T. (1995). Cognitive theory and therapy. In E. E. Beckham & W. R. Leber (Eds.), *Handbook of depression* (pp. 329–351). New York: Guilford Press.

Salkovskis, P. M. (1985). Obsessional–compulsive problems: A cognitive-behavioral analysis. *Behaviour Research and Therapy, 23,* 571–583.

Salkovskis, P. M., & Harrison, J. (1984). Abnormal and normal obsessions: A replication. *Behaviour Research and Therapy, 22,* 549–552.

Sanders, G. S. (1981). Driven by distraction: An integrative review of social facilitation theory and research. *Journal of Experimental Social Psychology, 17,* 227–251.

Shiffrin, R. M., & Schneider, W. (1977). Controlled and automatic human information processing: II. Perceptual learning, automatic attending, and a general theory. *Psychological Review, 84,* 127–190.

Simons, A. D., Garfield, S., & Murphy, D. (1984). The process of change in cognitive therapy and pharmacotherapy for depression. *Archives of General Psychiatry, 41,* 45–51.

Simons, A. D., Lustman, P. J., Wetzel, R. D., & Murphy, G. E. (1985). Predicting response to cognitive therapy of depression: The role of learned resourcefulness. *Cognitive Therapy and Research, 9,* 79–89.

Smyth, J. M. (1998). Written emotional expression: Effect sizes, outcome types, and moderating variables. *Journal of Consulting and Clinical Psychology, 63,* 174–184.

Spinhoven, P., & van der Does, A. J. W. (1999). Thought suppression, dissociation and psychopathology. *Personality and Individual Differences, 27,* 877–886.

Swann W. B., Jr., & Pittman, T. S. (1977). Initiating play activity of children: The moderating influences of verbal cues on intrinsic motivation. *Child Development, 48,* 1128–1132.

Sweeney, P. D., Anderson, K., & Bailey, S. (1986). Attributional style in depression: A meta-analytic review. *Journal of Personality and Social Psychology, 50,* 974–991.

Teasdale, J. D. (1996). Clinically relevant theory: Integrating clinical insight with cognitive science. In P. M. Salkovskis (Ed.), *Frontiers of cognitive therapy* (pp. 26–47). New York: Guilford Press.

Teasdale, J. D., & Barnard, P. J. (1993). *Affect, cognition, and change: Re-modeling depressive thought.* Hillsdale, NJ: Erlbaum.

Teasdale, J. D., Segal, Z., & Williams, M. G. (1995). How does cognitive therapy prevent depressive relapse and why should attentional control (mindfulness) training help? *Behavior Research and Therapy, 33,* 25–39.

Thera, N. (1962). *The heart of Buddhist meditation.* New York: Weiser.

van den Hout, M., Merckelbach, H., & Pool, K. (1996). Dissociation, reality monitoring trauma, and thought suppression. *Behavioural and Cognitive Psychotherapy, 24,* 97–108.

Wang, A., & Clark, D. A. (2002). Haunting thoughts: The problem of obsessive mental intrusions. *Journal of Cognitive Psychotherapy, 16,* 193–208.

Watson, D., & Kendall, P. C. (1989). Common and differentiating features of anxiety and depression: Current findings and future directions. In P. C. Kendall & D. Watson (Eds.), *Anxiety and depression: Distinctive and overlapping features* (pp. 493–508). San Diego, CA: Academic Press.

Wegner, D. M. (1989). *White bears and other unwanted thoughts.* New York: Viking/Penguin.

Wegner, D. M. (1994). Ironic processes of mental control. *Psychological Review, 101,* 34–52.

Wegner, D. M. (1997). When the antidote is the poison: Ironic mental control processes. *Psychological Science, 8,* 148–150.

Wegner, D. M., Eich, E., & Bjork, R. A. (1994). Thought suppression. In D. Druckman & R. A. Bjork (Eds.), *Learning, remembering, believing: Enhancing human performance* (pp. 277–293). Washington, DC: National Academy Press.

Wegner, D. M., & Erber, R. (1992). The hyperaccessibility of suppressed thoughts. *Journal of Personality and Social Psychology, 63,* 903–912.

Wegner, D. M., Erber, R. E., & Zanakos, S. (1993). Ironic processes in the mental control of mood and mood-related thought. *Journal of Personality and Social Psychology, 65,* 1093–1104.

Wegner, D. M., Schneider, D. J., Carter, S., & White, T. (1987). Paradoxical effects of thought suppression. *Journal of Personality and Social Psychology, 53,* 5–13.

Wegner, D. M., & Smart, L. (1997). Deep cognitive activation: A new approach to the unconscious. *Journal of Consulting and Clinical Psychology, 65,* 984–995.

Wegner, D. M., & Wenzlaff, R. M. (1996). Mental Control. In E. T. Higgins & A. W. Kruglanski (Eds.). *Social psychology: Handbook of basic principles.* New York: Guilford.

Wegner, D. M., & Zanakos, S. (1994). Chronic thought suppression. *Journal of Personality, 62,* 615–640.

Wells, A., & Papageorgiou, C. (1998). Relationships between worry, obsessive–compulsive symptoms and meta-cognitive beliefs. *Behaviour Research and Therapy, 36,* 899–913.

Wenzlaff, R. M. (1993). The mental control of depression: Psychological obstacles to emotional well-being. In D. M. Wegner & J. W. Pennebaker (Eds.), *Handbook of mental control* (pp. 238–257). Englewood Cliffs, NJ: Prentice Hall.

Wenzlaff, R. M., & Bates, D. E. (1998). Unmasking a cognitive vulnerability to depression: How lapses in mental control reveal depressive thinking. *Journal of Personality and Social Psychology, 75,* 1559–1571.

Wenzlaff, R. M., & Bates, D. E. (2000). The relative efficacy of concentration and suppression strategies of mental control. *Personality and Social Psychology Bulletin, 26,* 1200–1212.

Wenzlaff, R. M., & Grozier, S. A. (1988). Depression and the magnification of failure. *Journal of Abnormal Psychology, 97,* 90–93.

Wenzlaff, R. M., & Eisenberg, A. R. (2001). Mental control after dysphoria: Evidence of a suppressed, depressive bias. *Behavior Therapy, 32,* 27–45.

Wenzlaff, R. M., & LePage, J. P. (2000). The emotional impact of chosen and imposed thoughts. *Personality and Social Psychology Bulletin, 26*, 1502–1514.

Wenzlaff, R. M., & Luxton, D. D. (2003). The role of thought suppression in depressive rumination. *Cognitive Therapy and Research, 27*, 293–308.

Wenzlaff, R. M., Meier, J., & Salas, D. M. (2002a). Thought suppression and memory biases during and after depressive moods. *Cognition and Emotion, 16*, 403–422.

Wenzlaff, R. M., Rude, S. S., Taylor, C. J., Stultz, C. H., & Sweatt, R. A. (2001). Beneath the veil of thought suppression: Attentional bias and depression risk. *Cognition and Emotion, 15*, 235–252.

Wenzlaff, R. M., Rude, S. S., & West, L. M. (2002b). Cognitive vulnerability to depression: The role of thought suppression and attitude certainty. *Cognition and Emotion, 16*, 533–548.

Wenzlaff, R. M., & Wegner, D. M. (2000). Thought suppression. *Annual Review of Psychology, 51*, 59–91.

Wenzlaff, R. M., Wegner, D. M., & Klein, S. B. (1991). The role of thought suppression in the bonding of thought and mood. *Journal of Personality and Social Psychology, 60*, 500–508.

Wenzlaff, R. M., Wegner, D. M., & Roper, D. W. (1988). Depression and mental control: The resurgence of unwanted negative thoughts. *Journal of Personality and Social Psychology, 55*, 882–892.

Wicklund, R. A., & Brehm, J. W. (1976). *Perspectives on cognitive dissonance.* Hillsdale, NJ: Wiley.

Williams, J. M., & Nulty, D. D. (1986). Construct accessibility, depression and the emotional stroop task: Transient mood or stable structure? *Personality and Individual Differences, 7*, 485–491.

Wolpe, J. (1958). *Psychotherapy by reciprocal inhibition.* Stanford, CA: Stanford University Press.

Wolpe, J. (1973). *The practice of behavior therapy* (2nd ed.). Oxford, UK: Pergamon Press.

CHAPTER 4

UNWANTED INTRUSIVE THOUGHTS IN INSOMNIA

ALLISON G. HARVEY

Chronic insomnia is a prevalent psychological disorder that has severe consequences for the sufferer that include social, interpersonal, and occupational impairment. The aim of this chapter is to examine the extent to which intrusive and worrisome thought is important in the maintenance of insomnia. After defining intrusive thoughts, along with the related concepts of worry and rumination, I present a critical review of the evidence for the role of intrusive and worrisome thought in insomnia, both during the night *and* the day. I present and evaluate four theoretical explanations for the persistence of intrusive and worrisome thought in insomnia, including the impact of (1) beliefs about sleep, (2) metacognition, (3) strategies used to intentionally control or suppress unwanted thoughts, and (4) time distortion and sleep perception. Finally, the chapter specifies several clinical implications and future directions for research.

WHAT IS INSOMNIA?

Insomnia is a prevalent psychological health problem, with between 4 and 22% of people reporting chronic insomnia (Ancoli-Israel & Roth,

1999; Chevalier et al., 1999). The prevalence is higher among women (Espie, 1991; Morin, 1993) and older adults (Lichstein & Morin, 2000). People with insomnia suffer from more functional impairment, work absenteeism, impaired concentration and memory, and increased use of medical services (Roth & Ancoli-Israel, 1999). Further, there is evidence that insomnia significantly heightens the risk of having an accident (Ohayon et al., 1997) and significantly heightens the risk of subsequently developing another psychological disorder, particularly an anxiety disorder, depression, or substance-related disorder (see Harvey, 2001a, for review). Not surprisingly then, it is regarded as a serious public health problem with the direct and indirect costs associated with insomnia in the United States estimated between $30 billion and $35 billion (Chilcott & Shapiro, 1996).

The clinical use of the word *insomnia* does not refer to the occasional night of poor sleep that most people experience, especially in association with a stressful life event. Instead, the term *insomnia* refers to a difficulty, of at least 1 month's duration, that involves difficulty getting to sleep, maintaining sleep, or waking in the morning not feeling restored. For a diagnosis of "primary" insomnia according to the text revision of the fourth edition of *Diagnostic and Statistical Manual of Mental Disorders* (DSM-IV-TR; American Psychiatric Assoiacation, 2000), these disturbances must be severe enough to cause significant distress or impairment and must not be fully explained by another sleep disorder (e.g., sleep apnea or periodic limb movement disorder), mental disorder (e.g., bipolar disorder and generalized anxiety disorder), substance use (e.g., caffeine, some antidepressant medications, and especially the selective serotonin reuptake inhibitors), or illness (e.g., asthma and pain).

Insomnia is often comorbid with other psychological disorders especially depression, anxiety, and substance abuse (see Harvey, 2001a; McCrae & Lichstein, 2001, for review). In such cases it is sometimes clear that the insomnia is "secondary" to the so-called primary disorder and that treatment should be targeted at the primary disorder. However, more often than not the relationship between insomnia and the other disorder is more complex and not best captured by the primary versus secondary distinction (Harvey, 2001a). Instead, the insomnia and the other disorder are typically mutually maintaining. To give just one example, there is evidence that an intervention for insomnia and nightmares, for individuals diagnosed with posttraumatic stress disorder (PTSD), not only reduces sleep disturbance but also reduces the severity of PTSD symptomatology (Krakow et al., 2001). This finding is consis-

tent with the suggestion that insomnia, nightmares, and PTSD are mutually maintaining because the insomnia arises due to hyperarousal and
fear of falling asleep and experiencing a nightmare. But the insomnia results in sleep deprivation which, in turn, leads to impaired daytime functioning. These are conditions that are not conducive to the processing
and resolution of trauma memories but instead may substantially increase anxiety (for review, see Harvey, Jones, & Schmidt, 2003; Rothbaum & Mellman, 2001). Although yet to be empirically tested, I would
contend that the thought processes discussed in this chapter are relevant
to primary insomnia, as well as insomnia that is comorbid with another
medical or psychological health problem.

DEFINITION OF UNWANTED INTRUSIVE THOUGHTS

Intrusions are spontaneous, unwanted, unbidden, uncontrollable, and
discrete thoughts, images or urges that are attributed to an internal origin (Rachman 1981; Wells & Morrison 1994). From this definition note
that intrusive thoughts can occur as a verbal thought (words and sentences), an image (pictures), or an urge (a desire to do something/engage
in a particular act). While some intrusions are easily dismissed, under
certain circumstances they will trigger *worry* and *rumination* (e.g.,
Freeston & Ladouceur, 1993; Salkovskis, 1985; Wells, 2000; see also
Harvey, Watkins, Mansell & Shafran, 2004). Specifically, if the intrusion
is appraised as indicating danger or as being particularly personally relevant it is likely to result in worry and rumination.

The term *worry* refers to "a chain of thoughts and images, negatively affect-laden and relatively uncontrollable" (Borkovec, Robinson,
Pruzinsky, & DePree, 1983, p. 10). Empirical investigations have shown
that worry mainly occurs as verbal thought, as opposed to images (e.g.,
Borkovec & Inz, 1990). The term *rumination* has been used to refer to
the repetitive focusing on the "causes, meanings and consequences" of
one's feelings and symptoms (Nolen-Hoeksema, 1991, p. 567). As rumination has mostly been used to describe recurrent thought in the context
of depression and worry has often been used to describe recurrent
thought in the context of generalized anxiety disorder (GAD), two separate empirical literatures have developed that each seek to understand
the cause and consequences of either worry or rumination. However, in
a recent debate the notion that worry and rumination are distinct
thought phenomena has been challenged, with several researchers sug-

gesting that worry and rumination are overlapping or even identical processes (e.g., Fresco, Frankel, Mennin, Turk, & Heimberg, 2002; Segerstrom, Tsao, Alden, & Craske, 2000). Although the debate is not yet resolved, as insomnia is often comorbid with both GAD and depression (Harvey, 2001a; McCrae & Lichstein, 2001), it is likely that both worry and rumination will be relevant to investigations of thought phenomena in the context of insomnia. Taken together, intrusions, worry, and rumination are closely related terms, with intrusions referring to the initial trigger thought that may, under certain circumstances, initiate an ongoing thought process in the form of worry or rumination.

Since the investigations of Borkovec and colleagues in the early 1980s, it has been proposed that insomnia "is often the result of an inability to turn off intrusive, affectively-laden thoughts and images at bedtime" (Borkovec et al., 1983, p. 9). Clinical observation indicates that a majority of individuals suffering from insomnia complain that they cannot get to sleep and/or maintain sleep because of unwanted intrusive thoughts and worries (Borkovec, 1982). Given that these observations were made over two decades ago it is perhaps surprising to find that a detailed empirical analysis of unwanted intrusive and worrisome thoughts, in the context of insomnia, is in the early stages of development. For example, the field has not yet distinguished between the various thought phenomena described earlier (i.e., intrusive thoughts, worry, and rumination). Accordingly, in this chapter we discuss the literature pertaining to *unwanted intrusive and worrisome thought*, a phrase that reflects the absence of clear distinctions in the field to date.

UNWANTED INTRUSIVE THOUGHTS AND WORRY DURING THE NIGHT

A review of the literature indicates that research on the intrusive and worrisome thoughts experienced by patients with insomnia first occurred in the early 1980s and then reemerged in the early 1990s, from which point on there has been a steady stream of empirical data attesting to the importance of this clinical phenomena. This growth in interest has been spurred by the inclusion of intrusive and worrisome thinking in several theoretical models of the maintenance of insomnia (e.g., Borkovec, 1982; Espie, 2002; Harvey, 2002a; Lundh, 1998; Lundh & Broman, 2000; Morin, 1993). In this section, the empirical evidence that has accrued relating to thought processes that occur during the night are reviewed within three categories, divided according to the methodology employed: exploratory methods, correlational data and experimental data.

Exploratory Methods

In the now classic study, Lichstein and Rosenthal (1980) inquired among a sample of 296 individuals with insomnia whether cognitive or somatic arousal was the main determinant of their insomnia. Cognitive arousal was 10 times more likely to be cited, relative to somatic arousal. Results obtained from administering the Sleep Disturbance Questionnaire (SDQ; Espie, Brooks, & Lindsay, 1989) to patients with insomnia are consistent with Lichstein and Rosenthal's findings. The SDQ involves rating each of 12 statements for the extent to which they are relevant to "your typical sleep pattern." The key result of interest is that across the 12 statements, the items that refer to intrusive and worrisome thoughts, such as "My mind keeps turning things over" and "I am unable to empty my mind," are the ones most often endorsed by patients with insomnia (Espie et al., 1989; Harvey, 2000). In other words, these studies indicate that the majority of patients with insomnia perceive intrusive and worrisome thought as the main causal factor in their sleep disturbance.

Several research groups have conducted a content analysis of intrusive and worrisome thoughts during sleep induction (i.e., while trying to fall asleep). Table 4.1 summarizes these studies. As evident from the table, intrusive thoughts and worry about sleep and attempts to problem solve emerge as the major topics that people with insomnia think about during the pre-sleep period.

A number of methodological issues arise from this research. First, the initial three studies in Table 4.1 (Fichten et al., 1998; Harvey, 2000; Watts, Coyle, & East, 1994) involved an interview or questionnaire that required the participants to retrospectively recall to what extent they thought about a predetermined list of topics as they were trying to fall asleep. Unfortunately, each of the three studies employed a different list of topics. Hence, it is difficult to directly compare the results across the studies. This disadvantage and the limitations inherent to retrospective recall are overcome by the latter three studies that directly sampled the content of thinking during sleep induction. Kuisk, Bertelson, and Walsh (1989) conducted brief interviews at 4-minute intervals during the presleep period whereas Wicklow and Espie (2000) and Nelson and Harvey (2003) sent voice-activated recorders home with the participants and asked them to verbalize the content of their thoughts whenever they

TABLE 4.1. Studies Documenting the Content of Intrusive and Worrisome Thoughts during Sleep Onset

Authors	Watts et al. (1994)	Harvey (2002)	Fitchen et al. (1998)	Kuisk et al. (1989)	Wicklow & Espie (1999)	Nelson & Harvey (2003)
Participants	1. Worried insomniacs ($n = 28$) 2. Nonworried insomniacs ($n = 10$) 3. Worried noninsomniacs ($n = 11$) 4. Nonworried noninsomniacs ($n = 30$)	1. Individuals with insomnia ($n = 30$) 2. Good sleepers ($n = 30$)	Over 55 years of age: 1. Poor sleepers ($n = 122$) 2. Good sleepers ($n = 189$)	1. Normal sleepers ($n = 8$) 2. Objective insomnia ($n = 8$) 3. Subjective insomnia ($n = 8$)	Patients with insomnia ($n = 21$)	1. Patients with insomnia ($n = 20$) 2. Good sleepers ($n = 20$)
Type of study	Questionnaire	Interview	Questionnaire	Direct sampling	Direct sampling	Direct sampling of images
Statistical method	Principal components analysis	Between group chi-square tests with an adjusted p value to control for multiple comparisons	Principal components analysis	Content analysis then analyses of variance to measure three hypotheses.	Content analysis of audiorecorded material	Content analysis of audiorecorded material
Total number of participants	79	60	445	24	21 participants over three nights	30 participants

(continued)

TABLE 4.1. Studies Documenting the Content of Intrusive and Worrisome Thoughts during Sleep Onset

Authors	Watts et al. (1994)	Harvey (2002)	Fitchen et al. (1998)	Kuisk et al. (1989)	Wicklow & Espie (1999)	Nelson & Harvey (2003)
Results	Six factors: 1. Mental activity and rehearsal 2. Thoughts about sleep 3. Family and long-term concerns 4. Positive plans and concerns 5. Somatic preoccupations 6. Work and recent concerns	Insomnia group reported *more*: 1. Worry about not getting to sleep 2. General worries 3. Solving problems 4. Focus on the time 5. Focus on noises in the house Insomnia group reported *less*: 6. Focus on nothing in particular	Three factors: 1. Generalized positive thinking 2. Generalized negative thinking 3. Thoughts related to sleep	The objective insomnia group experienced more frequent cognitive activity compared to the subjective insomnia group. Both insomnia groups experienced more negative thoughts compared to the normal sleepers.	1. Rehearsal/ planning/ problem solving 2. Sleep and its consequences 3. Reflection on quality of thoughts 4. Arousal status 5. External noise 6. Autonomic experiences 7. Procedural factors 8. Rising from bed	Relative to the good sleeper group, the insomnia group reported: 1. Fewer random/ nonconnected thoughts 2. More thoughts about intimate relationships 3. More thoughts about sleep

had difficulty falling asleep. These direct sampling studies are particularly welcome additions to the literature as they are likely to increase the validity of the findings.

The second issue concerns the size of the samples employed. Note that for the Harvey (2000) study, the sample size was insufficient to enable the completion of a factor analysis. Further, in the Watts et al. (1994) study the sample size was not large enough to conduct a separate factor analysis on the insomnia sample. The only study that recruited a large enough sample to conduct a reliable factor analysis was the Fichten et al. (1998) study, but these researchers recruited "poor sleepers" rather than patients with insomnia. As such, the generalizability of these findings to an insomnia sample is yet to be determined.

Correlational Studies

A number of studies have reported a significant positive correlation between measures of presleep cognitive activity and sleep-onset latency (e.g., Fichten et al., 1998; Kelly, 2002; Nicassio, Mendlowitz, Fussell, & Petras, 1985; Van Egeren, Haynes, Franzen, & Hamilton, 1983). That is, the more unwanted intrusive and worrisome thoughts that people report the longer it takes for sleep onset. These studies extend the exploratory findings discussed in the previous section by demonstrating a statistical association between intrusive and worrisome thought and sleep. In an interesting extension to these studies, patients with insomnia who reported a tendency toward stress-related intrusive thoughts also reported poorer sleep quality (Hall et al., 2000). In this study, the tendency toward stress-related intrusive thoughts was measured by the Impact of Event Scale.

However, it should be noted that not all studies have found a correlation between cognitive activity and sleep. Sanavio (1988) reported a low correlation (0.09) between a measure of presleep thought, the Presleep Intrusive Cognitions Inventory, and self-reported sleep latency. As well, Van Egeren et al. (1983) found that the content of presleep thought was significantly correlated with subjectively estimated time taken to fall asleep but was not correlated with objective estimates of time taken to fall asleep (i.e., polysomnography). One likely account of these discrepant findings is that both the Sanavio (1988) and Van Egeren et al. (1983) studies tested the correlation between measures of the *content* of presleep thought rather than the *frequency* of presleep thought. Note that the distinction made in the Van Egeren et al. (1983) study, between the correlation with subjective sleep estimates (by self-report in the morning on waking) versus objective sleep estimates (by actigraphy or polysom-nography), is important to explore in future correlational research.

Experimental Studies

While the studies reviewed thus far are consistent with the hypothesis that unwanted intrusive and worrisome thought functions to maintain insomnia, studies documenting self-attributed cause, self-reported thought content, and correlations do not, in isolation, constitute strong evidence for a causal relationship between intrusive and worrisome thought and insomnia. However, empirical support is greatly strengthened by experi-mental manipulations of unwanted intrusive and worrisome thought. The relevant experimental studies can be divided into two groups: (1) those that aim to "activate" or increase intrusive and worrisome thought and (2) those that seek to "deactivate" or decrease intrusive and worri-some thought. The empirical work in this area is impressive because re-searchers have used a variety of research *contexts* and *samples* and by doing this they provide convergent evidence for the importance of intru-sive and worrisome thoughts in the maintenance of insomnia. Examples of the variety of contexts employed are an afternoon nap in a sleep labo-ratory, sleeping at night in a sleep laboratory, and sleeping at night in own home. Examples of the variety of samples employed are individuals who meet full diagnostic criteria for insomnia and are currently treat-ment seeking, individuals meeting full diagnostic criteria for insomnia but are recruited from the college population, poor sleepers, and good sleepers experimentally manipulated into a "state" of insomnia. In the section that follows, the studies that report the effect of manipulating unwanted intrusive and worrisome thought, as the participants are try-ing to get to sleep, are critically reviewed.

Experimentally Increasing Intrusive and Worrisome Presleep Thought

Gross and Borkovec (1982) manipulated the likelihood of experiencing intrusive and worrisome thought by informing one group of good sleep-ers, immediately before an afternoon nap, that they would have to give a speech. The group told that they would have to give a speech took sig-nificantly *longer* to fall asleep, relative to the control group who were not threatened with giving a speech. The authors interpreted this finding as indicating that the speech threat led to an increase in worry, which, in turn, resulted in poorer sleep. However, a limitation of this study was that a direct check of the assumption that the speech threat increased intrusive and worrisome thought was not included.

Lichstein and Fanning (1990) compared night time sleep in two samples of students, one with insomnia and the other who were good sleepers. A polygraph malfunction was staged to heightened participants' alertness to the possibility that they might be accidentally shocked. Following the manipulation, the insomnia group exhibited significantly higher skin conductance responses while trying to get to sleep, relative to those in the good sleeper group. On the basis that skin conductance is a correlate of cognitive arousal, the authors speculated that this increase reflected anxious worry/rumination in the sample with insomnia. Similar to the Gross and Borkovec study, a limitation was the absence of an independent check on the presence of worry/rumination. Also, sleep was not measured hence it is not possible to examine the impact of cognitive arousal on sleep onset.

Tang and Harvey (2004a) experimentally manipulated good sleepers to experience anxious or neutral cognitive arousal during the presleep period prior to an afternoon nap. The participants were staff and students recruited from the university population. Following Gross and Borkovec (1982), anxious cognitive arousal was activated by a speech threat whereas the activation of neutral cognitive arousal consisted of informing participants that they would be asked to write an essay on waking. Manipulation checks indicated that both the speech threat and the essay task increased cognitive activity equally but only the speech threat group experienced an increase in anxiety. However, both groups reported taking longer to fall asleep (sleep-onset latency; SOL), relative to a no manipulation control condition, but the two cognitive arousal groups (anxious versus neutral) did not differ on self-reported SOL.

Hall, Buysse, Reynolds, Kupfer, and Baum (1996) recruited undergraduate students who scored in the upper and lower range on a measure of tendency to experience intrusive thoughts. The study was conducted in the sleep laboratory during the night. Just prior to participants' bedtime, an experimental manipulation was administered in which half the participants were told that the following morning they would be asked to read magazines while the other half were told that the following morning they would be asked to give a speech. The group who were told that they would have to give a speech experienced more intrusive thought relating to the task whilst trying to fall asleep and during awakening throughout the night. Furthermore, stress-related intrusive thought was associated with longer time taken to fall asleep and more awakenings throughout the night (i.e., poorer sleep continuity). Perhaps surprisingly, a tendency to experience intrusive thoughts did not predict the frequency of intrusions during the experiment or sleep parameters. Unfortunately the researchers did not report how they assessed intrusive thoughts throughout the night. Nevertheless, the question of whether more enduring trait differences in intrusive thoughts might influence the situational intrusions that occur while trying to fall asleep is worthy of further investigation.

Experimentally Decreasing Intrusive and Worrisome Presleep Thought

Employing a sample of patients with insomnia, two studies reported that manipulations that distract the individual from intrusive and worrisome presleep cognitive activity significantly *shortened* sleep-onset latency (Haynes, Adams, & Franzen, 1981; Levey, Aldaz, Watts, & Coyle, 1991). The distracting task employed by Haynes et al. (1981) involved assigning participants moderately difficult arithmetic problems to solve, whereas Levey et al. (1991) interrupted the normal flow of thoughts by having subjects subvocalize the word *the* at a rate that competes with cognitive activity. Note that a limitation of the Levey et al. (1991) study was that it was an informal report involving a series of single-case studies with no control group to establish that the improvements reported were not simply a function of expectancy or demand characteristics.

In a third study, Harvey and Payne (2002) recruited undergraduate students who met diagnostic criteria for insomnia. The participants were randomly allocated to one of three conditions: instructions to distract from intrusive and worrisome thought using imagery ("imagery distraction group"), general instructions to distract without specific instructions about how to distract ("general distraction group"), or no instructions. The group that was given instructions to distract using imagery fell asleep more quickly and reported fewer, less frequent, and less distressing presleep cognitive activity compared to the "no instruction" group. The authors explained this finding by suggesting that the "imagery distraction" task occupied sufficient attentional resources to keep the individual from reengaging with thoughts, worries, and concerns during the presleep period.

Summary

There is now considerable evidence that patients with insomnia experience unwanted intrusive and worrisome thought during sleep onset and that the majority of patients attribute their sleep disturbance to a "racing mind." We also know that experimental manipulations that *increase* presleep cognitive activity result in an *increase* in the subjective estimation of time taken to fall asleep and that experimental manipulations that *decrease* presleep cognitive activity result in a *decrease* in SOL. Although this evidence clearly indicates that intrusive and worrisome thoughts are likely to be important in perpetuating insomnia, one caveat is that many of the studies were conducted with analogue samples or in laboratory settings. While such studies are important for providing convergent evidence, for establishing more rigorous methodology, and for investigating new concepts (Stopa & Clark, 2001), the extent to which such findings can be directly generalized to the sample of interest—general practitioner-referred insomnia samples—should be established via one of two methods. First, these findings need replication with treatment-seeking patient samples. Second, further empirical research is needed to determine whether the characteristics of intrusive and worrisome thought experienced by an analogue sample (e.g., good sleepers manipulated into a "state" of insomnia) varies quantitatively or qualitatively from the sleep disturbance of treatment seekers. It is likely that analogue and clinical intrusions occur along a continuum, given the literature documenting that intrusions (e.g., Purdon & Clark, 1993; Rachman & de Silva, 1978) and worry (e.g., Wells & Morrison, 1994) are very commonly experienced by participants in nonpatient samples.

Two of the studies reviewed in this section administered experimental manipulations that induced neutral cognitive activity. These studies are useful for determining whether neutral cognitive activity is as potent a sleep deterrent as worrisome cognition. In the Tang and Harvey (2004a) study one of the conditions involved telling good sleepers, prior to an afternoon nap session, that they would have to write an essay on waking. A manipulation check confirmed that this task increased cognitive activity but did not increase anxiety. The manipulation resulted in the participants reporting that they took longer to experience sleep. The time taken to fall asleep by this group was the same as the time for those in a comparison group who were given a speech threat. In the Haynes et al. (1981) study, good sleepers and patients with insomnia were given an arithmetic task to complete while trying to fall asleep, at night, in the sleep laboratory. The result was that the good sleeper group took longer to fall asleep whereas the insomnia group took less time to fall asleep, relative to their own baseline, established over two nights. Together these findings raise the possibility that the valence of the cognitive activity (neutral vs. worrisome) may have an impact on the sleep of good sleepers and patients with insomnia differently, with good sleepers experiencing poorer sleep when neutral cognitive activity is increased but patients with insomnia experiencing better sleep. Perhaps good sleepers are not accustomed to experiencing cognitive activity while trying to get to sleep so any increase (whether neutral or worrisome) is problematic. In contrast, neutral cognitive activity, for patients with insomnia, may serve as a distractor from worrisome cognitive activity. Of course, this interpretation relies on the assumption that arithmetic tasks generate neutral cognitive activity. A limitation of the Haynes et al. (1981) study was that a check for this assumption was not included in the protocol.

Unfortunately, no studies could be located that investigated different types of negative cognitive activity. In other words, worry, rumination, and intrusions have not yet been distinguished. Furthermore, it is also important to note that all the studies reviewed in this section focused on the initial presleep period, when people first get into bed and turn out the light at the beginning of the nighttime sleep period. Although there is no reason to believe that the results found will not also function to impair the return of sleep, this issue has yet to be empirically investigated.

UNWANTED INTRUSIVE THOUGHTS
AND WORRY DURING THE DAY

It is increasingly recognized that processes operating during the daytime are important to the maintenance of insomnia (e.g., Espie, 2002; Means, Lichstein, Epperson, & Johnson, 2000; Morin, 1993). In fact, I have argued elsewhere that daytime processes are equally important to nighttime processes in the maintenance of insomnia (Harvey, 2002a). It is this perspective that has hypothesized that excessive worrisome thinking about sleep and other topics contributes to a vicious cycle that maintains insomnia at night *as well as* tiredness, fatigue, and anxiety during the day. Here is one example of a daytime vicious cycle. On waking, people with insomnia often worry that they have not obtained sufficient sleep. This worry, in turn, triggers arousal and distress, monitoring for sleep-related threats (e.g., lapses in concentration and low mood), and the use of counterproductive safety behaviors (e.g., taking the day off work and napping). Each of these processes contributes to the maintenance of insomnia; worry, arousal, and distress drain attentional resources and interfere with satisfying and effective daytime performance (e.g., Sarason, 1984). Monitoring increases the detection of ambiguous cues (e.g., feelings of tiredness) that are then misinterpreted ("I mustn't have slept enough") (Clark, 1997), and the use of safety behaviors, such as taking the day off work to nap, maintains the belief that "if I feel awful on waking it means I haven't slept enough and that I should take the day off work so as to catch up on sleep" (Harvey, 2002b). To date, the role that these various daytime cognitive, behavioral, and affective processes play in the maintenance of insomnia remains to be empirically tested.

The only study that might constitute a measure of daytime thought processes in insomnia tested the prediction that, relative to good sleepers, patients with insomnia catastrophize more, which, in turn, is associated with increased negative affect and heightened perception of threat (Harvey & Greenall, 2003). A "catastrophizing interview" was administered to 30 patients with chronic insomnia and 30 good sleepers. Adapting a procedure that had been used with patients with an anxiety disorder (Vasey & Borkovec, 1992), sometimes referred to as the downward-arrow technique, the participants were asked, "What is it that worries you about nights when you have problems getting to sleep?" Where A denotes the answer to the latter question the participant was then asked, "What is it that worries you about A?" Where B denotes the answer the participant gave to this second question, the participant was then asked, "What is it that worries you about B?" (See Figure 4.1 for an example of the procedure.) This procedure continues until either participants say they have no more answers or until they repeat a similar answer three times. The participants were then asked to rate, for each response, the likelihood that it would *actually* occur from 0 "not at all likely" to 10 "extremely likely." These ratings were referred to as the "likelihood ratings." Consistent with predictions, the insomnia patients generated more catastrophes about the consequences of not sleeping and gave higher likelihood ratings relative to the good sleepers. For the insomnia group, but not the good sleepers, participating in the catastrophizing interview was associated with increased anxiety and discomfort. Although the authors suggested that this study might capture something of the thought processes and internal dialogue of patients with insomnia when they are lying in bed, the research was conducted during the daytime so the results may be more applicable to the thought processes that characterize patients with insomnia during the day. It is also possible

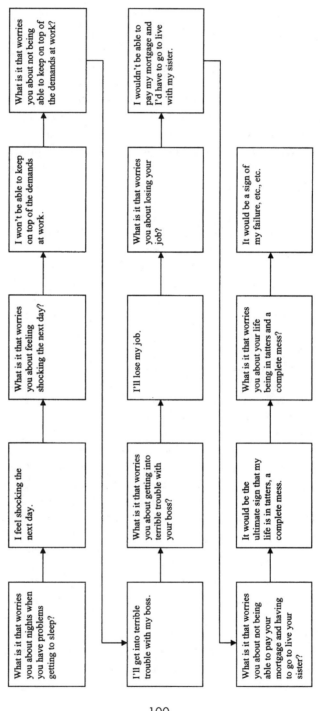

FIGURE 4.1. An example of the procedure of the Catastrophizing Interview used by Harvey and Greenall (2003).

that this paradigm captures intrusive thought, as opposed to worry and rumination, and hence may be useful for future research that seeks to differentiate between different cognitive phenomena.

THEORETICAL EXPLANATIONS FOR THE PERSISTENCE OF UNWANTED INTRUSIVE THOUGHTS

The unwanted intrusive thoughts that characterize a range of psychological disorders may persist because of three types of processes; "(a) pre-existing ideas, beliefs or schemas, (b) faulty appraisal of the intrusion and (c) futile efforts to intentionally control or suppress unwanted cognitions" (Clark, 2001, p. 125). In this section, I discuss these three aspects of unwanted intrusive thoughts in insomnia for their role in the persistence of insomnia. I also discuss one further explanation that is specific to insomnia: the role of intrusive and worrisome thought in distorting perception of sleep. Note at the outset that these are not mutually exclusive explanations but rather may all contribute to the persistence of unwanted thoughts to some varying degree.

Beliefs about Sleep

Following the pioneering work of Morin (1993), several theoretical models of insomnia have specified a role for unhelpful beliefs about sleep in the development and maintenance of sleep disturbance (Espie, 2002; Harvey, 2002a; Lundh, 1998; Lundh & Broman, 2000). In one of the first empirical studies on beliefs in insomnia, Morin and colleagues found that (1) older adults with insomnia were less realistic than good sleepers about how much sleep they require, (2) they strongly endorsed statements relating to the negative consequences of insomnia, and (3) they were more likely to attribute their insomnia to external and stable causes (Morin, Stone, Trinkle, Mercer, & Remsberg, 1993). These findings were later replicated by Fins et al. (1996).

A recent cognitive model of insomnia hypothesized that holding unhelpful beliefs about sleep will serve to exacerbate intrusive and worrisome thought during both the day and night (Harvey, 2002a). Following is an example of unhelpful beliefs about sleep exacerbating intrusive and worrisome thought during the day. A person who believes that he or she must get at least 8 hours of sleep each and every night will, during a period of sleep disturbance when only 4 hours of sleep per night is obtained, suffer more daytime intrusive and worrisome thoughts about the consequences of the poor sleep for his or her health in the future and for his or her ability to cope with work. An example of unhelpful beliefs about sleep that exacerbate intrusive and worrisome thought during the night would be a person who believes that nighttime sleep must be unbroken to be truly restorative. If that person experiences nights during which he or she wakes up once or twice, he or she might find it hard to fall back to sleep because of worry about the impact of the broken sleep on the following day. This hypothesis about the link between unhelpful beliefs about sleep and intrusive and worrisome thought, although intuitive, remains to be empirically tested.

Metacognition

As mentioned earlier in this chapter, one influence over whether an intrusive thought is selected for further attention, in the form of worry or rumination, is the appraisal and response to the intrusion (e.g., Freeston & Ladouceur, 1993; Salkovskis, 1985; Wells, 2000). This type of cognitive phenomena can be considered to be metacognition, which refers to the thoughts and beliefs that people hold about their thoughts as well as the processes that are involved in keeping track of, appraising, and controlling their thoughts (Flavell, 1979). To date, the topic of metacognition has not been addressed in the insomnia literature except one study that was designed to investigate the role of beliefs about the utility of presleep worry in insomnia. This study was based on Well's (1995) concept of "metaworry" and positive beliefs about worry. In this study the Utility of Pre-sleep Worry Questionnaire (UPWQ) was administered to individuals with insomnia (n = 31) and good sleepers (n = 31) (Harvey, 2003b). The UPWQ is comprised of 36 positive belief statements and 24 negative belief statements. The results indicated that while the insomnia and good sleeper group did not differ on negative beliefs about worrying in bed, patients with insomnia endorsed more positive beliefs about the benefits of worrying in bed, relative to the good sleepers. An example of a positive belief was that worry in bed "helps to sort out/put things in order in my mind," whereas an example of a negative belief was that worry in bed "makes me feel confused."

After completing the ratings of the positive belief statements, the participants were asked to review their endorsed items and rate the extent to which they found thinking while lying in bed actually helps them to achieve the goal stated in the question or whether they end up abandoning the goal in order to get to sleep. It is interesting to note that relative to good sleepers, the insomnia group exhibited a larger discrepancy between their *expectation* of what can be achieved by worrying in bed and what they actually *achieve*. In other words, the patients with insomnia held positive beliefs about the utility of worrying in bed but admitted that the goal inherent to the positive belief statement (e.g., worry in bed helps me prepare for the future) is rarely achieved. One explanation for this finding is that like patients with other psychological disorders, individuals with insomnia may have a bias toward processing information that is consistent with their beliefs and dismissive of, or fail to notice, disconfirmatory evidence. This study provides preliminary evidence to suggest that the role of metacognition in the maintenance of intrusive and worrisome thought in insomnia is likely to be a worthwhile line of investigation.

Control of Intrusive Thoughts

Thought Suppression

Given that most patients with insomnia perceive that their "racing mind" is causally related to their problems with sleep (e.g., Lichstein & Rosenthal, 1980), it seems inevitable that they will *do* something in an attempt to prevent, modify, or suppress the thoughts that they perceive to be interfering with their sleep. In this section it is suggested that the vast literature published following Wegner and colleague's classic "white bear" studies have direct relevance for the maintenance of insomnia (Wegner, 1989). Specifically, it has led to the proposal that the ironic effects of thought suppression are a mechanism for the etiology and persistence of unwanted intrusions (Salkovskis, 1989; Wegner, 1989).

Wegner (1994) accounted for the counterproductive effects of thought suppression by suggesting that the level of mental control enjoyed by an individual at any one time is a function of the joint action of a monitoring and operating process. Termed the *ironic process theory*, it maintains that attempts to suppress involve (1) an operating process that directs attention toward a thought other than the unwanted one and (2) a monitoring process that searches for failures to achieve the desired state. In many circumstances these interrelated processes work in tandem to successfully achieve suppression. However, there are a number of situations in which the balance is undermined, resulting in the unwanted thought intruding into consciousness. First, Wegner (1994) proposed that because the monitoring process takes less cognitive effort than the operating process, the ironic effect will be readily observed under conditions of cognitive load. Second, the operating and monitoring processes can both engage in a feature-positive search (looking for the presence of the target) or a feature-negative search (looking for the absence of the target). Given that the latter is harder than the former (Newman, Wolff, & Hearst, 1980), a task that involves looking for the absence of a target thought is likely to be unsuccessful. Conversely, a task that involves distracting from one thought on to a specific alternative target thought may well be successful. Three studies highlight the importance of this theory to sleep and insomnia.

Ansfield, Wegner, and Bowser (1996) instructed good sleepers to either fall asleep as quickly as possible or to fall asleep whenever they desired. In addition, participants were either allocated to a high (listening to marching music) or low (new age music) cognitive load condition. The group given the most cognitively demanding task (high load + being instructed to fall asleep quickly) had the most difficulty falling asleep.

In another study, individuals with insomnia and good sleepers were either instructed to suppress or not to suppress one issue/problem/thought while trying to get to sleep (Harvey, 2003b). On the night of the study, the participants who were told to suppress reported that they took longer to fall asleep and rated their sleep quality as poorer compared to participants given nonsuppression instructions. This finding suggests that attempting to suppress a thought adversely affects both (1) self-reported SOL and (2) sleep quality. This effect was detected for both the good sleepers and the patients with insomnia. Contrary to previous work (Wegner, 1989), there was no paradoxical increase in the frequency of the suppressed thought. While there are a number of possible explanations for this negative finding, one explanation may be the narrow focus of the thought-suppression instructions. In this study the participants were asked to choose and suppress only *one* issue/problem/thought and the measure of thought frequency only measured the frequency of this one issue/problem/thought. It is possible that participants successfully suppressed the selected issue/problem/thought by thinking about other issues/problems/thoughts. Future research should ask participants to suppress a broader range of thoughts and include measures of all presleep cognitive activity.

As described earlier, instructions to distract using imagery resulted in falling asleep more quickly and reporting less frequent presleep cognitive activity (Harvey & Payne, 2002). Another interpretation of this study is that it involved an investigation of the impact of instructing people with insomnia to engage in a feature-positive task (interesting and engaging imagery). Based on Wegner's theory, a feature-positive search should be associated with reduced intrusive and worrisome thought and, as a consequence, shorter time taken to fall asleep. Consistent with this prediction, on the night of the experiment the "imagery distraction" group reported taking less time to fall asleep and rated their presleep thoughts, worries, and concerns as less uncomfortable and distressing compared to those of both of the control groups. These results suggest that a feature-positive search facilitated sleep onset and reduced the discomfort associated with intrusive and worrisome thoughts.

As thought suppression is only one of a range of strategies that people may use in an attempt to manage and control unwanted thought, it will be necessary for future research to measure the effect of attempting thought control via a broader range of strategies. In an attempt to begin preparing for such experiments, the Thought Control Questionnaire (TCQ), designed by Wells and Davies (1994), has been adapted for use with patients with insomnia. This questionnaire, the TCQ-Insomnia (TCQ-I), was administered to 30 individuals with insomnia and 30 good sleepers (Harvey, 2001b). The results indicated that suppression, reappraisal, and worry were employed significantly more by participants with insomnia compared with good sleepers. The use of suppression is consistent with one of the experimental studies discussed earlier (Harvey, 2003b). While reappraisal may be an effective daytime strategy ensuring effective resolution of daytime hassles and concerns, it makes intuitive sense that engaging in similar processes at night might interfere with sleep onset. The finding relating to worry is consistent with previous work characterizing individuals with insomnia as particularly vulnerable to worry and neuroticism (Borkovec, 1982). Interestingly, preliminary evidence indicates that social control and replacement strategies may be used effectively to manage unwanted thoughts.

To summarize the results reviewed in this section, the evidence thus far is consistent with the proposal that the attempt to suppress unwanted thoughts is associated poorer sleep, although the specific link between thought suppression and increased thought intrusion has yet to be established. Findings with the TCQ-I suggests that social control and replacement may be more successful than suppression, reappraisal, and worry, although experimental manipulations of these variables is needed.

Imagery Control

A parallel literature has emerged that focuses on the control of imagery. As described at the beginning of this chapter, unwanted intrusive thoughts can occur as visual images or as verbal thought. Imagery control forms the basis of an important theoretical explanation of the persistence of worry in GAD (Borkovec, Ray, & Stöber, 1998). This perspective draws on three sets of findings: (1) that worry is comprised mostly of uncontrollable, negative affect-laden verbal thoughts rather than visual images (e.g., Freeston, Dugas, & Ladouceur, 1996); (2) that verbal thought about an emotional topic elicits less cardiovascular response compared to images of the same emotional topic (Vrana, Cuthbert, & Lang, 1986); and (3) that physiological response is required for successful emotional processing (Foa & Kozak, 1986). Based on these findings, Borkovec et al. (1998) proposed that thinking about an emotional topic in verbal mode results in a drop in physiological response, which in turn leads to an inhibition of emotional processing and the maintenance of an emotionally charged topic. Conversely, the translation of a concern into an image is suggested to increase physiological response in the short term but will ultimately facilitate successful processing and the resolution of the emotion (Borkovec et al., 1998). Application of this theorizing to insomnia leads to the hypothesis that because presleep worry includes "the presence of active, picture-like images" (Coates et al., 1982), perhaps patients with insomnia spontaneously disengage from images to think about the same topic in verbal thought thereby preventing emotional processing and contributing to the fuelling of intrusive and worrisome thought (Harvey, 2002a). Two published investigations have tested this proposal.

First, in an investigation of the imagery experienced during the presleep period, in the natural home environment, 20 patients with insomnia and 20 good sleepers recorded when an image came to their mind by pressing a handheld counter (Nelson & Harvey, 2003). They then provided an oral description of the image and indicated whether the image was "pleasant," "unpleasant," or "neutral." This information was recorded on a voice-activated tape recorder. Table 4.1 presents the content of the presleep imagery. In addition, the findings indicated that the insomnia group experienced more negatively valenced presleep images but a lower number of images overall, relative to the good sleeper group. As negative imagery is likely to be associated with physiological and affective activation (Vrana et al., 1986), perhaps this activation motivates the quick and reflexive termination of images (hence the lower number of images overall reported by the insomnia group) in order to switch thought to the verbal mode.

Taking this line of investigation a step further, in an experimental manipulation of imagery control, individuals with insomnia were exposed to a stressor (speech threat) just prior to getting into bed and were instructed to think about the speech and its implications in either images (image group, n = 14) or verbal thought (verbal group, n = 17) (Nelson & Harvey, 2002). These results indicated that in the short term, the image group reported more distress and arousal relative to the verbal group. In the longer term, the image group estimated that they fell asleep more quickly and, the following morning, reported less anxiety and more comfort about giving the speech compared to the verbal group.

These two sets of findings are consistent with Borkovec et al.'s (1998) observations about the role of imagery in GAD, and they indicate that imagery control may contribute to the maintenance of excessive presleep worry (Harvey, 2002a).

Perception of Sleep

There is one final possible mechanism by which unwanted intrusive and worrisome thought might contribute to the maintenance of insomnia. This explanation relates to the influence of information processing on time perception and the perception of sleep.

It is known that time estimation increases with an increase in the number of information units processed (e.g., Cantor & Thomas, 1977) and that patients with insomnia tend to overestimate how long it takes to fall asleep and underestimate how much sleep is obtained overall (e.g., see Perlis, Giles, Mendelson, Bootzin, & Wyatt, 1997, for review). Thus, it is proposed that distortions in time estimation during the presleep period may be a direct result of intrusive and worrisome thought whilst trying to fall asleep (Borkovec, 1982; Harvey, 2002a). In support of this hypothesis, several studies have reported a significant positive correlation between cognitive arousal while trying to get to sleep and distorted perception of sleep (Wicklow & Espie, 2000; Van Egeren et al., 1983). Further, Tang and Harvey (2004a) reported that activating worry in good sleepers (via a speech threat) resulted in significantly more distorted perception of sleep, relative to a no-instruction control group. Further, Broomfield and Espie (2003) interpreted their finding that paradoxical intention instructions (i.e., go to bed but try to stay awake) improved the sleep perception of insomnia patients by reducing sleep anxiety and the associated sleep-related intrusions. In sum, unwanted intrusive thoughts and worry may contribute to insomnia by causing a person to perceive that he or she obtained much less sleep than actually obtained. The adverse knock-on effects of this perception are twofold (Harvey, 2002a). First, perceiving a sleep deficit (whether one is present or not) will fuel intrusive and worrisome thought about not acquiring enough sleep and the impact of this on health and daytime functioning. This worry will, in turn, lead to the second consequence of impairing the individual's ability to fall asleep because worry and the accompanying anxiety are antithetical to sleep onset.

CLINICAL IMPLICATIONS

A number of implications can be drawn from the research discussed for developing more effective psychological treatments for insomnia. Our research group at the Oxford Centre for Insomnia Research and Treatment is midway through an evaluation of a treatment that includes many of the processes highlighted in this section. One of the key questions we have found to be important to address in treatment is *why* the patient is experiencing excessive and unwanted intrusive and worrisome thought. This chapter has taken four perspectives on why intrusive and worrisome thought persists in insomnia. The following section considers the possible treatment implications of each of these areas of research.

Beliefs about Sleep

Does the patient hold beliefs about sleep and insomnia that fuel intrusive and worrisome thought? Does the patient hold beliefs about the impact of daytime tiredness that reinforce unwanted distressing thoughts? If so, an intervention that focuses on altering unhelpful beliefs is warranted. In most randomized controlled trials of cognitive-behavioral therapy for insomnia, unhelpful beliefs about sleep are targeted by providing corrective education about sleep requirements and circadian rhythms (e.g., Edinger, Wohlgemuth, Radtke, Marsh, & Quillian, 2001).

We have supplemented this didactic intervention with behavioral experiments (see Ree & Harvey, 2004). A behavioral experiment involves arranging real-life experiences (in session or between sessions) that provide a crystal-clear and memorable demonstration to the patient that the perception or belief is not plausible. The behavioral experiment allows the patient to derive corrective feedback from the experience (e.g., Beck, 1995; Clark, 1999).

Metacognition

Does the person hold positive beliefs about the benefit of worry? If so, we assess for these beliefs using the UPWQ, which was described earlier.

To intervene, we draw on a combination of behavioral experiments designed to test the beliefs and the evaluation of the beliefs using more conventional cognitive restructuring tactics (e.g., Beck, 1995).

Management of Intrusive Thoughts

Is the person actively avoiding/suppressing thoughts and emotions all day? If the latter, then we start by giving the patient direct experience of the adverse effects of thought suppression by conducting, within the session, Wegner's white bear experiment. This experiment involves asking patients to close their eyes and try very hard not to think about a big white fluffy polar bear. After 5 minutes of attempting suppression, patients typically report that the suppression of white bear images is impossible. This experience is a compelling example of the adverse consequences of suppression. In addition, several other treatment approaches currently under development can be tailored to reduce attempted thought suppression or cognitive avoidance.

1. *Abandon attempts to control intrusive and worrisome thought.* Whether it is realistic to expect patients with insomnia to abandon the control and suppression of thought remains to be seen, but perhaps a glimmer of hope may rest in a treatment approach that encompasses acceptance- (Hayes, Strosahl, & Wilson, 1999) and mindfulness-based stress reduction (Segal, Williams, & Teasdale, 2002). These approaches emphasize an awareness of and acceptance of thoughts combined with a reduction in cognitive avoidance. A pilot study of this strategy with insomnia patients was recently reported by Lundh and Hindmarsh (2002). Forty individuals diagnosed with insomnia were asked to keep a sleep diary for 1 week, as a baseline measure of each participants' sleep pattern. The participants were then taught to use a "metacognitive observation exercise" while trying to get to sleep which involved, observing "their own thoughts, feelings and body sensations, without trying to change these in any way" with the aim of encouraging a "mindful observation of cognitive and emotional processes" (Lundh & Hindmarsh, 2002, p. 233). Over the following week the participants were asked to use this metacognitive observation exercise as they were trying to fall asleep. A comparison of the baseline week and the week in which the participants used the metacognitive observation exercise indicated that the latter was associated with falling asleep more quickly and obtaining more sleep. Although this study was limited by (1) the absence of a control group to rule out the possibility that the findings were an

artefact of keeping a sleep diary (Morin, 1993) and (2) the absence of checks of adherence (i.e., checks to ensure the participants did engage in the metacognitive observation exercise), the findings suggest that this line of research is worth pursing.

2. *Aim for the opposite of mental control.* This strategy involves eliminating all avoidance of unwanted thoughts and, instead, actually approaching the thoughts (Beever, Wenzlaff, Haynes, & Scott, 1999). In the context of insomnia this might take the form of simply letting the thoughts come or, capitalizing on the Nelson and Harvey (2002) findings, perhaps patients could be trained to purposively form an image of the unwanted thought with a view to promoting emotional processing and resolution. In a similar vein, a writing intervention (Pennebaker, 1997) in which individuals are encouraged to write about their unwanted thoughts may also reduce avoidance and promote approach and the processing of emotional material prior to bed. An analogue pilot study with poor sleepers suggests that this type of intervention may be beneficial (Harvey & Farrell, 2003), although a replication yielded null results (Harvey, Bugg, & Tang, 2003).

3. *Provide the operating process with a feature positive search to draw attention away from unwanted thoughts.* Some evidence for this possibility has been provided in the study already described where people with insomnia reported shorter SOL and less uncomfortable presleep intrusions when they imagined an interesting and engaging scene that was selected by the patient (Harvey & Payne, 2002). However, as the advantage associated with imagery distraction was only detected on one night, there are concerns about the durability of the effect (Harvey & Payne, 2002). Accordingly, we tend to limit use of imagery distraction to a behavioral experiment to test and disconfirm beliefs commonly held by patients with insomnia that "the thoughts that I have during the night are not in my control" and that this is indicative of "danger" (i.e., "something going wrong biologically" or "that I am going crazy").

Perception of Sleep

Do intrusive and worrisome thoughts lead to distorted perception of sleep? If so, we use a behavioral experiment that involves showing the patient the discrepancy between his or her subjective estimate of sleep and an objective estimate of sleep. The objective estimate of sleep that we use is actigraphy, which is a wristwatch device that contains a miniaturized piezoelectric acceleration sensor that detects and stores motor information along with actual clock time. The data are quickly and easily downloaded into software that generates an easily interpretable estimation of the sleep–wake cycle. This behavioral experiment is associated with reduced anxiety and preoccupation with sleep and more accurate sleep estimates (Tang & Harvey, 2004b).[1]

FUTURE RESEARCH

Research relating to the management of intrusions and worry in insomnia clearly constitutes an exciting and fruitful domain for future research. Many issues remain to be addressed. At the most fundamental level, research is required to differentiate intrusive thoughts from worry and rumination. Further, it will be necessary to test the hypothesis that when insomnia patients appraise an intrusion as personally threatening, a secondary process of worry and rumination will be triggered. The consequence of this chain of events for the emotional and behavioral symptoms of insomnia is another interesting avenue of investigation. It will also be important to carefully determine the specific characteristics of intrusive thoughts in insomnia including (1) to what extent intrusive thoughts occur as images rather than verbal thoughts, (2) are the intrusions of events past or future events/concerns, (3) to what extent they are experienced as controllable and intrusive, (4) to what extent are the intrusions repetitive, and (5) are they considered personally acceptable or unacceptable?

Experimental manipulations to determine which thought control strategies are counterproductive and whether any strategies are helpful for controlling unwanted thoughts are a crucial future direction. The experimental evidence reviewed in this chapter suggests that intrusive and worrisome thoughts are causally involved in the maintenance of insomnia and thus it is important to determine how widely they are experienced by patients (i.e., individual differences in the experience of intrusive thoughts). Such research is likely to have implications for indicating whether all patients, or just a subgroup, are likely to benefit from treatment components that target intrusive and worrisome thought. If found to be almost a universal cause of insomnia, then discussion will be needed to determine whether intrusive and worrisome thought should be included as part of the diagnostic criteria for insomnia.

Debate continues as to the processes that predispose, precipitate, and maintain insomnia (Spielman & Glovinsky, 1997). The extent to

---

[1]Ree and Harvey (2004) describe an alternative experiment, that makes the same point, if no equipment is available to provide an objective sleep estimate.

which intrusive and worrisome thoughts contribute to each of these three causal stages remains to be addressed in future research. In this chapter we have mainly focused on the role of intrusive and worrisome thought in maintaining insomnia.

As already highlighted, another important consideration is that research to date has almost exclusively explored sleep-onset insomnia. Nothing is known about the thought processes that occur during awakenings in the middle of the night. Also, thought processes that occur during the daytime are a completely new area for investigation. This is likely to be an important research issue given the possibility that intrusive and worrisome thought during the day may play a critical role in the maintenance of insomnia (Harvey, 2002a).

CONCLUSION

This chapter has critically examined the empirical literature on intrusive and worrisome thought in insomnia and concluded that the evidence for the importance of these cognitive phenomena in maintaining sleep disturbance *at night* is compelling. The hypothesis that intrusive and worrisome thoughts during the *daytime* are important in the persistence of insomnia is highlighted but remains to be empirically evaluated. Several theoretical explanations for the persistence of intrusive and worrisome thought in insomnia have been proposed, including (1) the role of beliefs about sleep, (2) metacognition, (3) the control of intrusive thoughts and (4) the role of time distortion and sleep perception. Finally, this chapter has explored the clinical implications of this literature and specified future directions for research in this area.

ACKNOWLEDGMENTS

I am grateful to Melissa Ree for helpful treatment-orientated discussions. This work was supported by the Wellcome Trust (Grant No. GR065913MA).

REFERENCES

American Psychiatric Association. (2000). *Diagnostic and statistical manual of mental disorders* (4th ed., text rev.). Washington, DC: Author.
Ancoli-Israel, S., & Roth, T. (1999). Characteristics of insomnia in the United

States: Results of the 1991 National Sleep Foundation Survey. I. *Sleep, 22*(Suppl. 2), S347–S353.

Ansfield, M. E., Wegner, D. M., & Bowser, R. (1996). Ironic effects of sleep urgency. *Behaviour Research and Therapy, 34,* 523–531.

Beck, A. T. (1976). *Cognitive therapy and the emotional disorders.* New York: Penguin.

Beck, J. S. (1995). *Cognitive therapy: Basics and beyond.* New York: Guilford Press.

Beever, C. G., Wenzlaff, R. M., Haynes, A. M., & Scott, W. D. (1999). Depression and the ironic effects of thought suppression: Therapeutic strategies for improving mental control. *Clinical Psychology: Science and Practice, 6,* 133–148.

Borkovec, T. D. (1982). Insomnia. *Journal of Consulting and Clinical Psychology, 50,* 880–895.

Borkovec, T. D., & Inz, J. (1990). The nature of worry in generalized anxiety disorder: A predominance of thought activity. *Behaviour Research and Therapy, 28,* 153–158.

Borkovec, T. D., Ray, W. J., & Stober, J. (1998). Worry: A cognitive phenomenon intimately linked to affective, physiological, and interpersonal behavioral processes. *Cognitive Therapy and Research, 22,* 561–576.

Borkovec, T. D., Robinson, E., Pruzinsky, T., & DePree, J. A. (1983). Preliminary exploration of worry: Some characteristics and processes. *Behavior Research and Therapy, 21,* 9–16.

Broomfield, N. M., & Espie, C. A. (2003). Initial insomnia and paradoxical intention: An experimental investigation of putative mechanisms using subjective and actigraphic measurement of sleep. *Behavioural and Cognitive Psychotherapy, 31,* 313–324.

Cantor, N. E., & Thomas, E. A. C. (1977). Control of attention in the processing of temporal and spatial information in complex visual patterns. *Journal of Experimental Psychology and Human Perceptual Performance, 3,* 243–250.

Chevalier, H., Los, F., Boichut, D., Bianchi, M., Nutt, D. J., Hajak, G., et al. (1999). Evaluation of severe insomnia in the general population: results of a European multinational survey. *Journal of Psychopharmacology, 13*(Suppl. 1), S21–S24.

Chilcott, L. A., & Shapiro, C. M. (1996). The socioeconomic impact of insomnia: An overview. *Psychoeconomics, 10*(Suppl. 1), 1–14.

Clark, D. A. (2001). Unwanted mental intrusions in clinical disorders: An introduction. *Journal of Cognitive Psychotherapy: An International Quarterly, 16,* 161–178.

Clark, D. M. (1999). Anxiety disorders: Why they persist and how to treat them. *Behaviour Research and Therapy, 37,* S5–S27.

Clark, D. M. (1997). Panic disorder and social phobia. In D. M. Clark & C. G. Fairburn (Eds.), *Science and practice of cognitive behaviour therapy* (pp. 119–154). Oxford, UK: Oxford University Press.

Coates, T. J., Killen, J. D., George, J., Marchini, E., Silverman, S., & Thoresen, C. E. (1982). Estimating sleep parameters: A multitrait–multimethod analysis. *Journal of Consulting and Clinical Psychology, 50,* 345–352.

Edinger, J. D., Wohlgemuth, W. K., Radtke, R. A., Marsh, G. R., & Quillian, R. E. (2001). Cognitive behavioral therapy for treatment of chronic primary insomnia: A randomized controlled trial. *Journal of the American Medical Association, 285,* 1856–64.

Espie, C. A. (1991). *The psychological treatment of insomnia.* London: Wiley.

Espie, C. A. (2002). Insomnia: Conceptual issues in the development, persistence, and treatment of sleep disorder in adults. *Annual Review of Psychology, 53,* 215–243.

Espie, C. A., Brooks, D. N., & Lindsay, W. R. (1989). An evaluation of tailored psychological treatment of insomnia. *Journal of Behaviour Therapy and Experimental Psychiatry, 20,* 143–153.

Fichten, C. S., Libman, E., Creti, L., Amsel, R., Tagalakis, V., & Brender, W. (1998). Thoughts during awake times in older good and poor sleepers—The self-statement test: 60+. *Cognitive Therapy and Research, 22,* 1–20.

Fins, A. I., Edinger, J. D., Sullivan, R. J., Marsh, G. R., Dailey, D., Hope, T. V., et al. (1996). Dysfunctional cognitions about sleep among older adults and their relationship to objective sleep findings. *Sleep Research, 25,* 242.

Flavell, J. H. (1979). Metacognition and cognitive monitoring: A new area of cognitive developmental inquiry. *American Psychologist, 34,* 906–911.

Foa, E. B., & Kozak, M. J. (1986). Emotional processing of fear: Exposure to corrective information. *Psychological Bulletin, 99,* 20–35.

Freeston, M. H., Dugas, M. J., & Ladouceur, R. (1996). Thoughts, images, worry and anxiety. *Cognitive Therapy and Research, 20,* 265–273.

Freeston, M. H., & Ladouceur, R. (1993). Appraisal of cognitive intrusions and response style: replication and extension. *Behaviour Research and Therapy, 31,* 181–191.

Fresco, D. M., Frankel, A. N., Mennin, D. S., Turk, C. L., & Heimberg, R. G. (2002). Distinct and overlapping features of rumination and worry: The relationship of cognitive production to negative affective states. *Cognitive Therapy and Research, 26,* 179–188.

Gross, R. T., & Borkovec, T. D. (1982). The effects of a cognitive intrusion manipulation on the sleep onset latency of good sleepers. *Behaviour Therapy, 13,* 112–116.

Hall, M., Buysse, D. J., Nowell, P. D., Nofzinger, E. A., Houck, P., Reynolds, C. F., et al. (2000). Symptoms of stress and depression as correlated of sleep in primary insomnia. *Psychosomatic Medicine, 62,* 227–230.

Hall, M., Buysse, D. J., Reynolds, C. F., Kupfer, D. J., & Baum, A. (1996). Stress-related intrusive thoughts disrupt sleep-onset and continuity. *Sleep Research, 25,* 163.

Harvey, A. G. (2000). Pre-sleep cognitive activity: A comparison of sleep-onset insomniacs and good sleepers. *British Journal of Clinical Psychology, 39,* 275–286.

Harvey, A. G. (2001a). Insomnia: Symptom or diagnosis? *Clinical Psychology Review, 21*, 1037–1059.

Harvey, A. G. (2001b). I can't sleep, my mind is racing! An investigation of strategies of thought control in insomnia. *Behavioural and Cognitive Psychotherapy, 29*, 3–12.

Harvey, A. G. (2002a). A cognitive model of insomnia. *Behaviour Research and Therapy, 40*, 869–893.

Harvey, A. G. (2002b). Identifying safety behaviors in insomnia. *Journal of Nervous and Mental Disease, 190*, 16–21.

Harvey, A. G. (2003a). Beliefs about the utility of pre-sleep worry: an investigation of individuals with insomnia and good sleepers. *Cognitive Therapy and Research, 27*, 403–414.

Harvey, A. G. (2003b). The attempted suppression of pre-sleep cognitive activity in insomnia. *Cognitive Therapy and Research, 27*, 593–602.

Harvey, A. G., Bugg, A., & Tang, N. K. Y. (2003). *Does emotional processing promote better sleep in chronic insomnia?* Paper presented at the 37th annual convention of the American Association for Behavior Therapy, Boston, MA.

Harvey, A. G., & Farrell, C. (2003). The efficacy of a Pennebaker-like writing intervention for poor sleepers. *Behavioral Sleep Medicine, 1*, 115–124.

Harvey, A. G., & Greenall, E. (2003). Catastrophic worry in insomnia. *Journal of Behavior Therapy and Experimental Psychiatry, 34*, 11–23.

Harvey, A. G., Jones, C., & Schmidt, A. D. (2003). Sleep and Posttraumatic Stress Disorder: A review. *Clinical Psychology Review, 23*, 377–407.

Harvey, A. G., & Payne, S. (2002). The management of unwanted pre-sleep thoughts in insomnia: Distraction with imagery versus general distraction. *Behaviour Research and Therapy, 40*, 267–277.

Harvey, A. G., Watkins, E., Mansell, W., & Shafran, R. (2004). *Cognitive behavioural processes across psychological disorders: A transdiagnostic approach to research and treatment.* New York: Oxford University Press.

Hayes, S. C., Strosahl, K. D., & Wilson, K. G. (1999). *Acceptance and commitment therapy: An experiential approach to behavior change.* New York: Guilford Press.

Haynes, S. N., Adams, A., & Franzen, M. (1981). The effects of presleep stress on sleep-onset insomnia. *Journal of Abnormal Psychology, 90*, 601–606.

Kelly, W. E. (2002). Worry and sleep length revisited: Worry, sleep length and sleep disturbance ascribed to worry. *Journal of Genetic Psychology, 163*, 296–304.

Krakow, B., Johnston, L., Melendrez, D., Hollifield, M., Warner, T. D., Chavez-Kennedy, D., et al. (2001). An open-label trial of evidence-based cognitive behavior therapy for nightmares and insomnia in crime victims with PTSD. *American Journal of Psychiatry, 158*, 2043–2047.

Kuisk, L. A., Bertelson, A. D., & Walsh, J. K. (1989). Presleep cognitive hyperarousal and affect as factors in objective and subjective insomnia. *Perceptual and Motor Skills, 69*, 1219–1225.

Levey, A. B., Aldaz, J. A., Watts, F. N., & Coyle, K. (1991). Articulatory suppression and the treatment of insomnia. *Behaviour Research and Therapy, 29,* 85–89.

Lichstein, K. L., & Fanning, J. (1990). Cognitive anxiety in insomnia: An analogue test. *Stress Medicine, 6,* 47–51.

Lichstein K. L., & Morin, C. M. (2000). *Treatment of late-life insomnia.* Sage: California.

Lichstein, K. L., & Rosenthal, T. L. (1980). Insomniacs' perceptions of cognitive versus somatic determinants of sleep disturbance. *Journal of Abnormal Psychology, 89,* 105–107.

Lundh, L-G. (1998). Cognitive-behavioural analysis and treatment of insomnia. *Scandinavian Journal of Behaviour Therapy, 27,* 10–29.

Lundh, L-G., & Broman, J-E. (2000). Insomnia as an interaction between sleep-interfering and sleep-interpreting processes. *Journal of Psychosomatic Research, 49,* 299–310.

Lundh, L-G., & Hindmarsh, H. (2002). Can meta-cognitive observation be used in the treatment of insomnia? A pilot study of a cognitive-emotional self-observation task. *Behavioural and Cognitive Psychotherapy, 30,* 233–236.

McCrae, C. S., & Lichstein, K. L. (2001). Secondary insomnia: Diagnostic challenges and intervention opportunities. *Sleep Medicine Reviews, 5,* 47–61.

Means, M. L., Lichstein, K. L., Epperson, M. T., & Johnson C. T. (2000). Relaxation therapy for insomnia: Nighttime and day time effects. *Behaviour Research and Therapy, 38,* 665–678.

Morin, C. M. (1993). *Insomnia: Psychological assessment and management.* New York: Guilford Press.

Morin, C. M., Stone, J., Trinkle, D., Mercer, J., & Remsberg, S. (1993). Dysfunctional beliefs and attitudes about sleep among older adults with and without insomnia complaints. *Psychology and Aging, 8,* 463–467.

Nelson, J., & Harvey, A. G. (2002). The differential functions of imagery and verbal thought in insomnia. *Journal of Abnormal Psychology, 111,* 665–669.

Nelson, J., & Harvey, A. G. (2003). Pre-sleep imagery under the microscope: A comparison of patients with insomnia and good sleepers. *Behaviour Research and Therapy, 41,* 273–284.

Newman, J. P., Wolff, W. T., & Hearst, E. (1980). The feature-positive effect in adult human subjects. *Journal of Experimental Psychology: Human Learning and Memory, 6,* 630–650.

Nicassio, P. M., Mendlowitz, D. R., Fussell, J. J., & Petras, L. (1985). The phenomenology of the pre-sleep state: The development of the Pre-Sleep Arousal Scale. *Behaviour Research and Therapy, 23,* 263–271.

Nolen-Hoeksema, S. (1991). Responses to depression and their effects on the duration of depressive episodes. *Journal of Abnormal Psychology, 100,* 569–582.

Ohayon, M. M., Guilleminault, C., Paiva, T., Priest, R. G., Rapoport, D. M., Sagales, T., et al. (1997). An international study on sleep disorders in the general population: Methodological aspects of the use of the Sleep-EVAL system. *Sleep, 20,* 1086–1092.

Pennebaker, J. W. (1997). Writing about emotional experiences as a therapeutic process. *Psychological Science, 8*, 162–166.

Perlis, M. L., Giles, D. E., Mendelson, W. B., Bootzin, R. R., & Wyatt, J. K. (1997). Psychophysiological insomnia: The behavioural model and a neurocognitive perspective. *Journal of Sleep Research, 6*, 179–188.

Purdon, C., & Clark, D. A. (1993). Obsessive intrusive thoughts in nonclinical subjects. 1. Content and relationship with depressive, anxious and obsessional symptoms. *Behaviour Research and Therapy, 31*, 713–720.

Rachman, S. (1981). Part 1: Unwanted intrusive cognitions. *Advances in Behaviour Research and Therapy, 3*, 89–99.

Rachman, S., & de Silva, P. (1978). Abnormal and normal obsessions. *Behaviour Research and Therapy, 16*, 233–248.

Ree, M. J., & Harvey, A. G. (2004). Behavioural experimental in chronic insomnia. In J. Bennett-Levy, G. Butler, M. J. V. Fennell, A. Hackmann, M. Mueller, & D. Westbrook (Eds.), *The Oxford handbook of behavioural experiments* (pp. 287–308). Oxford, UK: Oxford University Press.

Roth, T., & Ancoli-Israel, S. (1999). Daytime consequences and correlates of insomnia in the United States: Results of the 1991 National Sleep Foundation Survey. II. I. *Sleep, 22*(Suppl. 2), S354–S358.

Rothbaum, B. O., & Mellman, T. A. (2001). Dreams and exposure therapy in PTSD. *Journal of Traumatic Stress, 14*, 481–490.

Salkovskis, P. M. (1985). Obsessional–compulsive problems: A cognitive-behavioural analysis. *Behaviour Research and Therapy, 25*, 571–583.

Salkovskis, P. M. (1989). Cognitive-behavioral factors and the persistence of intrusive thoughts in obsessional problems. *Behaviour Research and Therapy, 27*, 677–682.

Sanavio, E. (1988). Pre-sleep cognitive intrusions and treatment of onset-insomnia. *Behaviour Research and Therapy, 26*, 451–459.

Sarason, I. G. (1984). Test anxiety, stress, and social support. *Journal of Personality, 49*, 101–114.

Segal, Z. V., Williams, J. M. G., & Teasdale, J. D. (2002). *Mindfulness-based cognitive therapy for depression: A new approach to preventing relapse.* New York: Guilford Press.

Segerstrom, S. C., Tsao, J. C., Alden, L. E., & Craske, M. G. (2000). Worry and rumination: Repetitive thought as a concomitant and predictor of negative mood. *Cognitive Therapy and Research, 20*, 13–36.

Spielman, A. J., & Glovinsky, P. B. (1997). Diagnostic interview and differential diagnosis for complaints of insomnia. In M.R. Pressman & W.C. Orr. *Understanding sleep: The evaluation and treatment of sleep disorders* (pp. 125–160). Washington DC: American Psychological Association.

Stopa, L., & Clark, D. M. (2001). Social phobia: Comments on the viability and validity of an analogue research strategy and British norms for the Fear of Negative Evaluation Questionnaire. *Behavioural and Cognitive Psychotherapy, 29*, 423–430.

Tang, N., & Harvey, A. G. (2004a). Effects of cognitive arousal and physiological arousal on sleep perception. *Sleep, 27,* 69–78.

Tang, N. K. Y., & Harvey, A. (2004b). Correcting distorted perception of sleep in insomnia: A novel behavioural experiment? *Behaviour Research and Therapy, 42,* 27–39.

Van Egeren, L., Haynes, T. W., Franzen, M., & Hamilton, J. (1983). Presleep cognitions and attributions in sleep-onset insomnia. *Journal of Behavioural Medicine, 6,* 217–232.

Vasey, M. W., & Borkovec, T. D. (1992). Catastrophising assessment of worrisome thoughts. *Cognitive Therapy and Research, 16,* 505–519.

Vrana, S. R., Cuthbert, B. N., & Lang, P. J. (1986). Fear imagery and text processing. *Psychophysiology, 23,* 247–253.

Watts, F. N., Coyle, K., & East, M. P. (1994). The contribution of worry to insomnia. *British Journal of Clinical Psychology, 33,* 211–220.

Wegner, D. M. (1989). *White bears and other unwanted thoughts: Suppression, obsession and the psychology of mental control.* New York: Viking.

Wegner, D. M. (1994). Ironic processes of mental control. *Psychological Review, 101,* 34–52.

Wells, A. (1995). Meta-cognition and worry: A cognitive model of generalised anxiety disorder. *Behavioural and Cognitive Psychotherapy, 23,* 301–320.

Wells, A. (2000). *Emotional disorders and metacognition: innovative cognitive therapy.* Wiley, Chichester.

Wells, A., & Davies, M. I. (1994). The thought control questionnaire: a measure of individual differences in the control of unwanted thoughts. *Behaviour Research and Therapy, 32,* 871–878.

Wells, A., & Morrison, A. P. (1994). Qualitative dimensions of normal worry and normal intrusive thoughts. *Behaviour Research and Therapy, 32,* 867–870.

Wicklow, A., & Espie, C. A. (2000). Intrusive thoughts and their relationship to actigraphic measurement of sleep: Towards a cognitive model of insomnia. *Behaviour Research and Therapy, 38,* 679–694.

CHAPTER 5

WORRY, INTRUSIVE THOUGHTS, AND GENERALIZED ANXIETY DISORDER

The Metacognitive Theory and Treatment

ADRIAN WELLS

Worry is a type of thinking that possesses features of intrusive thoughts and thus has special significance to the topic of this volume. It can be viewed as triggered by the sudden entrance into consciousness of distressing intrusive thoughts or images. It is a pervasive cognitive process that occurs across a wide range of disorders and it has been linked to cognitive vulnerability to psychological dysfunction (Wells & Matthews, 1994). Worry is a predominant feature of generalized anxiety disorder (GAD), which has been conceptualized as the most "normal" anxiety disorder, similar to high trait anxiety (Rapee, 1991). Because worry may be a contributor to the development and maintenance of a wide range of psychological disorders, an analysis of worry should have implications both for increasing our understanding of pathological processes and mechanisms and for developing therapy techniques.

In this chapter I review the nature of worry and use the metacognitive model of GAD as a basis for understanding underlying psychological factors involved in the development and persistence of pathological intrusive thoughts in the form of worry. The model provides a basis of extrapolation concerning mechanisms involved in other types of perseverative thoughts, such as those found in posttraumatic stress disorder and obsessional disorder, and thus some of this chapter is also devoted to these wider considerations.

THE NATURE OF WORRY

Although there are different varieties of intrusive thoughts and there is much in common between these varieties, nonetheless there are also some important differences. Rachman (1981) provided an early definition of intrusions, characterizing them as interrupting ongoing activity and being spontaneous, unwanted, and difficult to control. It is now clear that many types of thought fit into this broad characterization or possess some of these features, including worry, obsessions, ruminations, flashbacks, negative automatic thoughts, self-statements, and so on. I have commented previously (Wells, 1994) that it is unclear whether these terms refer to similar or very different types of mental event. Before we examine some of the studies that have compared the features of different types of intrusive thoughts, it will be helpful to begin with a broad definition of worry as this is the intrusion that is of central concern in this chapter.

The scientific study of worry can be traced to the topic of test anxiety (e.g., Wine, 1971). Here theorists noted that anxiety in performance situations could be divided into a cognitive and somatic component, labeled *worry* and *emotionality*. Research on these two components revealed that the worry component is associated with task interference marked by poorer task performance.

Later, largely due to the work of Borkovec and colleagues (e.g., Borkovec, Robinson, Pruzinsky, & DePree, 1983), worry became a topic for enquiry in clinical psychology. But this was not without some controversy. In particular, O'Neill (1985) argued that a separate construct of worry was unnecessary as it was merely the cognitive component of anxiety and there would be minimal benefit in separating this from anxiety.

Borkovec et al. (1983) defined worry in the following way:

> Worry is a chain of thoughts and images, negatively affect-laden and relatively uncontrollable; it represents an attempt to engage in mental problem-solving on an issue whose outcome is uncertain but contains

the possibility of one or more negative outcomes; consequently, worry relates closely to fear processes. (p. 10)

Summarizing a number of definitions of worry Macleod, Williams, and Bekerian (1991) conclude that common to these definitions are the following characteristics: "Worry is a cognitive phenomenon, it is concerned with future events where there is uncertainty about the outcome, the future being thought about is a negative one, and this is accompanied by feelings of anxiety" (p. 478).

Developments in clinical theory of pathological worrying have led to refinements and elaborations to the definition of worry. An important aspect of worry highlighted in the work of Borkovec and colleagues is that it involves a predominance of verbal–linguistic activity over imaginal activity (Borkovec & Lyonfields, 1993; Borkovec & Inz, 1990). This distinction is important in Borkovec's cognitive model of GAD in which patients are thought to be using worry as a form of distraction from more upsetting types of thoughts such as fearful imagery. Developments in theory of GAD point to subclassifications of worry types depending on their nature and function. In particular, Wells (1994, 1997) distinguishes between the occurrence of worry and the negative appraisal of worry based on metacognitive beliefs about the activity. The distinction is made between Type 1 worry, which is worry about external events and noncognitive internal events, and Type 2 worry, which is worry about worrying. Taking into account these empirical and theoretical developments I have proposed the following definition of worry to capture these features:

> Worry is a chain of catastrophising thoughts that are predominantly verbal. It consists of the contemplation of potentially dangerous situations and of personal coping strategies. It is intrusive and controllable although it is often experienced as uncontrollable. Worrying is associated with a motivation to prevent or avoid potential danger. Worry itself may be viewed as a coping strategy but can become the focus of an individuals concern. (Wells, 1999, p. 87)

This definition is intended to capture several important features of worry: its *style*, which involves chains of verbal thought; its *content*, which involves catastrophizing about danger and thinking about coping responses; and its *functional aspects* as a coping/avoidance strategy. In addition the definition emphasizes that while worry is actually controllable it is subjectively experienced as *uncontrollable*. Thus, there is a dissociation between actual controllability and appraised controllability. Finally, the last part of the definition captures the distinction between Type 1 and Type 2 worry.

IS WORRY DIFFERENT FROM OTHER INTRUSIONS?

Not all intrusions, it would seem, are created equal. Recent analyses have focused on comparing worry with other types of intrusive thoughts. In this section I briefly review the similarities and differences that appear to exist between worry and obsessions and between worry and depressive thoughts.

Turner, Beidel, and Stanley (1992) reviewed the literature on worry and intrusive thoughts to examine differences between these cognitive events. They concluded that several differences could be identified:

1. Worry themes are typically related to normal daily experience whereas obsessions include themes of dirt, contamination, and so on.
2. The majority of patients with GAD are able to identify either internal or external triggers for worry, whereas the majority of obsessional patients seem unable to identify triggers.
3. Worry usually occurs as verbal thought whereas obsessions can occur as thoughts, images, or impulses.
4. Worry does not appear to be resisted as strongly as obsessions and it is perceived as less intrusive.
5. The content of clinical worries, unlike clinical obsessions, is not perceived as unacceptable.

Unfortunately at the time of their review there were no studies directly comparing worry with other types of intrusions.

In the first study to examine worry and obsessions in a nonpatient sample, Wells and Morrison (1994) asked nonclinical participants to monitor for two naturally occurring worries and two obsessions and then rate these events on several dimensions. Compared to obsessions, worry was rated as longer in duration, more verbal (less imagery), more realistic, less involuntary, and associated with a greater compulsion to act. These thoughts did not differ significantly along dimensions of: intrusiveness, controllability, dismisability, how distracting they were, how attention grabbing, how much distress they caused, and the amount they were resisted. These results support the predominance of verbal activity in the worry process; however, they do not accord with Turner et al.'s (1992) conclusions that worry is resisted less than obsessions and is less intrusive, at least for nonpathological subtypes of these mental events. Further evidence of the separate nature of worry and intrusive thoughts comes from Gross and Eifert (1990). They found that items assessing disapproval of worry and of intrusive thoughts loaded on separate factors, supporting the idea that worry can be separated from intrusive thoughts.

Clark and Claybourn (1997) used a number of rating scales to assess process dimensions of worry and obsessive thoughts in a nonpatient sample. Compared to obsessional thoughts, worry was found to be significantly more focused on the consequences of negative events, was more distressing, caused more worry about feeling distressed, was more likely to lead to effective solutions for everyday problems, was more likely to be associated with checking, and caused more interference with daily living. It may be of some significance to note that in this study and in the Wells and Morrison (1994) study worry was associated more with behavioral responses (compulsions to act, checking) than obsessions were. One possibility is that worry acts as an interface between obsessions and neutralizing behaviors. Thus, normal obsessions are more likely to develop into pathological obsessive–compulsive disorder, when the occurrence of obsessional intrusions is followed by a period of worry leading to neutralizing responses as a means of controlling worry or persistent negative thinking.

An important feature that appears to discriminate worry from obsessional thoughts is the relationship that these thoughts have with the concept of self (American Psychiatric Association, 2000). Obsessional thoughts are experienced as ego-dystonic (i.e., repugnant and uncharacteristic of the self), a feature distinguishing them from other types of intrusion such as worry and depressive rumination (Purdon & Clark, 1993). Purdon and Clark (1999) propose that obsessional thoughts are ego-dystonic because they are inconsistent with perceptions of the self and important personal value systems. As we see later in this chapter, worry especially in the context of GAD may be perceived as threatening, not because of inconsistencies with the self-view but because individuals believe it is dangerous in other respects. According to the metacognitive model of GAD, worry, unlike obsessional thoughts, is seen as characteristic of the self and as possessing a number of advantages.

Other studies have sought to explore the differences between anxious and depressive thinking, without explicitly focusing on worry as the mode of anxious thought (e.g., Clark, 1992). Clark and de Silva (1985) observed in a nonclinical sample that anxious thoughts were rated as significantly greater in emotional intensity than depressive thoughts. Anxious and depressive thoughts emerged as separate factors in a factor analysis of responses, suggesting that they were differentiable phenomena. Papageorgiou and Wells (1999) used a self-monitoring methodology and examined process and metacognitive characteristics of worry and depressive thoughts in nonpatients. These thoughts showed much overlap, but some differences did emerge. Worry was rated as more verbal, associated with a greater compulsion to act, greater effort at problem solving, and greater confidence in problem solving than depressive thinking. Depressive thoughts had a greater past orientation than worry. These thoughts did not differ on many dimensions, including intrusiveness and controllability. For worry, greater anxiety was correlated with less dismisability, greater distraction by the thought, a greater compulsion to act on the thought, greater metaworry, and more attention to the thought, when depression was partialed out.

In summary, a number of phenomenological differences between types of thoughts have been identified. The classification and discrimination of thoughts is worthwhile because of the potential contribution it can make to the accurate identification of disorders characterized by particular types of intrusion. Moreover, some varieties of thought may have an impact on other thought types in a manner that contributes to the development of psychological disorder and recovery from disorder. For example, Borkovec and Inz (1990) and Roemer and Borkovec (1993) have suggested that individuals shift attention to verbal conceptual activity as a means of avoiding distress and somatic arousal associated with the intrusion of negative imagery into consciousness. In the next section I examine evidence for such relationships in more detail, and we see how using worry as a form of avoidance or control of other intrusions may have ramifications for emotional processing following stress. Later in this chapter I also examine how it is not only the occurrence of worry but also the appraisal of worry (thoughts about thoughts) that leads to deleterious emotional reactions. The idea that appraisal of thoughts is central to some disorders is a feature of models of obsessive–compulsive disorder (OCD) (Salkovskis, 1985; Rachman, 1997; Purdon & Clark, 1999; Wells, 1997), posttraumatic stress disorder (Wells, 2000), and GAD (Wells, 1995).

THE EFFECT OF WORRY ON OTHER INTRUSIONS

Borkovec and colleagues have proposed a theory of GAD in which patient's use worry as distraction from more upsetting thoughts that occur in the form of images. However, worry is negatively reinforced by these anxiety-reducing consequences, leading to diminished controllability of the activity (e.g., Borkovec & Inz, 1990). Aside from patients with GAD, studies with the Thought Control Questionnaire (TCQ; Wells & Davies, 1994) show that there are more general individual differences in the use of worry as a control strategy.

One of the implications of using worry as a mental control or cognitive avoidance strategy is that it may interfere with normal adaptation and emotional processing that normally require the processing of images. We have been evaluating a metacognitive model of posttraumatic stress disorder (PTSD) (Wells & Sembi, in press-a, in press-b) in which verbal perseverative activity in the form of worry/rumination is one of the factors that increases the risk of prolonged stress reactions by blocking natural cognitive adaptation processes. Data from several studies support the idea that worry contributes to intrusive images and PTSD following exposure to stress. Butler, Wells, and Dewick (1995) exposed participants to a stressful film about a workshop accident. They then instructed participants to settle down (control condition), image the events of the film, or worry in verbal form about events in the film for four minutes after viewing it. Participants asked to worry reported significantly more intrusive images related to the film over a subsequent 3-day period than did participants in the other groups. In a larger study, Wells and Papageorgiou (1995) used four different postfilm manipulations intended to vary in the extent to which they blocked emotional processing or lead to a "tagging" of memories about the film. They showed that the highest frequency of intrusive images during a 3-day period after viewing the film occurred in participants asked to worry for 4 minutes after viewing the film.

A link between worry and trauma reactions has been demonstrated in research with the TCQ. The TCQ (Wells & Davies, 1994) is a self-report measure of individual differences in the tendency to use five different types of strategy to control distressing thoughts. The strategies are worry, punishment, reappraisal, social control, and distraction. The tendency to use worry or punishment is positively associated with emotional vulnerability (Wells & Davies, 1994; Reynolds & Wells, 1999). Warda and Bryant (1998) found that patients with acute stress disorder used more worry and punishment than did patients without ASD. More recently, Holeva, Tarrier and Wells, (2001), explored the prospective predictors of PTSD following road traffic accidents. In this study the use of worry to control thoughts predicted the presence of PTSD between 4 and 6 months after the accident when the presence of stress symptoms at time 1 was controlled.

In addition to the incubation of intrusive images following stress and an apparent role in the development of posttraumatic stress reactions, the tendency to use worry as a thought control strategy also appears to be associated with obsessive–compulsive symptoms. Amir, Cashman, and Foa (1997) found that in contrast to control subjects, patients with OCD used significantly more punishment and worry thought control strategies. However, to date studies have not directly tested whether worry intensifies obsessional thoughts and/or compulsions. If it does, it would be reasonable to expect that obsessions would be more frequent or severe in patients with GAD. Schut, Castonguay, and Borkovec (2001) examined the frequency of obsessions and compulsions in diagnosed patients with GAD. Only two patients met full criteria for an additional diagnosis of OCD. 24.3% of the sample reported compulsions and 12.6% reported obsessions. The most common compulsion was checking. Abramowitz and Foa (1998) examined participants from the DSM-IV field trial of OCD (n = 381) and divided them into two groups: (1) OCD and no GAD, (2) both OCD and GAD. The comorbidity rate was 20%. While the presence of GAD did not elevate OCD symptoms, it was associated with more pathological responsibility and indecisiveness. Thus, it appears that the severity of obsessional symptoms is not related to the presence of GAD. However, we cannot partial out any effects that may be due specifically to worry in the absence of GAD.

The data suggest that while worriers show some negative reactions to intrusive thoughts, and worry and obsessions are correlated, worry does not appear to be associated with an increase in obsessional symptoms. There is some indication that it may be associated more with compulsive behavior such as checking. Consistent with this view, Wells and Morrison (1994) found that worry was associated with a significantly greater compulsion to act than obsessions in a nonclinical sample. Tallis and de Silva (1992) found that worry was more consistently associated with checking and doubting than washing and slowness. The latter authors suggest that the association emerges from the functional similarity between worry and checking and that both represent a form of avoidance of imminent danger.

Although worry may not be associated with an increase in obsessions, there is evidence to support the idea that worry may increase the frequency of more general negative thought intrusions. When asked to focus on a simple task such as breathing, worriers report a lower ability to remain focused and more frequent distractions by negative thoughts than did nonworriers (Borkovec et al., 1983). Furthermore, the duration of worry appears to affect the frequency of intrusive thoughts. Borkovec et al. (1983) asked high- and low-worry subjects to engage in 30, 15, or 0 minutes of worry and then asked them to focus on their breathing for a further 5 minutes. During the breathing task, thought content reports were obtained every minute. Compared to nonworriers, the worriers reported more anxiety and depression, less task-focused attention, and more negative thoughts during the breathing task. When worrier and nonworrier data were combined, it revealed that for the 15-minute worry period, negative thought intrusions increased, while for the 0 and 30-minute groups, distractions decreased. These results suggest that brief periods of worrying can increase subsequent negative thinking. It has been suggested that worry acts like fear, in that brief exposures can increase fear while longer exposures lead to fear extinction.

In summary, worry appears to be associated with a range of negative emotional and cognitive outcomes. There is some suggestion that worry may be particularly problematic following exposure to stress. As well there seems to be some specificity of relationships between worry and obsessive–compulsive symptoms in that worry appears to be associated most with checking behavior. While worrying may exacerbate stress-related imagery, increase PTSD, and lead to more distractions by some forms of negative thoughts, it does not appear to be associated with an increased frequency of obsessions. However, no studies have manipulated worry and directly assessed the effect on the frequency, salience, intensity, and distress of obsessional thoughts. Future studies should aim to test effects of this kind.

The effects of worry may be limited to intrusions linked to emotional processing mechanisms and ego-syntonic negative thoughts rather than to the mechanisms underlying ego-dystonic thoughts that characterize OCD. Perhaps, the covert and overt neutralizing (rumination) that exists in obsessional disorders preempts cognitive capacity to the extent that unhelpful worry processes are displaced in these particular cases. However, it would be potentially worthwhile to investigate if covert and/or overt neutralizing resulted in incubation or blocked emotional processing effects that have been found for worry.

METACOGNITION AND THE CONTROL
OF INTRUSIVE THOUGHTS

Metacognition refers to the cognitive factors that appraise, control, and monitor thinking itself. Most cognitive activities are supervised and controlled by metacognitive operations. Thus, styles of thinking and the real or experienced uncontrollability and intrusiveness of thoughts will, in my view, only be understood by recourse to metacognitive levels of explanation. In the rest of this chapter I describe the metacognitive model of pathological worry in GAD and the metacognitive therapy derived from the model. However, I would like to preempt that discussion with a few brief words about dimensions of metacognition that are relevant for understanding clinical disorders and that will reappear in the GAD model.

In formulating metacognitive factors, distinctions are typically made between metacognitive knowledge (i.e., beliefs about thinking), metacognitive strategies (techniques people use to alter and monitor aspects of their cognition), and metacognitive experiences (appraisals of thoughts, the occurrence of feeling states). These dimensions of metacognition can be measured by recent self-report instruments. For example, the Metacognitions Questionnaire (MCQ; Cartwright-Hatton & Wells, 1997) assesses five dimensions on separate subscales: positive beliefs about worry, negative beliefs about thoughts concerning themes of uncontrollability and danger, cognitive confidence, beliefs about need to control thoughts, and cognitive self-consciousness (the tendency to focus attention on thought processes). Recently a shortened 30-item version of this instrument with the same factor structure has been devised (Wells & Cartwright-Hatton, 2004). The TCQ (Wells & Davies, 1994) measures five metacognitive strategies used to control distressing intrusive thoughts: worry, punishment, social control, reappraisal, and distraction. Worry and punishment appear to be reliably associated with emotional disorder.

To understand the factors that contribute to intrusive and uncontrollable thoughts I believe that it is necessary to understand the knowledge that individuals have about their own cognitive processes. This knowledge influences the strategies that people use to manage their own mental states and influences the emotional consequences of intrusive thoughts. Knowledge can be represented in the form of stable beliefs about thinking, such as the belief that it is advantageous to think in a certain way, or the belief that certain thoughts are harmful. Knowledge also exists as beliefs or theories about metacognitive feeling states.

Metacognitive feelings are important sources of data that influence behavior and judgment. For example, the feeling of knowing experience (closely linked to the tip-of-the-tongue effect) can lead to sustained attempts at memory retrieval. Metacognitive beliefs about feelings can provide a framework that leads individuals to use feeling states as a specific form of adaptive or misleading source of data about the self and world. For instance, in the metacognitive model of OCD (Wells, 1997, 2000), internal metacognitive experiences that are often feeling states are used as maladaptive criteria for deciding to initiate or terminate compulsive responses. Thus, feeling states and other specific internal criteria can provide individuals with data about the status of their cognitive system and also represent goals, which are part of the person's metacognitive plan or program for coping. For example, a patient with obsessional disorder was afflicted by intrusive thoughts about having committed a murder, which he had not done. To relieve his distress he repeatedly reviewed his memory for a period of his life and tried to recall all the details without any gaps in his memory. He interpreted gaps in memory as a sign that he could not be sure that he had not committed murder and the feeling of uncertainty was interpreted as a sign that he must have done it. Each memory search effort was terminated when the internal criteria of having a complete memory sequence and a feeling of "certainty" was achieved. As we see later, internal criteria are used by individuals with GAD as termination signals for the work of worrying.

THE METACOGNITIVE MODEL OF GAD

Figure 5.1 presents the metacognitive model of GAD. This model is intended to explain the difficult-to-control, excessive, distressing, and generalized nature of worry that characterizes patients with GAD. Individuals with GAD hold positive metacognitive beliefs about the use of worry as a coping strategy. Examples of such beliefs include the following: "worrying helps me cope, if I worry I'll be prepared, worrying keeps me safe." These beliefs are not unique to GAD and the model holds that most individuals have them. However, patients with GAD appear to use worry as a predominant means of coping with threat, suggesting that these beliefs are more closely linked to the invariable selection of worry as a coping strategy in these patients.

On encountering an intrusive thought, often in the form of a "What if . . . ?" question (e.g., "What if something goes wrong on holiday?"), the person with GAD activates positive beliefs about worry leading to

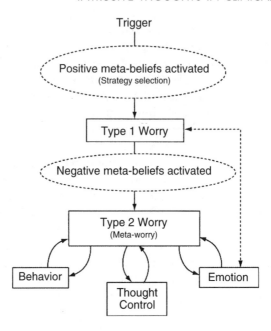

FIGURE 5.1. The metacognitive model of generalized anxiety disorder. From Wells (1997, p. 204). Copyright 1997 by John Wiley & Sons Limited. Reprinted by permission.

Type 1 worrying as a means of contemplating a range of negative outcomes and possible ways of coping. The Type 1 worry sequence consists of a chain of catastrophizing thoughts in which the person attempts to generate answers and coping responses until some internal goal that signals it is safe to stop worrying is achieved. The internal state varies but is often a feeling that one will be able to cope or an appraisal that most possibilities have been covered. Worrying may also be interrupted by competing external demands such as the necessity to engage in distracting activities, but patients often return to the "work of worry" until they feel able to cope with future calamities.

During the Type 1 worry sequence, negative beliefs about worry are activated. Negative beliefs in GAD fall into two broad domains concerning (1) the uncontrollability of worry, and (2) the dangers of worry for mental, physical or social well-being. Negative beliefs typically develop after positive beliefs, and it is their development that leads to a transition to pathological worry and GAD. Once negative beliefs become activated during Type 1 worry episodes, the person negatively appraises the occurrence of worry (i.e., the individual begins to worry about worry). This Type 2 worry (also known as metaworry) leads to several consequences that in turn lead to a persistence of GAD.

Metaworry is associated with an increase in negative emotions such as anxiety and sadness. These emotions are a problem because they can interfere with achieving an internal feeling state that signals that it is safe to stop worrying. Such emotions can be misinterpreted as a sign of failure to cope, thereby leading to sustained attempts at Type 1 worrying as a coping strategy. Emotional symptoms such as racing thoughts, somatic arousal responses, and loss of energy can be misinterpreted as evidence that worrying is causing harm, thereby reinforcing metaworry and negative beliefs. When symptoms are misinterpreted as a sign of imminent catastrophe such as mental breakdown, panic attacks can occur. Thus, the model can explain the co-occurrence of GAD with panic attacks.

The person with GAD engages in behavioral responses aimed at avoiding the dangers of worrying. There are many different behaviors such as reassurance seeking, avoidance of situations that might trigger worrying thoughts (such as people, places, and information), and information search such as surfing the Internet. There are three potential problems with these behaviors: (1) some behaviors provide conflicting, ambiguous, or incorrect information that creates uncertainty which acts as a further trigger for worrying; (2) behaviors such as seeking reassurance from others or avoiding situations removes an opportunity to discover that worrying can be effectively self-controlled rather than avoided or controlled by others; and (3) the effective cessation of worrying prevents the person from discovering that worrying is harmless. Furthermore, the nonoccurrence of catastrophe, such as mental breakdown, fails to be confirmed.

The person with GAD often engages in direct thought control strategies that are not helpful. Because of conflicting motivations concerning worry, on the one hand worry is considered to be helpful and on the other it is potentially dangerous. Individuals often attempt to overcome this conflict by trying not to think thoughts that might trigger worry. For instance, the person currently experiencing work stress will try not to think about work when away from the work situation. The problem with this is that such thought suppression attempts are not very effective and the ineffectiveness can be interpreted as evidence of loss of mental control. If, however, worrying is triggered, the person has conflicting motivations about interrupting the activity, as this would be similar to not attempting to cope. Therefore, the person does not actively and concertedly interrupt the worry process and is prone to conflict in control attempts. This prevents the individual from discovering that worry can be displaced and beliefs about uncontrollability are thereby maintained. Once again, however, the double bind of having two types of negative beliefs about worry (uncontrollability and danger) means that even when worry is interrupted, the person is prevented from discovering that worry is harmless because the catastrophe associated with worrying too much has been avoided.

EMPIRICAL SUPPORT FOR
THE METACOGNITIVE MODEL

Evidence from studies of nonpatients high in pathological worry and studies of nonpatients and patients meeting criteria for a diagnosis of GAD provide support for central features of the model. The empirical support is summarized as follows:

1. The model predicts that Type 2 worry should be a better predictor of pathological worrying such as that found in GAD than Type 1 worry frequency. Wells and Carter (1999), showed in nonpatients that Type 2 worry was positively associated with scores on the Penn State Worry Questionnaire, but Type 1 worry (social and health) was not significant. The variables were entered as simultaneous predictors in multiple regression analyses. This relationship was not affected by the inclusion of trait anxiety and ratings of the uncontrollability of worry in subsequent equations.

2. Wells (in press) used a measure of Type 2 worry assessing the danger dimension and omitting the uncontrollability dimension (to eliminate confounds with DSM-IV criteria for GAD) to examine differences between individuals meeting criteria for GAD and those with somatic anxiety or no anxiety. Individuals classified as meeting criteria for GAD reported significantly higher Type 2 worry scores than did other participants. Moreover, this difference remained when variability in Type 1 worry was controlled.

3. Wells and Carter (2001) found evidence of specificity of Type 2 worry and negative beliefs about worry to GAD. In a comparison of patients with GAD according to DSM-III-R, social phobia, panic disorder, or nonanxious controls, patients with GAD had significantly higher scores on Type 2 worry and significantly higher negative beliefs about worry compared with the other groups. In discriminant function analysis in which Type 1 worry domains and metacognitive factors were

entered, two functions emerged that were typified by Type 1 worry and negative metacognitions (combining Type 2 worry and negative beliefs about worry). Patients with GAD were discriminated from other patient groups by elevated negative metacognitions, while social phobia and panic patients were characterized by specific Type 1 worry domains.

4. In a prospective study of the predictors of GAD over a 12–15-week period, Nassif (1999) found that Type 2 worry and negative beliefs about worry concerning uncontrollability and danger measured at time 1 predicted the presence of GAD at time 2, when the presence of GAD at time 1 was controlled. These data provide some preliminary support for the causal status of negative metacognitions concerning worry in the development of GAD.

5. The model suggests that positive and negative beliefs about worrying may be associated with conflicting motivations to control or engage in worry. A study by Purdon (2000) provides evidence on this issue. She examined the situational effect of appraisals of worry in nonpatients. Negative appraisals correlated positively with trait measures of metaworry and negative metacognitive beliefs. Greater in-situation negative appraisals of worry were associated with greater anxiety. While negative appraisals of worry were associated with greater thought control, positive beliefs about worry were concurrent predictors of reduced motivation to get rid of thoughts.

6. Several studies have identified the presence of positive beliefs about worry in high worriers and patients with GAD (Borkovec & Roemer, 1995; Davey, Tallis, & Capuzzo, 1996; Cartwright-Hatton & Wells, 1997).

7. Research on thought suppression shows that attempts to control thoughts is rarely entirely effective (Purdon, 1999; Wegner, Schneider, Carter, & White, 1987) with mixed evidence that it may in some circumstances increase the frequency of thought targets. However, it should be noted that studies have not directly assessed such effects in GAD.

8. The relationship between pathological worry and negative metacognitions is not the result of overlaps between these dimensions and other types of intrusions, namely, obsessive–compulsive symptoms (Wells & Papageorgiou, 1998).

METACOGNITIVE THERAPY FOR GAD

The metacognitive model provides an explanation of the cognitive factors underlying problematic worry in GAD. The model explains the disappointing effects of existing treatments for GAD by suggesting that they do not modify the underlying metacognitions driving the problem. An implication is that treatment should focus on modifying negative metacognitions and the patient's tendency to use worry as a predominant means of coping and dealing with intrusions. Finally, the model suggests that cognitive vulnerability to GAD, and to psychological disturbance following stress, is linked to the presence of metacognitive beliefs; therefore, modification of such beliefs should increase resistance to future disorder. A metacognitive therapy based on the model has been developed and is undergoing evaluation. In this section I present a description of the basic treatment. For a more detailed account the reader is referred to Wells (1997, 2000).

Metacognitive therapy follows a specific sequence in which case conceptualization and socialization are followed by the targeting of negative beliefs about uncontrollability of worry. This is followed by targeting negative beliefs about the danger of worries and then challenging positive beliefs as a prerequisite for examining alternative strategies for dealing with cognitive intrusions and stress. Each of these phases is briefly described in turn.

Case Conceptualization and Socialization

At the beginning of treatment, a case conceptualization is constructed based on the model depicted in Figure 5.1. This process typically proceeds by reviewing a recent episode in which the patient was distressed by a period of worry. Identification of an episode is followed by a series of questions intended to elicit information for the relevant components in the case conceptualization. The therapist uses questions such as the following:

> "What was the trigger for your worrying? That is, what was the quick thought that started it off? [Probes: Did you have a negative 'what if . . . ?' type of thought? Did you have a thought that you could not cope? Did you experience a negative image?] When you had that thought, what did you worry about [Type 1 worry]?"

The therapist then explores the patient's emotional response:

> "When you had those worries, how did you feel emotionally? [Probe: Did you feel relaxed or tense/anxious?] What symptoms did you notice?"

Next the therapist elicits Type 2 worry and negative beliefs (note that the themes are the same).

> "When you felt that way, did you have any negative thoughts about your worry and the way you were feeling? [Probe: What thoughts did you have?] Did you think anything bad could happen if you continued to worry? [Probe: What's the worst that could happen?] If your worrying felt bad, why didn't you stop worrying [to elicit uncontrollability beliefs]?"

Next the therapist elicits positive beliefs about worry by asking the following questions:

> "Do you think there are any advantages to worrying? [Probe: Can worrying be useful in some ways?]"

Positive beliefs about worry may not be readily accessible at the outset of treatment in some cases. Under these circumstances the therapist should consult self-report scales such as the GADS (Wells, 1997) as a source of these beliefs. Alternatively, this part of the conceptualization may be left incomplete at the beginning of treatment and revisited later on at the appropriate time in therapy. Next, the therapist explores the nature of behavioral responses to worry:

> "Do you do anything to cope with worry? [Probes: What do you do? Do you ask for reassurance? Do you avoid people or situations that trigger worry? Do you search for information to put your mind at rest, etc.?] Do you ever use alcohol or other substances to control your worry?"

Finally, the therapist gives particular attention to thought control strategies and inquires about the use of thought suppression and failure to disengage the worry process.

> "Do you ever try not to think about certain things because it might trigger a worry? [Probe: What do you try not to think? Can you give me an example?] Do you ever decide not to worry once it has started? I don't mean that you try not to think about a worrying topic, but that you just decide not to worry even if you do think about a trigger?"

This line of questioning enables the therapist to construct a case conceptualization.

The next step is socialization to the model so that the patient can begin to develop an understanding of the factors that contribute to persistent and difficult to control worry. Socialization consists of describing the case conceptualization and discussing the linkages in the model. For instance, the therapist can ask patients how anxious they would feel if they no longer believed that worrying was uncontrollable and dangerous. This question illustrates how negative metacognitions contribute to the problem. One useful strategy is to ask hypothetical questions to demonstrate the role of metacognitions. Here the therapist asks the question: "If you believed that worrying was a necessary thing to do for survival, how much of a problem would worrying be?"

Following the initial phase of socialization, the therapist then introduces a thought suppression experiment to show how coping strategies such as suppression are not particularly helpful. The patient is asked to attempt not to think a target thought ("Try not to think about a green elephant") for 2 minutes. After this time the therapist asks what happened. Typically patients find they were unable to exclude the target thought and the therapist then asks what sense the patient makes of this in terms of the effects of trying to suppress worry triggers. Even if the patient was successful in achieving the task, the therapist can then ask: "So how successful are you at doing that with worrying thoughts?" The therapist then discusses the idea that suppression may be counterproductive, and that there may be alternative ways to respond to thoughts that trigger worry that enable the patient to move forward in challenging negative beliefs about worry.

The unhelpful role of other coping behaviors incorporated in the behaviors section of the model is also considered. Patients are asked, "How well are these strategies working? Have you eliminated your worry problem yet? Do you think these behaviors could be keeping the problem going?"

Challenging Uncontrollability Beliefs

Verbal reattribution techniques are employed initially to weaken beliefs about the uncontrollability of worry. A review of situations in which worry was displaced by competing activities is used as evidence that worrying is subject to control. Examples include the displacement of worrying by absorption in a task, by answering a telephone call, or by having to deal with an emergency. Following this stage the therapist introduces the "worry postponement experiment." Patients are asked to notice a cognitive intrusion that triggers worry and to postpone the worry process in response to the trigger until a specified time period later in the day. Later in the day the patient can use the worry period for a prespecified time of 15 minutes to further test the controllability of worry. However, the worry period is not compulsory and it should be emphasized that many patients decide not to use it or forget about their worry. In introducing worry postponement it is important that the therapist takes time to make the clear distinction between *suppression* and *suspension* of the subsequent worry process. The aim is not for the patient to suppress worrying thoughts and remove them from consciousness, but to decide not to engage the iterative catastrophizing sequence of Type 1 worry in response to the cognitive intrusion. The initial thought may remain in consciousness but the patient decides not to engage with it. Worry postponement is allocated as a daily homework experiment.

Next the therapist introduces the "loss of control experiment" in which the patient is asked to use the postponed worry period as an opportunity to try to deliberately lose control of worrying. Usually, attempts to try to lose control of worry are practiced first in the therapy session before they are undertaken as a homework assignment. Having tried to lose control of worry during a postponed worry period, the next step is to try to do so *in situ*. The patient is asked to try to lose control of worrying in response to a natural trigger. Throughout these procedures the therapist tracks the patient's level of belief in uncontrollability, and when it reaches zero, treatment moves on to dealing with beliefs about danger.

Challenging Beliefs about Danger

Negative metacognitive beliefs about danger are dealt with in a similar way to beliefs about uncontrollability. Verbal strategies are employed consisting of techniques such as questioning the evidence that worry can lead to physical or mental harm. The therapist helps the patient to see that there is little evidence that worrying is dangerous. For example, patients can be asked how many people they estimate to worry in their neighborhood, and of those people how many have developed health problems due to worry. Counterevidence should be examined, such as the existence of people that the patient knows who are worriers and yet have reached a good level of maturity. The mechanism by which worry leads to harm should be questioned. In particular, patients often equate

worry with the anxiety response, and the role of such a response in pro-
tecting the individual from danger should be highlighted. Some patients
equate worry with stress and because they believe stress is harmful they
use this equation to assume that worry is also harmful. The difference
between worry and stress should be highlighted as a means of decoup-
ling this unhelpful association. In addition, it should be pointed out that
psychological stress interacts with important person factors in producing
health outcomes and that there is not a simple, direct, or even strong association.

Negative beliefs about mental breakdown or physical harm resulting from worry are modified by behavioral experiment. The therapist
asks the patient to worry more in an attempt to produce clearly specified
negative outcomes of this kind. For example, a patient concerned that
worrying could lead to mental breakdown was asked what this would
look like. She replied that this would mean having schizophrenic symptoms such as hearing voices that were not really there. An experiment
was run in the therapy session to see if intense worrying would lead to
such an outcome. This was then attempted for homework the next time
the patient felt anxious and was worried.

Minisurveys provide a further experimental means of addressing
negative beliefs. Patients are asked to determine if other people whom
they know engage in worry, how often they worry, and if they are ever
bothered by worrying. A prediction is usually made prior to conducting
the experiment concerning how many people the patient predicts will report worrying. Patients are normally surprised to discover that a higher
proportion of people worry than predicted, and that many people have
worries that bother them. This strategy can be coupled with asking patients how normal they believe worrying to be, and its ubiquitous nature
can be used as further evidence against negative beliefs about the dangers of worrying (e.g., "Seventy percent of people worry often; do seventy percent of people go crazy?").

Modifying Positive Metacognitive Beliefs

Positive metacognitive beliefs are challenged by reviewing the evidence
and counterevidence for them, and by a variety of specific procedures. A
specific procedure consists of asking patients to engage in activities normally associated with worrying while deliberately increasing and decreasing worry. For example, when the person believes that worrying
assists performance at work, the abandonment of worry for 1 or 2 days
should lead to evidence of poorer performance. In contrast, the enhance-

ment of worry should lead to improved performance. Failure to find such effects are used to modify positive beliefs.

Strategy Shifts

Toward the end of treatment the therapist reviews with the patient alternative strategies for dealing with cognitive intrusions that trigger worrying. Alternatives include deciding to let worries go and generating alternative brief positive endings for "What if . . . ?" catastrophizing Type 1 worry sequences.

Relapse Prevention

Finally in treatment, the therapist works with the patient to construct a "therapy blueprint." This blueprint consists of an example of the case conceptualization, a list of the key negative and positive beliefs, and the evidence against them. It also consists of a written summary of alternative strategies for dealing with old and new worries in the future.

APPLICATION OF METACOGNITIVE THEORY TO OTHER DISORDERS OF INTRUSIONS

Metacognitive theory and treatment have applications beyond the domain of GAD. Although it is beyond the scope of this chapter to enter into discussion of these possibilities in any detail, I make brief reference here.

The GAD model described in this chapter is based on an information-processing model of psychopathology that we (Wells & Matthews, 1994) advanced some years ago. A central tenet of this model is that psychological disorder is based on a dysfunction in metacognition. This dysfunction gives rise to a generic cognitive attentional syndrome (CAS) that constitutes a central vulnerability to the development and persistence of psychological disorders. The CAS is characterized by metacognitive beliefs or "plans" (i.e., programs) for processing that lead to perseveration in cognition in the form of worry/rumination, attentional strategies of threat monitoring, and coping behaviours that fail to restructure maladaptive beliefs. This theoretical perspective has led to the development of specific metacognitive models and treatments of disorders as diverse as OCD (Wells, 1997, 2000), PTSD (Wells, 2000; Wells & Sembi, in press-a, in press-b), and major depressive disorder (Papageorgiou & Wells, 1999, 2003; Wells & Papageorgiou, 2003). Furthermore, the approach implies that it should be beneficial to develop nonspecific metacognitive-focused treatment strategies that directly target the CAS. These strategies aim at rewriting plans for processing by modifying attentional strategies that lock patients into disorder-congruent processing, and by strategies that allow patients to develop increased flexible control over cognition. Metacognitive therapy also aims to modify beliefs that lead to the selection and maintenance of perseverative styles of thinking and lead to the use of maladaptive internal sources of data as the basis for erroneous appraisals concerning the status of the self and the world.

The metacognitive model of OCD (Wells & Matthews, 1994; Wells, 1997, 2000) assumes that beliefs about the power and meaning of intrusive thoughts combined with beliefs about the need to control such thoughts and perform rituals contributes to anxiety and enhances the salience and frequency of cognitive intrusions. The metacognitive approach to PTSD (Wells, 2000; Wells & Sembi, in press-a, in press-b) is based on the principle that following stress, a natural inbuilt process is the formation of a metacognitive plan for guiding cognition and action in future encounters with stress. This plan is achieved by running mental simulations of dealing with the stress that was experienced. Once a plan is acquired, internal self-regulatory processes allow cognition to be retuned to the normal environment. However, metacognitive beliefs that guide attention to threat and lead to high levels of worry/ruminative activity, and avoidance of trauma-related thoughts, block normal simulation processes.

In the case of OCD, the treatment implications are that therapists should focus on challenging beliefs about the power and meaning of intrusive thoughts, as well as modify predictions concerning the consequences of not performing rituals. In addition, because the metacognitive knowledge base is viewed as existing at least partially in the form of plans for processing, it will be necessary to provide alternative cognitive and attentional plans that the patient can use to make judgments and guide behavior in problematic situations.

The implication of the metacognitive approach for treating PTSD is that the CAS should be removed so that natural emotional processing (mental simulations) can be reinstated. Dropping out of the CAS will involve training in flexible responding to intrusions, attentional redeployment to non-threat-relevant aspects of the environment during exposure, and strategies such as those in the treatment of GAD for reducing the frequency of worry and rumination.

SUMMARY AND CONCLUSIONS

Worry is a particularly important class of cognition that can be triggered by unwanted intrusive thoughts and itself has intrusive qualities. It is a central feature of GAD but may well be involved in the genesis of other forms of psychopathology. It has been conceptualized as a feature of a generic cognitive attentional syndrome in psychological disorder, and it seems likely that treatment techniques designed specifically to deal with worry will be beneficial in treating GAD and also in treating other disorders as well.

It is possible to differentiate worry from other varieties of intrusive thought—a distinction that can lead to exploring the effects of worry on other types of thinking. Worrying appears to have an effect on enhancing other types of intrusive thought, particularly negative thoughts, and stress-related intrusive images. Worry itself has been divided into two main types which represent general worry about noncognitive events (Type 1 worry) and worry about worrying and related cognitive intrusions (Type 2 worry).

The metacognitive approach provides a basis for understanding the development and persistence of pathological worry in GAD. Here negative metacognitive beliefs and positive beliefs are central in determining the development of excessive and difficult to control worry. This approach emphasizes the need to conceptualize and modify beliefs about worry rather than focusing on reality testing the content of individual worries or training in relaxation responses. The latter strategies do not necessarily provide unambiguous information that can lead to a revision of erroneous metacognitions.

Research and theory on metacognition can enhance our understanding of psychopathology processes and suggest alternative avenues of intervention for cognitive therapy of GAD and other disorders of cognitive intrusions. The metacognitive approach has the potential to provide a basis for the treatment of a range of psychological disorders.

REFERENCES

Abramowitz, J. S., & Foa, E. B. (1998). Worries and obsessions in individuals with obsessive–compulsive disorder with and without comorbid generalized anxiety disorder. *Behaviour Research and Therapy, 36,* 695–700.

American Psychiatric Association. (2000). *Diagnostic and statistical manual of mental disorders* (4th ed., text rev.). Washington, DC: Author.

Amir, N., Cashman, L., & Foa, E. B. (1997). Strategies of thought control in obsessive–compulsive disorder. *Behaviour Research and Therapy, 35,* 775–777.

Borkovec, T. D., & Inz, J. (1990). The nature of worry in generalised anxiety disorder: A predominance of thought activity. *Behaviour Research and Therapy, 28,* 153–158.

Borkovec, T. D., & Lyonfields, J. D. (1993). Worry: Thought suppression of emotional processing. In H. W. Krohne (Ed.), *Vigilance and avoidance* (pp. 101–118). Toronto: Mogrefe and Huber.

Borkovec, T. D., Robinson, E., Pruzinsky, T., & DePree, J. A. (1983). Preliminary exploration of worry: Some characteristics and processes. *Behaviour Research and Therapy, 21,* 9–16.

Borkovec, T. D., & Roemer, L. (1995). Perceived functions of worry among generalised anxiety subjects: Distraction from more emotionally distressing topics? *Journal of Behavior Therapy and Experimental Psychiatry, 26,* 25–30.

Butler, G., Wells, A., & Dewick, H. (1995). Differential effects of worry and imagery after exposure to a stressful stimulus: A pilot study. *Behavioural and Cognitive Psychotherapy, 23,* 45–56.

Cartwright-Hatton, S., & Wells, A. (1997). Beliefs about worry and intrusions: The Metacognitions Questionnaire and its correlates. *Journal of Anxiety Disorders, 11,* 279–315.

Clark, D. A. (1992). Depressive, anxious and intrusive thoughts in psychiatric patients and outpatients. *Behaviour Research and Therapy, 30,* 93–102.

Clark, D. A., & Claybourn, M. (1997). Process characteristics of worry and obsessive intrusive thoughts. *Behaviour Research and Therapy, 35,* 1139–1141.

Clark, D. A., & de Silva, P. (1985). The nature of depressive and anxious intrusive thoughts: Distinct or uniform phenomena? *Behaviour Research and Therapy, 23,* 383–393.

Davey, G. C. L., Tallis, F., & Capuzzo, N. (1996). Beliefs about the consequences of worrying. *Cognitive Therapy and Research, 20,* 499–520.

Gross, P. R., & Eifert, G. H. (1990). Components of generalized anxiety: The role of intrusive thoughts vs. worry. *Behaviour Research and Therapy, 28,* 421–428.

Holeva, V., Tarrier, N., & Wells, A. (2001). Prevalence and predictors of acute stress disorder and PTSD following road traffic accidents: Thought control strategies and social support. *Behavior Therapy, 32,* 65–84.

MacLeod, A. K., Williams, J. M. G., & Bekerian, D. A. (1991). Worry is reasonable: The role of explorations in pessimism about future personal events. *Journal of Abnormal Psychology, 100,* 478–486.

Nassif, Y. (1999). *Predictors of pathological worry.* Unpublished MPhil thesis, University of Manchester, UK.

O'Neill, G. W. (1985). Is worry a valuable concept? *Behaviour Research and Therapy, 23,* 479–480.

Papageorgiou, C., & Wells, A. (1999) Process and meta-cognitive dimensions of depressive and anxious thoughts and relationships with emotional intensity

[Special issue: Metacognition and cognitive behaviour therapy]. *Clinical Psychology and Psychotherapy, 6,* 156–162.

Papageorgiou, C., & Wells, A. (2003). An empirical test of a clinical metacognitive model of rumination and depression. *Cognitive Therapy and Research, 27,* 261–273.

Purdon, C. (1999). Thought suppression and psychopathology. *Behaviour Research and Therapy, 37,* 1029–1054.

Purdon, C. (2000, July). *Metacognition and the persistence of worry.* Paper presented at the annual conference of the British Association of Behavioural and Cognitive Psychotherapy, Institute of Education, London.

Purdon, C., & Clark, D. A. (1993). Obsessive intrusive thoughts in non-clinical subjects: I. Content and relation with depressive anxious and obsessional symptoms. *Behaviour Research and Therapy, 31,* 713–720.

Purdon, C., & Clark, D. A. (1999). Meta-cognition and obsessions [Special issue: Metacognition and cognitive behaviour therapy]. *Clinical Psychology and Psychotherapy, 6,* 102–111.

Rachman, S. J. (1997). A cognitive theory of obsessions. *Behaviour Research and Therapy, 36,* 793–802.

Rapee, R. M. (1991). Generalized anxiety disorder: A review and of clinical features and theoretical concepts. *Clinical Psychology Review, 11,* 419–440.

Reynolds, M., & Wells, A. (1999). The thought control questionnaire: Psychometric properties in a clinical sample, and relationship with PTSD and depression. *Psychological Medicine, 29,* 1089–1099.

Roemer, L., & Borkovec, T. D. (1993). Worry: Unwanted cognitive activity that controls unwanted somatic experience. In D. M. Wegner & J. W. Pennebaker (Eds.), *Handbook of mental control* (pp. 220–238). Upper Saddle River, NJ: Prentice Hall.

Salkovskis, P. M. (1985). Obsessional–compulsive problems: A cognitive-behavioural analysis. *Behaviour Research and Therapy, 23,* 571–583.

Schut, A. J., Castonguay, L. G., & Borkovec, T. D. (2001). Compulsive checking behaviors in generalized anxiety disorder. *Journal of Clinical Psychology, 57,* 705–715.

Tallis, F., & de Silva, P. (1992). Worry and obsessional symptoms: A correlational analysis. *Behaviour Research and Therapy, 30,* 103–105.

Turner, S. M., Beidel, D. C., & Stanley, M. A. (1992). Are obsessional thoughts and worry different cognitive phenomena? *Clinical Psychology Review, 12,* 257–270.

Warda, G., & Bryant, R. A. (1998). Cognitive bias in acute stress disorder. *Behaviour Research and Therapy, 36,* 1177–1183.

Wegner, D. M., Schneider, D. J., Carter, S., & White, T. (1987). Paradoxical effects of thought suppression. *Journal of Personality and Social Psychiatry, 53,* 5–13.

Wells, A. (1994). Attention and the control of worry. In G. C. L. Davey & F. Tallis (Eds.), *Worrying: Perspectives on theory, assessment and treatment* (pp. 91–114). Chichester, UK: Wiley.

Wells, A. (1995). Meta-cognition and worry: A cognitive model of generalised anxiety disorder. *Behavioural and Cognitive Psychotherapy*, *23*, 301–320.

Wells, A. (1997). *Cognitive therapy of anxiety disorders: A practice manual and conceptual guide*. Chichester, UK: Wiley.

Wells, A. (1999). A metacognitive model and therapy for generalized anxiety disorder. *Clinical Psychology and Psychotherapy*, *6*, 86–95.

Wells, A. (2000). *Emotional disorders and metacognition: Innovative cognitive therapy*. Chichester, UK: Wiley.

Wells, A. (in press). Assessment of meta-worry and relationship with DSM-IV GAD. *Cognitive Therapy and Research*.

Wells, A., & Carter, K. (1999). Preliminary tests of a cognitive model of GAD. *Behaviour Research and Therapy*, *37*, 585–594.

Wells, A., & Carter, K. (2001). Further tests of a cognitive model of generalized anxiety disorder: Metacognitions and worry in GAD, panic disorder, social phobia, depression, and nonpatients. *Behavior Therapy*, *32*, 85–102.

Wells, A., & Cartwright-Hatton, S. (2004). A short form of the metacognitions questionnaire: Properties of the MCQ-30. *Behaviour Research and Therapy*, *42*, 385–396.

Wells, A., & Davies, M. (1994). The Thought Control Questionnaire: A measure of individual differences in the control of unwanted thoughts. *Behaviour Research and Therapy*, *32*, 871–878.

Wells, A., & Matthews, G. (1994). *Attention and emotion. A clinical perspective*. Hove, UK: Erlbaum.

Wells, A., & Morrison, T. (1994). Qualitative dimensions of normal worry and normal intrusive thoughts: A comparative study. *Behaviour Research and Therapy*, *32*, 867–870.

Wells, A., & Papageorgiou, C. (1995). Worry and the incubation of intrusive images following stress. *Behaviour Research and Therapy*, *33*, 579–583.

Wells, A., & Papageorgiou, C. (1998). Relationships between worry and obsessive–compulsive symptoms and meta-cognitive beliefs. *Behaviour Research and Therapy*, *36*, 899–913.

Wells, A., & Papageorgiou, C. (2003). Metacognitive therapy for despressive rumination. In C. Papageorgiou & A. Wells (Eds.), *Depressive rumination: nature theory and treatment* (pp. 259–273). Chichester, UK: Wiley.

Wells, A., & Sembi. S. (in press-a). Metacognitive therapy for PTSD: A core treatment manual. *Cognitive and Behavioral Practice*.

Wells, A., & Sembi, S. (in press-b). Metacognitive therapy for PTSD: A preliminary investigation of a new brief treatment. *Journal of Behavior Therapy and Experimental Psychiatry*.

Wine, J. D. (1971). Test anxiety and the direction of attention. *Psychological Bulletin*, *76*, 92–104.

CHAPTER 6

THINKING IS BELIEVING

Ego-Dystonic Intrusive Thoughts
in Obsessive–Compulsive Disorder

DAVID A. CLARK
KIERON O'CONNOR

The phenomena of unwanted mental intrusions are particularly relevant to obsessive–compulsive disorder (OCD). Clinical obsessions can be viewed as an extreme form of unwanted intrusive thought, image, or impulse. Individuals with OCD report a subjective experience of obsessions that fits closely with our current understanding of unwanted intrusive thoughts (Clark, 2004; Rachman & Hodgson, 1980). Thus it is understandable that much of our present knowledge of unwanted intrusive cognition stems from research on OCD.

Rachman and de Silva (1978) reported the first investigation of whether obsessional thinking might actually occur in the general population. Their discovery that nonclinical individuals experience intrusive thoughts, images, and impulses that have similar content to clinical obsessions was important for suggesting a possible origin of clinical obsessions and a continuity between cognitive phenomena within the normal population and its clinical variant in OCD. Based on this finding, the later cognitive-behavioral theories of Salkovskis (1985, 1989a, 1999), Rachman (1997, 1998, 2003), and others (Clark, 2004; Freeston, Rhéaume, & Ladouceur, 1996; Obsessive Compulsive Cognitions Working Group, 1997) proposed that the development of clinical obsessions originated from the natural occurrence of unwanted and unacceptable mental intrusions. Cognitive-behavioral theorists argue that practically everyone experiences intrusive thought content that is indistinguishable from the content of clinical obsessions. Thus, nonclinical individuals can have a variety of ego-alien thoughts covering such themes as (1) dirt/contamination, (2) harm/injury to self or others, (3) doubt over their thoughts or actions, (4) whether they might commit some unacceptable sexual act, (5) violations of symmetry/exactness, (6) committing a moral violation, or (7) overtly verbalizing blasphemy (see also Clark & Rhyno, Chapter 1, this volume). According to contemporary cognitive-behavioral theories, whether such unwanted intrusive thoughts escalate in frequency and intensity to become clinical obsessions depends on how individuals evaluate or interpret (appraise) the cognition. However, the nature of "normal obsessions" has not been well-elaborated in cognitive-behavioral models of OCD.

In this chapter we provide a critical overview of cognitive-behavioral appraisal theories of obsessions. We begin by examining whether the link between "normal" and "abnormal" obsessions is as solid as assumed by cognitive-behavioral theorists. It is suggested that a consideration of inferential reasoning processes provides further clarification of the link between normal and abnormal obsessions. Although the cognitive-behavioral models of OCD focus on key cognitive products in the persistence (and possibly etiology) of obsessions, they tend to overlook important inferential processes that also play an important role in the pathogenesis of clinical obsessions. We propose an expanded conceptual model of obsessions that integrates Clark's (2004) cognitive control theory of obsessions with O'Connor's (O'Connor & Robillard, 1995; O'Connor, 2002) inferential model of obsessions. Empirical research relevant to this expanded view on obsessions is reviewed and treatment implications of this conceptualization are discussed. The chapter concludes by proposing key questions and future directions that research based on the present conceptualization might take to advance our understanding of nonclinical and clinical obsessive intrusive thoughts.

NORMAL AND ABNORMAL OBSESSIONS

Chapter 1 provided a review of the research documenting the occurrence of unwanted and unacceptable intrusive thoughts, images, and impulses in nonclinical populations. From his behavioral perspective on OCD, Rachman (1981) classified a thought, image, or impulse intrusive if (1) it interrupted ongoing activity, (2) was recognized as having an internal origin, and (3) was difficult to control. In addition, Rachman noted that there is a quality of "willful independence" to intrusive thoughts, such that they are a fairly abrupt and unwelcomed incursion into consciousness. Once an intrusive thought captures attentional resource it can be very difficult to remove or suppress. Rachman (1981) commented that the intrusive thoughts most relevant to obsessions are *unwanted* as opposed to the welcomed (wanted) mental intrusions that we might call inspiration. Also, like obsessions, unwanted intrusive thoughts have a repetitive quality that cannot be entirely attributed to external precipitants.

Several studies have indicated that unwanted intrusive thoughts with content similar to clinical obsessions are a universal experience shared by approximately 80–90% of populations without OCD (e.g., Clark & de Silva, 1985; Freeston, Ladouceur, Thibodeau, & Gagnon, 1991; Parkinson & Rachman, 1981; Purdon & Clark, 1993; Rachman & de Silva, 1978; Salkovskis & Harrison, 1984). These findings clearly indicate that nonclinical individuals have unwanted mental intrusions that are thematically similar to clinical obsessions, although they are much less frequent, distressing, and uncontrollable than their clinical counterpart (Rachman & Hodgson, 1980).

Although this research suggests that the vast majority of individuals have "normal obsessions," there is some evidence that the experience of "normal obsessions" in the general population may have been inaccurately portrayed (see also Clark & Rhyno, Chapter 1, this volume). For example, it is clear that not all obsessional content was equally represented in these nonclinical intrusive thoughts studies, with some of the more frequently endorsed intrusions more likely examples of anxious or maybe even depressive thinking (Clark & Purdon, 1995). As well, obsessions with overt compulsions were often underrepresented in these studies, especially the more bizarre overvalued ideation, and other intrusions reported by nonclinical individuals would now be recognized as mental tics (e.g., replaying mentally a song or phrase), which have a distinct etiology (O'Connor, 2001, 2004). More recently, we conducted a structured interview in which 50 nonclinical students were asked to report their most frequent and distressing unwanted intrusive thought. Only 11% of the unwanted intrusive thoughts involved themes consistent with clinical obsessions. Instead, the overwhelming majority of intrusive thoughts involved anxious or worrisome thought content (Clark, Wang, Markowitz, & Purdon, 2002). Nevertheless, Purdon and Clark (1993) did find that the majority of nonclinical individuals report occasional occurrences of unwanted intrusive thoughts that have a clear thematic relation to clinical obsessions.

Researchers and clinicians might have more success in identifying truly obsessive-like unwanted intrusive thoughts, images, or impulses if they took into consideration both the form and content of the unwanted thought. Obsessions can be differentiated from other negative cognitive phenomena by certain characteristics such as their intrusive quality, unacceptability, subjective resistance, uncontrollability, and ego-dystonicity (Clark, 2004). It is this latter characteristic that deserves special mention in the present context.

It is quite clear that the content of normal or abnormal obsessions plays an important role in how the individual interprets or appraises the intrusion. Rachman (1998) acknowledges that there is a close interplay between the content of a person's obsession and whether or not he or she attaches excessive personal significance to the cognition. Intrusive thoughts that are *ego-dystonic* (i.e., contrary to or inconsistent with one's sense of self as reflected in core personal values, ideals, and moral attributes) will draw particular attention and processing priority (Clark, 2004; Purdon, 2001; Purdon & Clark, 1999; Rachman, 1998). These thoughts threaten a person's self-view because they are contrary to cherished goals, values, and sense of self. It is this uncharacteristic or ego-alien quality of the thought that imbues it with special personal significance and importance. In fact, the repeated occurrence of these ego-dystonic intrusions may cause individuals to question their true character (Purdon, 2001). This is illustrated in the case example of the person with obsessional ruminations who became very distressed by the intrusive thought, "Did I molest a child while I was in the public washroom?" This repugnant intrusive thought caused considerable distress because the individual viewed sexual abuse of children a horrific crime that is entirely inconsistent with his self-view as a highly moral, caring individual. The appraisal, "Could I be the type of person who could violate children?" is an important question that endows the intrusion with special personal significance. Evaluating unwanted intrusive thoughts, images, and impulses in light of whether they represent a threat to personal goals and values will help differentiate obsessive intrusive thoughts from other types of negative cognitions.

Apart from the content of the obsessive intrusive thoughts, there is also the question of the form the thought takes, which is not well captured in simple statements of its theme or content. As several authors from Janet (1903) onward have noted, doubt is an important quality of obsessional thoughts, particularly when talking of obsessions associated with overt checking or washing compulsions (e.g., "perhaps the oven is left on" and "maybe my hands are dirty"). However, this doubting seems not to take the form of a genuine questioning doubt (e.g., "I wonder if it will rain tomorrow" and "Maybe this time next year I could be in London"). It rather takes the form of an *inference of doubt* about an actual state of affairs. An inference is essentially a plausible proposition about a possible state of affairs, itself arrived at by reasoning but which forms the premise for further deductive/inductive reasoning. Furthermore, the doubt is not posed in a spirit of impartial enquiry (e.g., "Now, did I leave the stove on or did I not? Let's weigh up the probabilities either way and see what evidence best supports the hypotheses."). The inference of doubt is already emotionally charged and leads to a spiraling chain of second possibilities, all, of course, negative. In fact, we can quite distinctly identify two thought components to the doubt: (1) the primary inference of doubt ("Maybe the stove is on") and (2) its consequences or secondary inference ("If the stove is on, the house will catch fire, I'll lose everything and etc. . . ."). It is this latter secondary inference that contemporary appraisal models of OCD tend to focus on rather than the original primary inference of doubt.

Specifying a primary and secondary inference of doubt can help explain the idiosyncratic and inconsistent nature of obsessional thinking. That is, an analysis of the clinical obsession or intrusive thought in terms of a primary and secondary inference of doubt can elucidate how a particular thought, image, or impulse acquires obsessive properties. For example, a person suffering from contamination fears constantly has the same doubt about germs landing on her skin ("maybe airborne microbes have transferred onto my skin"). However, she is not afraid to touch plastic bags or shop counters or to breathe in air for fear of microbes, even though, objectively speaking, these activities could be equally infectious. An analysis in terms of the primary (i.e., "maybe airborne microbes have transferred onto my skin") and secondary (i.e., "I might then develop a terrible rash on my skin") inference of doubt can explain why this person is so distressed by the thought of airborne germs landing on her skin but is not distressed by touching objects in her natural environment. In sum, an initial doubt or primary inference which is emotionally charged and personally significant is an important characteristic of the obsessive intrusive thought that orients the person toward engaging in the faulty primary and secondary appraisals proposed in contemporary cognitive-behavioral theories of OCD.

FROM INTRUSION TO OBSESSION:
THE DEVELOPMENT OF CLINICAL OBSESSIONS

Figure 6.1 presents a schematic diagram that specifies the various cognitive processes that may be involved in the escalation of unwanted, ego-dystonic intrusive thoughts into more frequent, persistent, and severe clinical obsessions. The proposed model draws on the theoretical contributions of the appraisal theories of Salkovskis (1985, 1999), Rachman (1997, 1998, 2003), and Clark (2004), as well as the inferential confusion model of O'Connor (Aardema & O'Connor, 2003; O'Connor, 2002; O'Connor & Robillard, 1995). We next discuss the various cognitive processes and products involved in the pathogenesis of obsessions according to their role and conceptual status within the model.

Vulnerability Factors

Given the nearly universal experience of unwanted ego-dystonic intrusive thoughts in the general population coupled with the relatively low incidence of OCD, it is obvious that risk for the development of obsessional illness is not equally distributed across the population. Clearly some individuals are more vulnerable to the development of OCD than are other individuals. However, there are no prospective studies on psychological factors that increase susceptibility to the development of obsessional symptoms (McNally, 2001). A number of theorists have speculated on the type of early-childhood experiences and critical learning incidents that might lead to the development of maladaptive beliefs about responsibility, threat, and the importance of thoughts that could in turn heighten one's sensitivity to particular ego-dystonic mental intrusions (e.g., Rachman, 1997, 2003; Salkovskis, Shafran, Rachman, & Freeston, 1999). Yet, empirical evidence for these causal pathways to obsessions has not been obtained.

In Figure 6.1 we present five personality and cognitive constructs that might heighten susceptibility to unwanted ego-dystonic intrusive thoughts. Three of these constructs, high negative affect, anxious apprehension, and ambivalent self-evaluation, are broad concepts that no doubt increase vulnerability to anxiety disorders generally. Watson and Clark (1984) proposed that the personality/mood disposition of *high negative affect*, characterized by a tendency to experience frequent and intense negative thoughts and feelings, increases susceptibility to a variety of negative emotional states. Barlow (2002) theorized that a tendency for *elevated levels of anxious apprehension* is due to the interac-

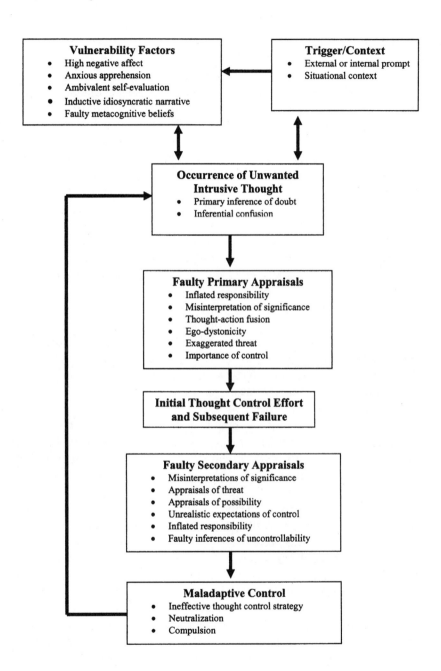

FIGURE 6.1. Integrated inferential and appraisal model of obsessions.

tion of a generalized biological predisposition for nervousness or emotionality, a psychological vulnerability for a diminished sense of control, and a specific psychological vulnerability that causes people to focus anxious apprehension on a specific object or event. Guidano and Liotti (1983) suggested that individuals prone to obsessional thinking might have a conflictual, uncertain, and *fragile self-image* that causes them to seek perfection and certainty.

The two remaining vulnerability constructs, *inductive idiosyncratic narrative* and *metacognitive beliefs,* may be vulnerability constructs that play a more specific role in the etiology of obsessions. The primary inferences that characterize obsessional thinking (see discussion later) are supported by an inductively generated idiosyncratic narrative that employs one or several devices to elicit a state of obsessional doubt. These reasoning errors contribute to the formation of the inductive narrative, which itself creates the primary doubting inference that is evident in obsessions. Table 6.1 presents the reasoning errors identified within an OCD-relevant inductive idiosyncratic narrative.

The role of the inductive narrative in the development of obsessional thinking is illustrated in the following clinical example. A person with OCD recounts an inductive narrative which convinces her that her hands could be dirty (*primary inference of doubt*) and so she must wash her hands. "So, I say to myself: Well, my kids were playing outside and like I know it's dirty outside (*selective use of fact*). I've seen the dirt on the pavement and I think they may have touched something dirty (*category error*), like picked up something from the street, dirty paper or dog shit, and then I say well if they're dirty then I'm going to be dirty (*apparently comparable events*) and I'm going to make the house dirty, and I imagine the house dirty and me with my dirty hands, so I start to feel dirty (*imaginary sequence*). So I go in and wash and I can't stop, you know, it's like a voice in my head, saying over and over again, you're dirty, even though you're washing and you see nothing (*distrust of normal senses*), you could still be dirty (*inverse inference*)."

In this example the person with OCD infers on the basis of a purely subjectively generated narrative that her hands could be dirty and then acts "as if" the hands are dirty in the absence of any visible proof. The person then tries to remove an imaginary doubt by real washing, but because the imaginary discourse and real sense information are in two separate realms, she can never succeed. Furthermore, because the senses are distrusted, repetition can only feed the imaginary discourse of doubt rather than provide new information. This confusion of a subjective discourse with reality, complete with some or all of the foregoing reasoning

TABLE 6.1. Reasoning Errors That Characterize the Inductive Idiosyncratic Narrative of Obsessional Thought

Reasoning error	Definition
Category errors	Confusing two logical or ontically distinct properties or objects (e.g., "If this white table is dirty, it means the other white table could need cleaning").
Apparently comparable events	Confusing two distinct events separated by time, place and/or causal agency (e.g., "My friend often drives off and leaves his garage door open, so mine could be left open").
Selective use of out-of-context facts or misplaced concreteness	Abstract facts are inappropriately applied to specific personal contexts (e.g., "Microbes do exist so therefore there might be microbes infecting my hand").
Purely imaginary sequences	Making up convincing stories and living them (e.g., "I can imagine the waves entering my head so they could be infecting my brain").
Inverse inference	Inferences about reality precede rather than follow observation of reality (e.g., "A lot of people must have walked on this floor, therefore it could be dirty").
Distrust of normal perception	Disregarding the senses in favor of going deeper into reality (e.g., "Even though my senses tell me there's nothing there, I know by my intelligence that there might be more than I can see").

errors, is termed *inferential confusion*. People with OCD, however, do not appear to have any problems perceiving or sensing reality (Constans, Foa, Franklin, & Matthews, 1995), it seems rather that the certainty of correctly perceived sense information is replaced by doubt generated through "inferential confusion," thereby resulting in the belief that "maybe" a state of affairs is possible despite contradictory evidence from the senses.

The OCD-relevant inductive narrative is constructed from facts or ideas that have no bearing on present reality (O'Connor & Robillard, 1995). The following are examples of OCD fictional narratives (i.e., inductive idiosyncratic narratives) derived from faulty reasoning and leading to a confusion of inference (see O'Connor, 2002). A woman repeatedly checks only the front door for fear that her cat might escape even though this has never happened, although the cat did escape through the back door, which she never checks. A pharmacist compulsively recounts pills but not her labeling of medication even though she has made mistakes in labeling but never in counting pills. As evident from these examples, the inductive inferential narratives are mental models that are not only derived from faulty reasoning but when activated naturally lead to the faulty inference of doubt that characterizes obsessions.

Another type of schematic thinking that may be particularly applicable to the development of obsessions is the presence of maladaptive *metacognitive beliefs*. An important part of the capacity to monitor and regulate our information processing system is the ability to "think about thinking" or what Flavell (1979) termed *metacognition*. As part of this capacity for metacognition, individuals will develop beliefs about the function, meaning, and controllability of their cognitive apparatus. In OCD, like other anxiety disorders, individuals may hold a number of maladaptive beliefs about the function and meaning of unwanted ego-dystonic intrusive thoughts (obsessions) that make them more inclined to misinterpret the significance of certain unwanted mental intrusions (Wells, 1997; Wells & Mathews, 1994). For example, individuals who believe that unexpected intrusive thoughts are a reflection of one's true nature, that bad thoughts can lead to bad deeds (thought–action fusion), or that it is entirely possible, even desirable, to exercise strict control over one's mental life will be more vulnerable to an escalation in unwanted, ego-dystonic intrusive thoughts because these beliefs will increase the likelihood that they will appraise the intrusion as a personally significant and threatening occurrence. Like other types of dysfunctional schemas, maladaptive metacognitive beliefs are a product of childhood experiences and critical learning incidents as an adolescent and adult.

Although we have proposed a number of enduring personality, cognitive, and reasoning characteristics that may increase susceptibility to obsessional thinking, ego-dystonic intrusions or obsessions rarely, if ever, occur in a vacuum. Parkinson and Rachman (1981) found that even nonclinical individuals could identify an external trigger to 69% of their intrusive thoughts, and Rachman and Hodgson (1980) noted that most, but not all, obsessions are triggered by external cues and stresses. O'Connor (2002) argued that intrusive thoughts or obsessions are triggered in response to a percept of an external or internal prompt or event. In OCD with overt compulsions, perception of an external stimulus (i.e., "seeing a sharp knife on the kitchen counter") may trigger an obsessive thought (i.e., "what if I snap and stab my child?"). For obsessional rumination without overt compulsion, an internal percept (i.e., "thoughts of God") might trigger an obsessive thought (i.e., "what if I committed the unforgivable sin against God?"). The percept of an internal or external stimulus is not the obsession but rather the trigger that elicits the obsessive or unwanted intrusive thought.

Occurrence of the Intrusion

The inference model of OCD is particularly helpful in elucidating the nature of the obsession itself (Aardema & O'Connor, 2003; O'Connor, 2002; O'Connor & Robillard, 1995). According to this model, obsessions always involve an element of doubt that is inherently emotionally charged and personally significant. This initial doubt is termed the *primary inference*. In the case of obsessions with overt compulsions, the inference about a state of affairs is logically implied in a thought–action sequence. For example, if I'm scrubbing a toilet clean, then there must be a primary inference concerning the possibility of the toilet being unclean which motivates the cleaning. Thus the obsessional thought occurs as a calculated end point or conclusion based on (1) an external/internal percept, (2) activation of relevant vulnerability factors that include an idiosyncratic inductive narrative, and (3) a faulty inferential process.

Because of the apparent logical sequence between primary and secondary inferences and behavior, it is convenient to represent the development of inferences in the template of formal logic. A familiar form of deductive logic would be as follows: (1) food can be put on clean plates; (2) this plate is clean; so (3) I can put the food on it. In classic deductive logic, a conditional premise, A, qualifies a case, B, which leads to a corollary, C. Inductive logic, on the other hand, takes the form of generalizing on the basis of experience: (1) this plate has that mark; (2) plates with that mark break easily; (3) this plate could easily break. Here an instance or case A is seen as part of an experienced category B, which subsequently leads to a corollary C. This corollary could then of course become the premise of another logical sequence, and so on. Faulty conclusions then may be a result of faulty inference processes or faulty premises.

In everyday life, people are heavily influenced by many factors other than the formal rules of deduction and induction when they make inferences. The primary inferences in OCD are also supported by an inductively generated idiosyncratic narrative.

Inferential confusion arises when all narrative models available to the person on which to draw inferences convince the person to live "as if" he or she were, for example, dirty even without visible proof. A chain of learned inductive inferences and associations convinces the person to infer that a possible state of affairs exists, and to act on this primary inference despite the information from his or her senses. The doubting inference arises from the internally generated narrative in the complete absence of accompanying empirical sense-driven information. In fact, and this is important therapeutically, the senses are generally ignored by the doubt. The senses may have already rendered the person "certain" that there is no danger, but the doubt from the internally generated narrative trumps this "certainty" and replaces it with the primary doubting inference "maybe." In extreme cases the person can almost enter an imaginary dissociated state, particularly if the obsessional ideas involve so-called "fusions" (thought–action, thought–event, thought–object fusion) where imagination plays a decisive role in rendering remote events more probable—for example, thinking of an accident will make its occurrence more probable (O'Connor & Aardema, 2003). The end result is an ego-dystonic intrusive thought or obsession expressed as a primary doubting inference that confuses a subjective narrative of possibility with sense-based evidence from reality ("maybe I contracted HIV by touching that doorknob," "did I completely turn off the stove when I left the house," "what if I lose control and harm someone," "did I harm a child while using the public washroom").

Primary Appraisals of Intrusions

Whereas the inferential model is helpful in positing a faulty reasoning process that may be involved in the genesis of ego-dystonic intrusive thoughts, the cognitive appraisal theories of Salkovskis, Rachman, and others are most useful in explaining the escalation and persistence of ego-dystonic intrusive thoughts, images, and impulses into clinical obsessions. The basic premise of the appraisal models is that whether or not an unwanted intrusive thought develops into a clinical obsession depends on how it is appraised and whether it is associated with a neutralization response. If the intrusive thought is erroneously appraised as personally significant and threatening, some attempt will be made to control the thought, thereby neutralizing distress or the imagined negative consequences associated with the unwanted cognition. Thus faulty appraisals and reliance on neutralization, compulsions, or other control strategies are the two main processes that lead to an escalation of unwanted intrusive thoughts into obsessions. Although in the short term neutralization may lead to a reduction in distress and an increase in perceived control, over the longer term the faulty appraisals and control strategies will elevate the salience of the mental intrusion and lead to an increase in its frequency.

A number of faulty appraisals have been proposed as pivotal to the persistence of obsessions including inflated responsibility (Salkovskis, 1985, 1989, 1999), misinterpretations of significance (Rachman, 1997, 1998, 2003), overimportance of thought, overestimation of threat, importance of control, intolerance of uncertainty, and perfectionism (Obsessive Compulsive Cognitions Working Group, 1997). It is beyond the scope of this chapter to present a detailed account of each theory. Salkovskis and Rachman have written extensively about their cognitive-behavioral perspectives on OCD, and Clark (2004) presents a comprehensive critical review of each model.

Salkovskis (1985, 1989, 1999) argues that it is not the intrusive thought itself that is the problem but, rather, the meaning that is attached to it. When intrusive thoughts are misinterpreted as signifying that an individual is personally responsible to prevent some anticipated crucial negative outcome from occurring to self or others, then the intrusions will become more salient, accessible, and distressing (Salkovskis & Wahl, 2003). The role of inflated responsibility appraisals is readily apparent in harming/aggression and doubting obsessions. Examples would be the person with intrusive thoughts about running down pedestrians with his car who believes he must neutralize this thought in order to protect others, the individual with obsessions of contamination who believes she must ensure that she does not pass on this contamination to others, or the person with obsessional doubts over locking doors who believes he will be responsible for allowing the house to be burglarized. In each of these cases, an appraisal of inflated personal responsibility will lead to some effort to neutralize or control the intrusive thought, which in turn contributes to an escalation of its frequency and intensity.

Rachman (1997, 1998, 2003) proposes a slightly different, though related, faulty appraisal process in the escalation of obsessional thinking. The central tenet is that obsessions are caused by a "catastrophic misinterpretation of the significance of one's intrusive thoughts/images/ impulses" (Rachman, 1998, p. 385). Misinterpretations of significance involve the erroneous view that an intrusive thought is an indication of something meaningful about one's character. As well, this meaning usually involves some threat or dire consequences for the self or others. Rachman (1998) stated that unwanted intrusive thoughts can escalate into clinical obsessions only if they are misinterpreted as personally significant and as signifying a threat to self or others. An example of the role of catastrophic misinterpretations of significance is evident in the university student who felt compelled to read and reread passages from his textbooks whenever he had the intrusive thought "I don't know this section of the chapter perfectly." This obsessive thought was considered highly significant and threatening because the student believed that without perfect memorization he would fail the exam.

Rachman (1997, 1998, 2003) noted that other cognitive appraisal processes, such as thought–action fusion bias (the tendency to equate thoughts with actions) and inflated responsibility, will increase the likelihood of misinterpretations of significance. In addition, neutralization (and compulsions) and the use of excessive thought control may bring temporary relief, but indirectly these response strategies preserve the causal misinterpretations and anticipated negative consequences of the intrusive thought.

The Obsessive Compulsive Cognitions Working Group (OCCWG, 1997), a group of 46 researchers who conducted a series of collaborative studies on the cognitive basis of OCD, proposed additional faulty appraisals that may be involved in the pathogenesis of obsessions. These included the evaluation of intrusive thoughts as (1) overly important ("because I am thinking this way, it must be important"), (2) highly threatening ("if I continue to think this way, something terrible is going to happen"), (3) requiring complete control ("I've got to stop thinking this way"), (4) necessitating a high level of certainty ("I need to be certain that nothing bad will happen"), and (5) associated with a state of perfection ("I can't stop thinking about this until I do it perfectly"). When individuals hold these faulty appraisals and beliefs about unwanted intrusive thoughts, they will engage in neutralization, compulsive rituals, and other futile thought control strategies which themselves only serve to perpetuate the ego-dystonic or obsessive thought.

Secondary Appraisals of Control

As illustrated in Figure 6.1, a primary inference (intrusive thought) which elicits a faulty appraisal process will naturally lead to some effort to control the unwanted thought and its associated distress or imagined outcome. However, even under the best of circumstances, intentional suppression or control of thoughts is far from perfect. In fact, intentional control of unwanted thoughts paradoxically may lead to a subsequent increase in the to-be-suppressed thought, especially after suppression efforts cease (Wegner, 1994; Wenzlaff & Wegner, 2000). The end result is that initial attempts to control an unwanted thought or obsession will most likely fail with the eventual return of the unwanted thought into conscious awareness. The return of the intrusive thought will then trigger a secondary appraisal process in which the individual evaluates the consequences of not exerting complete control over the obsession.

Recently Clark (2004) suggested a number of faulty appraisals that may be involved in a person's evaluation of his or her failure to control an unwanted intrusive thought or obsession. Individuals who are susceptible to obsessional thinking might misinterpret their unsuccessful thought control efforts as highly significant and threatening. The perceived failure to achieve adequate control over the unwanted intrusive thought might be interpreted as a highly significant failure that could eventually lead to dire negative consequences for the self or others. Vulnerable individuals may also believe that near perfect suppression or prevention of an unwanted train of thoughts is not only possible (i.e., appraisal of possibility) but in fact highly desirable and may be even necessary. As well, the obsession-prone individual may perceive a high degree of personal responsibility for ensuring control over his or her mental faculties and may arrive at a number of faulty inferences about the consequences of failed control over the intrusive thought. Examples of faulty inferences of control based on actual clinical cases include the following: "If I can't control unwanted sexual thoughts, then I might lose control over my sexual behavior," or "If I can't control unwanted intrusive thoughts, then I must be a weak and vulnerable person who is capable of losing control." Notice that these faulty inferences of control resemble the errors of reasoning that we initially described in the ontogenesis of the inductive narrative that contributes to the emergence of unwanted, egodystonic intrusive thoughts. Often the faulty inferences of control take the form of "if–then" clauses in which success or failure to control or dismiss an unwanted thought is viewed as an important sign or test.

EMPIRICAL EVIDENCE
FOR THE INTEGRATED MODEL

The conceptual model for the pathogenesis of obsessions presented in Figure 6.1 is an amalgamation of ideas proposed by O'Connor and colleagues (Aardema & O'Connor, 2003; O'Connor, 2002; O'Connor & Robillard, 1995) and Clark and colleagues (Clark, 2004; Clark & Purdon, 1993; Purdon & Clark, 1999). A number of concepts are involved in the proposed model, and for some of these constructs, empirical support is beginning to emerge. Empirical evidence can be found for concepts such as (1) external precipitants; (2) the occurrence of unwanted ego-dystonic intrusive thoughts; (3) faulty primary appraisals of significance, responsibility, and overestimated threat; (4) and the reliance on neutralization and other dysfunctional control strategies in the etiology and persistence of clinical obsessions. It is beyond the scope of this chapter to attempt to review this fairly extensive literature. The interested reader is referred to recent theoretical and empirical reviews offered by Clark (2004), Frost and Steketee (2002), Salkovskis and Wahl (2003), and Rachman (2003).

There are two critical elements in the current model that are not found in other cognitive-behavioral conceptualization of obsessions. What evidence is there that the unwanted intrusive thoughts, images, and impulses that form the basis of clinical obsessions can be expressed in terms of a faulty primary inference? Is there any empirical support for the assertion that faulty inductive reasoning and inferential confusion are critical processes in the production of obsessive-like intrusive thoughts? And, second, what evidence is there that faulty secondary appraisals of control are involved in the persistence of obsessional thinking?

Evidence for Primary Inferences in OCD

It is not known at the present time whether the reasoning errors proposed for the genesis of obsessional intrusions are genuine errors, rhetorical devices, or cognitive deficits. In other words, when asked to produce the inductive narrative behind the primary inference (i.e., obsessional intrusion), is the person simply producing a justification for the obsessional conviction already in place or are there genuine reasoning biases that produce the doubt? Experimental research so far leads us to suspect it is a genuine inferential confusion. Levels of anxiety, for example, increase as the obsessional narrative is recounted and decrease when an alternative narrative discounts the obsessional narrative (O'Connor, 2002), which one would not expect if the narrative was simply justifying a prexisting high anxiety level. People with OCD do show a tendency to doubt reality and invest more in imagined alternatives than both controls and other anxiety disorders (Pélissier & O'Connor, 2002). This finding has been replicated over both OCD relevant and neutral tasks (Pélissier & O'Connor, 2003).

Figure 6.2 shows a typical example of how doubt in a reality-based statement can be increased more in an obsessional client than in a control participant, by introduction of successive alternative hypothetical possibilities challenging the original statement. However, it seems that

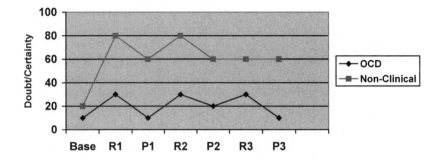

FIGURE 6.2. Effects of reality-based information (R1 to R3) and possibility-based information (P1 to P3) on levels of doubt/certainty in a subject with OCD and a nonclinical subject. Data from Aardema, O'Connor, and Pélissier (2004).

despite the susceptibility to imaginary narratives, people with OCD do employ normal inference processes in non-OCD situations. The susceptibility to doubt has been attributed to disconfirmation bias in OCD (Dar, Bush, Hermesh, Taub, & Fux, 2000; Dudley & Over, 2003) perhaps due to a chronic lack of confidence. But clearly more empirical research is required to establish the specificity of these reasoning errors to OCD. Also, it is still not known whether these reasoning errors and inferential doubt are applicable to all types of obsessional thoughts, images, and impulses or whether they are a cause or consequence of the obsessional state.

Secondary Appraisals of Control in OCD

There is fairly consistent empirical evidence that individuals with OCD score significantly higher than do nonobsessional clinical and nonclinical comparison groups on self-report measures of importance and need to control obsessions (e.g., Sookman, Pinard, & Beck, 2001; Steketee, Frost, & Cohen, 1998). Other studies have found that measures of control beliefs and appraisals correlate significantly with measures of obsessional symptoms (e.g., Clark, Purdon, & Wang, 2003; Steketee et al., 1998; see Emmelkamp & Aardema, 1999, for contrary findings).

The strongest support for the role of control appraisals and beliefs in OCD can be found in studies that used the Interpretations of Intrusions Inventory (III) and the Obsessive Beliefs Questionnaire (OBQ). Both of these measures were developed by the OCCWG and represent the most extensively validated self-report measures of faulty appraisals and beliefs in OCD. The III contains a subscale that measures faulty appraisals of control over unwanted intrusive thoughts, whereas the OBQ has six subscales that assess dysfunctional beliefs relevant for OCD. Two of these subscales assess beliefs about the importance of thoughts and need to control unwanted intrusive thoughts or obsessions. In two separate studies involving approximately 250 individuals with OCD (study 1, n = 101; study 2, n = 248), items dealing with appraisals (i.e., III) and beliefs (i.e., OBQ) about control were significantly correlated with OCD symptom measures, and the OCD group scored significantly higher on the III and OBQ control scales than did nonobsessional anxious and nonclinical comparison groups (OCCWG, 2001, 2003). Using an Italian version of the OBQ and III, Sica et al. (2003) confirmed that individuals with OCD scored significantly higher on the III and OBQ Control subscales than did a group with generalized anxiety disorders and a nonclinical control group. Julien, O'Connor, and Todorov (2003) found that individuals with obsessional ruminations without overt compulsions scored significantly higher on OBQ Control than did patients with washing compulsions and, to a lesser extent, individuals with checking rituals.

Few studies have yet to directly investigate the role of thought control appraisals in the persistence of ego-dystonic intrusive thoughts and obsessions. Individuals with OCD report more attempts to control their unwanted ego-dystonic intrusive thoughts with less perceived success than do nonclinical persons (Ladouceur et al., 2000). In addition individuals with OCD are more likely to use ineffective thought control strategies such as worry or punishment and less likely to use a more effective control approach such as distraction than are anxious and nonclinical comparison groups (Abramowitz, Whiteside, Kalsy, & Tolin, 2003; Amir, Cashman, & Foa, 1997). Purdon (2001) found that appraisals of failed thought control predicted self-reported effort to suppress unwanted thoughts in a thought suppression experiment, and that dysfunctional beliefs about control interacted with suppression effort to predict subsequent success in suppressing reoccurrence of unwanted thoughts (Purdon, 1997). Finally, Tolin, Abramowitz, Hamlin, and Synodi (2002) reanalyzed their findings from a thought suppression experiment and discovered that the OCD group made stronger internal attributions for failure to control unwanted target thought intrusions than did the anxious or nonclinical comparison groups.

Together these initial findings suggest that appraisals and beliefs about the importance and perceived consequence of failure to control unwanted ego-dystonic intrusive and obsessive thoughts may play an important role in the pathogenesis of obsessions. However, many issues remain unresolved, including a clear specification of the exact nature of the faulty secondary appraisal process in OCD, how this appraisal process affects the frequency and severity of obsessions, the relation of faulty control appraisals to neutralization and compulsive rituals, and the specificity of these cognitive processes to OCD.

TREATMENT IMPLICATIONS
OF THE INTEGRATED MODEL

In recent years considerable interest has been generated in the application of cognitive intervention strategies for the treatment of OCD, especially obsessions. A number of behavioral researchers have advocated the integration of cognitive strategies with more standard exposure and response prevention in the treatment of obsessional symptoms (Clark, 2004; Freeston, Léger, & Ladouceur, 2001; Rachman, 1998, 2003; Salkovskis & Warwick, 1988; van Oppen & Arntz, 1994). This new cognitive-behavioral therapy (CBT) for OCD is derived from the fundamental assumptions and constructs of the cognitive appraisal models previously described in this chapter.

The CBT approach to treatment uses both cognitive and behavioral intervention tactics to achieve symptomatic relief by modifying inferential doubt, faulty appraisals and beliefs, and the dysfunctional neutralization responses that maintain obsessional thinking. Table 6.2 presents the main treatment components of CBT that are more or less emphasized in different cognitive-behavioral treatment protocols for OCD. Before continuing, it is worth noting that exposure and response prevention (ERP) is still a critical treatment element that features prominently in cognitive-behavioral treatment protocols (e.g, Freeston & Ladouceur, 1997; Rachman, 2003; Salkovskis, 1999; Salkovskis & Wahl, 2003). ERP is still the only psychological intervention that is considered a well-established treatment for OCD, whereas cognitive therapy has attained the more provisional designation of a probably efficacious treatment (Chambless et al., 1998). In "Expert Consensus Guidelines for Treatment of Obsessive–Compulsive Disorder" (March, Frances, Carpenter, & Kahn, 1997), ERP was judged the optimal behavioral treatment for both obsessions and compulsions, with cognitive intervention providing additional benefit by targeting OCD beliefs and possibly improving compliance with ERP.

A number of books, chapters, and review articles have recently been

TABLE 6.2. Therapeutic Components of Cognitive-Behavioral Treatment of OCD

Education on the appraisal model
A cognitive explanation based on the role of faulty appraisals and neutralization is presented for the persistence of OC symptoms and associated distress. This provides the client with a rationale for the treatment that follows.

Identification and differentiation of appraisals and intrusions
Individuals are taught to identify the primary way they misinterpret the importance or significance of their obsessions. It is critical that clients learn to distinguish between the obsession or intrusion itself, and their cognitive reaction to the intrusion (i.e., their appraisal of the unwanted thought).

Cognitive restructuring strategies
Individuals are taught how to use standard cognitive techniques to question the maladaptive appraisal of the obsession.

Alternative appraisals of the obsession
Emphasis is placed on the development of a more adaptive, less anxiety-provoking interpretation of the occurrence and/or content of an unwanted intrusive thought.

The role of compulsive ritual, neutralization, and avoidance
Clients are given instruction in exposure and response prevention in order to reduce the impact of compulsions, neutralization and avoidance on the persistence of the obsession.

Behavioral experimentation
Behavioral assignments are given that test out the faulty appraisals and beliefs associated with the obsession. The aim of these experiments is to provide the client with experiences that will lead to an abandonment of maladaptive reactions to the obsession and the acceptance of healthier responses.

Modifying self-referent and metacognitive beliefs
Core beliefs about the significance and control of unwanted intrusive thoughts must be addressed as part of treatment maintenance.

Relapse prevention
Before terminating treatment, response to symptom relapse and recurrence is addressed.

Note. From Clark (2004). Copyright 2004 by The Guilford Press. Reprinted by permission.

published which provide a detailed description of CBT for obsessions and compulsions (Clark, 2004; Freeston et al., 2001; Rachman, 2003; Salkovskis & Wahl, 2003). In this chapter we briefly discuss two aspects of CBT that may have been overlooked in previous cognitive-behavioral treatment descriptions; the modification of the faulty inductive narrative and inferential confusion that characterizes obsessional thinking, and the correction of secondary misappraisals of control.

Inference-Based Treatment

The ultimate aim of inference-based therapy is to replace the doubting narrative with confidence in the senses. Like other cognitive-behavioral approaches, inference-based therapy seeks to detach the person from the reality value and importance of the intrusive thought. However, rather than identifying a thought as just a thought, intervention at the level of the inferential confusion targets the narrative that convinces the person that a hypothetical possibility is a real (even if small) likelihood. In other cases the clinician will want to identify the crossover point where the person enters an imaginary world of possibility and the obsessional doubt becomes "lived in." From this, subsequent rituals and other neutralizations are a natural consequence of a confusion between an imaginary and a real problem. Next we summarize a number of critical steps that must be taken to modify the primary and secondary inferential doubt in OCD. A more detailed description can be found elsewhere (O'Connor & Robillard, 1999).

1. *Elicit the primary and secondary inferences and the accompanying narrative.* The first step is to examine in more detail the narrative supporting convictions in the primary inference. The primary inference may be a summary statement. "I may be contaminated," but its force is far better captured by the narrative perpetuating the conviction. One limitation of the inference approach is that this primary inference may not be immediately transparent because the person is caught up with images of the consequences of the inference (secondary inferences). Also it is true that people with OCD often report no external consequences to their primary inferences, particularly with ordering rituals (e.g., perhaps this object is not correctly placed). Frequently, however, there are internal consequences to how people feel about themselves.

2. *Clarify the source of the narrative and reasoning errors.* The next stage after eliciting the narratives associated with key premises is to examine the source of information in the narratives. Generally the

source of "knowledge" in the narrative comes from unreliable remote sources (i.e., hearsay, memory, irrelevant facts, nonpertinent associations, imaginary sequences, and apparently similar events), but never from actual experience or proof. The remoteness of these sources to the actual here and now is emphasized. After examining the narrative in detail, the aim is for the client to agree that the stories are subjective and largely imaginary and not based on actual proof (even if they still give the story credibility).

3. *Highlight discrepancies between OCD risk perception and normal risk perception.* At this point we look more intensively at inference processes in non-OCD domains of life. The aim is to highlight discrepancies in the extent to which information from the senses is credited in OCD and non-OCD situations; thus highlighting the subjective and imaginary nature of OCD inferences and the inverse inference process. Generally in non-OCD cases people use senses (sight, touch, smell, hearing, taste) to determine what is there, and then subsequently to draw inferences about meaning. This is not only distinct from but opposed to the OCD situation, where the five "senses" inform that there is no problem but the person nevertheless infers there must be a problem on the basis of the narrative (inverse inference). In fact, recital of the narrative is "antagonistic" to using the senses.

4. *Pinpoint the OCD self-referent theme.* Even if it does turn out that people with OCD are more prone to a reasoning style that produces erroneous inferences, we still need to explain idiosyncratic thematic content of the inferences, and we suggest this content relates ultimately to a self-referent theme. If someone infers "maybe I have lost something," it implies that the person considers him- or herself to be the type of person who could indeed lose something. Such self-referent themes seem to reflect a self-positioning with respect to the world and others and can often appear idiosyncratic and nuanced, but they are not easily classified as general beliefs. A self-referent theme (belief) underlies the likelihood of a situational trigger eliciting a particular doubt with its accompanying narrative. This viewpoint links in with the vulnerability factor of ambivalent self-reference.

5. *Illustrate the respective roles of reasoning errors in the narrative.* It is important to illustrate the power of the narrative to elicit strong emotions and behavior, and how inferences can be gripping even when we know they are unfounded and based on "inferential confusion." The power of the narrative can also be demonstrated by taking narratives using the habitual obsessional plots pertinent to the client and

then recounting an alternative narrative with an alternative plot to see how the narrative influences emotions and primary inferences.

So, for example, an alternative to the OCD narrative cited earlier in this chapter would be: "My kids were playing outside but they didn't deliberately touch dirty objects. The pavement has some dirt on it but they were not playing on the ground, and they are not deliberately picking up dirt. They are always careful to keep their hands clean when they come in the house. Just because my kids have been outside, it doesn't mean I am dirty unless I see dirt with my senses. If I don't see dirt, I can't feel dirt and I trust my senses not my imagination to see reality."

Constructing the alternative narrative is closely intertwined with discussing corresponding reasoning errors. The alternative narrative is not static and can be further elaborated over sessions as the person becomes less certain of the OCD narrative. In fact, in the client's exercise sheets, we include evaluation of levels of conviction in each element of the story. The aim is not that the client replaces the OCD narrative with a more realistic one but, rather, that the person realizes how the OCD story fuels the doubt and accompanying emotions and how changing the narrative modifies doubt. Because nothing else has changed except the narrative, the exercise pinpoints the subjective narrative and not reality as the source of the obsessional discomfort. As with other cognitive reasoning techniques, it is important that the narrative process does not itself become another form of neutralization.

6. *Using the narrative to reduce anxiety and conviction.* We now rehearse, within sessions, modification of the OCD narrative by replacing it with an alternative narrative for each obsessional doubt. The aim is to give further insight and credibility to the idea that the inferential confusion stems from the influence of the narrative and can only be changed by changing the narrative behind the inference. For this exercise to work, the alternative narratives have to be detailed and have to match every aspect of the obsessional narratives. Of course, the alternative narratives take a lot more effort to construct than the obsessional narratives because they are not automatic.

7. *Reality "sensing."* When in the OCD situation the person does not recount any narratives but resists onset of the primary obsessional inference on the basis that it is 100% subjective and replaces it with sense information drawn from the here and now. The rationale behind reality sensing is somewhat different from exposure and reality testing. In reality "sensing" the person employs an antagonistic logic, whereby instead of avoiding the situation or adding doubt into it by

going off into the narrative, the person defines reality by relying entirely on information from their five senses. As with other cognitive-behavioral therapies, it is very important to eliminate all avoidance and neutralization rituals, large and small, which impair using the senses, or whose rationale is justified by any aspect of the obsessional narrative.

Treatment of Secondary Appraisals of Control

The first step in dealing with faulty secondary appraisals of control is to teach clients how to identify their appraisals of control. The person with OCD can be asked a number of probing questions, such as "How important is it for you to control the obsession?" or "What worries you most if you can't get control over the unwanted thought?" These questions are intended to help clients learn how to evaluate their coping strategies and the perceived consequences of failing to control the obsession. The faulty secondary appraisals of control discussed previously should become apparent through Socratic questioning and homework assignments that sensitize clients to their automatic misappraisals of control.

Once the most prominent secondary control appraisals have been identified, cognitive and behavioral interventions can be designed to challenge the client's erroneous belief that control of the obsession is critical to overcoming the frequency and associated distress of the obsession. Various behavioral experiments can be designed to test whether thought control and neutralization efforts are indeed an effective way to deal with the obsession (for further discussion, see Clark, 2004; Rachman, 2003). For example, the client could be asked to keep a diary of the frequency and associated distress of the obsession. On certain days clients are asked to increase their effort to control the obsession, whereas on alternative days the client is instructed to relinquish thought control efforts. A comparison is made of the frequency and distress of the obsession across "control" and "noncontrol" days. The point of this intervention is to provide new information and experiences that refute the client's obsession-relevant appraisals and beliefs about the need to exert control over the obsession and to reinforce the healthier, more adaptive perspective that control is unnecessary and counterproductive in reducing obsessive–compulsive symptoms. In addition, ERP exercises will be critical to convincing the person with OCD that there is nothing to fear from the obsession and that the best way to reduce the distress of OCD is to "do nothing" in response to the obsession. However, to achieve these therapy objectives, it is important to directly challenge and refute the client's faulty appraisals about the need to control obsessions and avert the perceived negative consequences resulting from a failure to control unwanted, ego-dystonic intrusive thoughts, images, and impulses.

CONCLUSION AND FUTURE DIRECTIONS

In this chapter we have presented a cognitive-behavioral model for the etiology and persistence of clinical obsessions that draws on current cognitive appraisal theories of OCD and the inference-based model of O'Connor and colleagues (Aardema & O'Connor, 2003; O'Connor, 2002; O'Connor & Robillard, 1995). Like other cognitive-behavioral perspectives, clinical obsessions were viewed as originating from the same type of unwanted, ego-dystonic intrusive thoughts, images, and impulses that have been documented as naturally occurring phenomena in the general population. However, unlike a number of appraisal theories that take the occurrence of intrusive thoughts as their starting point, the current perspective has argued that preexisting general and specific vulnerability factors, as well as the activation of faulty induction reasoning processes, result in a faulty primary inference of doubt. It is the presence or absence of this primary inference of doubt that predetermines whether an unwanted ego-dystonic intrusive thought remains an isolated oddity within the stream of consciousness or possesses the capacity to elicit a cascading sequence of faulty primary and secondary appraisals of significance and control. A number of cognitive processes were highlighted that lead to a further escalation in the frequency, intensity, and uncontrollability of the ego-dystonic intrusive thought or obsession once the vulnerable person initiates a faulty inferential and appraisal process.

Based on the cognitive-behavioral model presented in Figure 6.1, a number of treatment recommendations were offered that focused, in particular, on correcting the faulty inferential processes and the erroneous secondary appraisals of control that characterize obsessional states. The cognitive and behavioral intervention tactics described are similar to the treatment innovations advocated in other CBT treatment protocols. The main difference in our approach is the focus or target of the intervention. We suggest that cognitive-behavioral treatment of obsessions may be improved by a greater focus on correcting the faulty inferential reasoning and secondary appraisals of control that are involved in the persistence and escalation of obsessional problems.

As evident by the brevity of our review of the empirical literature, much of what we have presented is conjecture based on clinical experience and some preliminary empirical findings. However, many important questions remain. Can all obsessional phenomena be construed in terms of an inference of doubt? Are the faulty inductive reasoning processes and erroneous primary and secondary appraisals cause, consequence, or epiphenomena in OCD? How OCD-specific are these cognitive processes in comparison to other anxiety disorders or even depression? What is the most accurate and reliable way to assess these phenomena? When we turn to the issue of treatment, will a greater emphasis on the correction of faulty inference and erroneous appraisals improve the effectiveness of psychological treatments for OCD? Is there any therapeutic benefits achieved from this greater cognitive emphasis? And, finally, is the proposed shift in treatment emphasis better suited for some types of obsessional problems than for others? Until research begins to address many of these fundamental questions, the conceptual framework and treatment recommendations described in this chapter must be considered tentative.

ACKNOWLEDGMENT

Work on this chapter was supported by a grant (No. 410-2001-0084) from the Social Sciences and Humanities Research Council of Canada awarded to David A. Clark.

REFERENCES

Aardema, F., & O'Connor, K. (2003). White bears that are not there: inference processes in obsession. *Journal of Cognitive Psychotherapy, 17,* 23–37.

Aardema, F., O'Connor, K. P., & Pélissier, M. C. (2004). *Quantifying doubt in OCD.* Manuscript in preparation, Centre de recherche Fernand-Seguin, Université de Montréal, Montréal, Québec.

Abramowitz, J. S., Whiteside, S., Kalsy, S. A., & Tolin, D. F. (2003). Thought control strategies in obsessive-compulsive disorder: A replication and extension. *Behaviour Research and Therapy, 41,* 529–540.

Amir, N., Cashman, L., & Foa, E. B. (1997). Strategies of thought control in obsessive–compulsive disorder. *Behaviour Research and Therapy, 35,* 775–777.

Barlow, D. H. (2002). *Anxiety and its disorders: The nature and treatment of anxiety and panic* (2nd ed.). New York: Guilford Press.

Chambless, D. L., Baker, M. J., Baucom, D. H., Beutler, L. E., Calhoun, K. S., Crits-

Christoph, P., et al. (1998). Update on empirically validated therapies. II. *The Clinical Psychologist, 51*, 3–16.

Clark, D. A. (2004). *Cognitive-behavioral therapy for OCD.* New York: Guilford Press.

Clark, D. A., & de Silva, P. (1985). The nature of depressive and anxious thoughts: Distinct or uniform phenomena? *Behaviour Research and Therapy, 23*, 383–393.

Clark, D. A., & Purdon, C. L. (1993). New perspectives for a cognitive theory of obsessions. *Australian Psychologist, 28*, 161–167.

Clark, D. A., & Purdon, C. L. (1995). The assessment of unwanted intrusive thoughts: A review and critique of the literature. *Behaviour Research and Therapy, 33*, 967–976.

Clark, D. A., Purdon, C., & Wang, A. (2003). The Meta-Cognitive Beliefs Questionnaire: development of a measure of obsessional beliefs. *Behaviour Research and Therapy, 41*, 655–669.

Clark, D. A., Wang, A., Markowitz, L., & Purdon, C. (2002, November). *A cognitive profile of mental control: Failure in non-clinical individuals.* Poster presented at the annual meeting of the Association for the Advancement of Behavior Therapy, Reno, NV.

Constans, J. I., Foa, E. B., Franklin, M. E., & Mathews, A. (1995). Memory for actual and imagined events in OC checkers. *Behaviour Research and Therapy, 33*, 665–671.

Dar, R., Rish, S., Hermesh, H., Taub, M., & Fux, M. (2000). Realism of confidence in obsessive-compulsive checkers. *Journal of Abnormal Psychology, 109*, 673–678.

Dudley, R. E. J., & Over, D. E. (2003). People with delusions jump to conclusions: A theoretical account of research findings on the reasoning of people with delusions. *Clinical Psychology and Psychotherapy, 10*, 263–274.

Emmelkamp, P. M. G., & Aardema, A. (1999). Metacognition, specific obsessive-compulsive beliefs and obsessive–compulsive behaviour. *Clinical Psychology and Psychotherapy, 6*, 139–145.

Flavell, J. H. (1979). Metacognition and cognitive monitoring: A new area of cognitive-developmental inquiry. *American Psychologist, 34*, 906–911.

Freeston, M. H., & Ladouceur, R. (1997). *The cognitive behavioral treatment of obsessions: A treatment manual.* Unpublished manuscript, École de psychologie, Université Laval, Québec, Canada.

Freeston, M. H., Ladouceur, R., Thibodeau, N., & Gagnon, F. (1991). Cognitive intrusions in a non-clinical population. I. Response style, subjective experience, and appraisal. *Behaviour Research and Therapy, 29*, 585–597.

Freeston, M. H., Léger, E., & Ladouceur, R. (2001). Cognitive therapy of obsessive thoughts. *Cognitive and Behavioral Practice, 8*, 61–78.

Freeston, M. H., Rhéaume, J., & Ladouceur, R. (1996). Correcting faulty appraisals of obsessional thoughts. *Behaviour Research and Therapy, 34*, 433–446.

Frost, R. O., & Steketee, G. (Eds.). (2002). *Cognitive approaches to obsessions and compulsions: Theory, assessment, and treatment.* Amsterdam: Elsevier Science.

Guidano, V. F., & Liotti, G. (1983). *Cognitive processes and emotional disorders : A structural approach to psychotherapy.* New York: Guilford Press.

Janet, P. (1903). *Les obsessions et la psychasthénie* (Vols. 1, 3, 2nd ed.). Paris: Alcan.

Julien, D., O'Connor, K. P., & Todorov, C. (2004). *The relation between belief domains and OCD subtypes.* Unpublished manuscript, Centre de recherché Fernand-Seguin, Montréal, Québec.

Ladouceur, R., Freeston, M. H., Rheaume, J., Dugas, M. J., Gagnon, F., Thibodeau, N., et al. (2000). Strategies used with intrusive thoughts: A comparison of OCD patients with anxious and community controls. *Journal of Abnormal Psychology, 109,* 179–187.

March, J. S., Frances, A., Carpenter, D., & Kahn, D. A. (1997). Expert consensus guideline for treatment of obsessive–compulsive disorder. *Journal of Clinical Psychiatry Suppl.*(4), 5–72.

McNally, R. J. (2001). Vulnerability to anxiety disorders in adulthood. In R. E. Ingram & J. M. Price (Eds.), *Vulnerability to psychopathology: Risk across the lifespan* (pp. 304–321). New York: Guilford Press.

Obsessive Compulsive Cognitions Working Group. (1997). Cognitive assessment of obsessive–compulsive disorder. *Behaviour Research and Therapy, 35,* 667–681.

Obsessive Compulsive Cognitions Working Group. (2001). Development and initial validation of the Obsessive Beliefs Questionnaire and the Interpretation of Intrusions Inventory. *Behaviour Research and Therapy, 39,* 987–1006.

Obsessive Compulsive Cognitions Working Group. (2003). Psychometric validation of the Obsessive Beliefs Questionnaire and the Interpretation of Intrusions Inventory: Part I. *Behaviour Research and Therapy, 41,* 863–878.

O'Connor, K.P. (2001). Clinical and psychological features distinguishing obsessive–compulsive and chronic tic disorders. *Clinical Psychology Review, 20,* 1–30.

O'Connor, K.P. (2002) Intrusions and inferences in obsessive–compulsive disorder. *Clinical Psychology and Psychotherapy, 9,* 38–46.

O'Connor, K. P. (in press). Comparing Tourette's syndrome and OCD. In J. S. Abramowitz & A. C. Houts (Eds.), *Handbook of controversial issues in obsessive compulsive disorder.* New York: Kluwer Academic Press.

O'Connor, K.P., & Aardema, F. (2003). Fusion or confusion in obsessive–compulsive disorder? *Psychological Reports, 93,* 227–232.

O'Connor, K.P., & Robillard, S. (1995). Inference processes in obsessive–compulsive disorder: Some clinical observations. *Behaviour Research and Therapy, 33,* 887–896.

O'Connor, K. P., & Robillard, S. (1999). A cognitive approach to the treatment of primary inferences in obsessive-compulsive disorder. *Journal of Cognitive Psychotherapy: An International Quarterly, 13*, 359–375.

Parkinson, L., & Rachman, S. (1981). Part II. The nature of intrusive thoughts. *Advances in Behaviour Research and Therapy, 3*, 101–110.

Pélissier, M.-C., & O'Connor, K. P. (2002). Deductive and inductive reasoning in obsessive-compulsive disorder. *British Journal of Clinical Psychology, 41*, 5–27.

Pélissier, M.-C., & O'Connor, K. P. (2003). *Inductive reasoning in OCD*. Paper presented at the annual meeting of the Association for the Advancement of Behavior Therapy, Boston.

Purdon, C. (1997). *The role of thought suppression and meta-cognitive beliefs in the persistence of obsession-like intrusive thoughts*. Unpublished doctoral dissertation, University of New Brunswick, Canada.

Purdon, C. (2001). Appraisal of obsessional thought recurrences: Impact on anxiety and mood state. *Behavior Therapy, 32*, 47–64.

Purdon, C., & Clark, D. A. (1993). Obsessive intrusive thoughts in nonclinical subjects. Part I. Content and relation with depressive, anxious and obsessional symptoms. *Behaviour Research and Therapy, 31*, 713–720.

Purdon, C. L., & Clark, D. A. (1999). Metacognition and obsessions. *Clinical Psychology and Psychotherapy, 6*, 102–110.

Rachman, S. J. (1981). Part I. Unwanted intrusive cognitions. *Advances in Behaviour Research and Therapy, 3*, 89–99.

Rachman, S. J. (1997). A cognitive theory of obsessions. *Behaviour Research and Therapy, 35*, 793–802.

Rachman, S. J. (1998). A cognitive theory of obsessions: Elaborations. *Behaviour Research and Therapy, 36*, 385–401.

Rachman, S. J. (2003). *The treatment of obsessions*. Oxford, UK: Oxford University Press.

Rachman, S. J., & de Silva, P. (1978). Abnormal and normal obsessions. *Behaviour Research and Therapy, 16*, 233–248.

Rachman, S. J., & Hodgson, R. J. (1980). *Obsessions and compulsions*. Englewood Cliffs, NJ: Prentice Hall.

Salkovskis, P. M. (1985). Obsessional–compulsive problems: A cognitive-behavioural analysis. *Behaviour Research and Therapy, 23*, 571–583.

Salkovskis, P. M. (1989). Cognitive-behavioural factors and the persistence of intrusive thoughts in obsessional problems. *Behaviour Research and Therapy, 27*, 677–682.

Salkovskis, P. M. (1999). Understanding and treating obsessive–compulsive disorder. *Behaviour Research and Therapy, 37*, S29–S52.

Salkovskis, P. M., & Harrison, J. (1984). Abnormal and normal obsessions—A replication. *Behaviour Research and Therapy, 22*, 1–4.

Salkovskis, P. M., Shafran, R., Rachman, S., & Freeston, M. H. (1999). Multiple pathways to inflated responsibility beliefs in obsessional problems: possible origins and implications for therapy and research. *Behaviour Research and Therapy*, *37*, 1055–1072.

Salkovskis, P. M., & Wahl, K. (2003). Treating obsessional problems using cognitive-behavioural therapy. In M. Reinecke & D. A. Clark (Eds.), *Cognitive therapy across the lifespan: Theory, research and practice* (pp. 138–171). Cambridge, UK: Cambridge University Press.

Salkovskis, P. M., & Warwick, H. M. C. (1988). Cognitive therapy of obsessive–compulsive disorder. In C. Perris, I. M. Blackburn, & H. Perris (Eds.), *Cognitive psychotherapy: Theory and practice* (pp. 376–395). Berlin: Springer-Verlag.

Sookman, D., Pinard, G., & Beck, A. T. (2001). Vulnerability schemas in obsessive–compulsive disorder. *Journal of Cognitive Psychotherapy: An International Quarterly*, *15*, 109–130.

Steketee, G. S., Frost, R. O., & Cohen, I. (1998). Beliefs in obsessive–compulsive disorder. *Journal of Anxiety Disorders*, *12*, 525–537.

Tolin, D. F., Abramowitz, J. S., Hamlin, C., & Synodi, D. S. (2002). Attributions for thought suppression failure in obsessive–compulsive disorder, *Cognitive Therapy and Research*, *26*, 505–517.

van Oppen, P., & Arntz, A. (1994). Cognitive therapy for obsessive-compulsive disorder. *Behaviour Research and Therapy*, *32*, 79–87.

Watson, D., & Clark, L. A. (1984). Negative affectivity: The disposition to experience aversive emotional states. *Psychological Bulletin*, *96*, 465–490.

Wegner, D. M. (1994). Ironic processes of mental control. *Psychological Review*, *101*, 34–52.

Wells, A. (1997). *Cognitive therapy of anxiety disorders: A practice manual and conceptual guide*. Chichester, UK: Wiley.

Wells, A., & Matthews, G. (1994). *Attention and emotion: A clinical perspective*. Hove, UK: Erlbaum.

Wenzlaff, R. M., & Wegner, D. M. (2000). Thought suppression. *Annual Review of Psychology*, *51*, 59–91.

CHAPTER 7

PSYCHOSIS AND THE PHENOMENON OF UNWANTED INTRUSIVE THOUGHTS

ANTHONY P. MORRISON

THE NATURE OF UNWANTED INTRUSIONS IN PSYCHOSIS

The psychopathology of intrusions in psychosis has received little attention from researchers, although there is a growing interest in cognitive approaches to understanding psychotic experience. Several cognitive models of psychosis explicitly include the concept of unwanted intrusive thoughts and have adopted a metacognitive approach to understanding the role that they play in the onset and maintenance of psychotic disorders (Freeman, Garety, Kuipers, Fowler, & Bebbington, 2002; Morrison, 2001; Morrison, Haddock, & Tarrier, 1995).

For the purposes of this chapter, I adopt a working definition of unwanted intrusive thoughts, based on existing definitions (Horowitz, 1975; Rachman, 1981): they are viewed as thoughts, images, or impulses that are experienced as unwanted and uncontrollable and interrupt ongoing activity. There is an important distinction to be made between such existing definitions and the more inclusive approach adopted here; that is, existing definitions emphasize that such intrusive thoughts

175

are recognized as the product of one's own mind and attributed to an internal source. I argue in this chapter that advances in the understanding of psychosis can be developed utilizing the concept of intrusive thoughts that are attributed to an external source, as well as those perceived as internally generated; as discussed later, many psychotic experiences have pronounced similarities with nonpsychotic intrusive thoughts, and it is possible to conceptualize the attribution of source for such intrusions as a separate appraisal process.

The heterogeneity of symptoms associated with the diagnosis of schizophrenia and other psychotic disorders, and associated difficulties concerning the reliability and validity of the diagnosis, has led a number of authors to suggest that research examining the etiology and treatment of psychosis should focus on individual symptoms rather than broadly defined clinical syndromes (Bentall, 1990; Persons, 1986). This chapter, therefore, focuses on "positive" psychotic experiences, which are often viewed as the defining symptoms of the syndrome of schizophrenia. These symptoms include (1) auditory hallucinations or hearing voices (audible thoughts, a discussion or argument about the patient or voices describing the patient's ongoing activity), (2) persecutory delusions (the patient believes that an external agent is trying to cause him or her harm), (3) ideas of reference (they believe an external agent to be talking about them), (4) somatic passivity experiences (they experience bodily sensations as being caused by an external agent), (5) thought insertion (the patient experiences thoughts as being put in his or her mind by an external agent), (6) thought withdrawal (the patient experiences thoughts being removed by an external agent), and (7) thought broadcast (the patient experiences his or her thoughts as being transmitted to other people). Thought disorder (or speech/language disorder, including tangential thinking and word salad) is also considered.

There are several similarities between psychotic phenomena and unwanted intrusive thoughts (UITs). Garety and Hemsley (1994) found that many patients with delusional beliefs scored highly (8 or more out of 10) on characteristics that are commonly associated with UITs (e.g., resistance [69%] and interference [47%]). It has also been noted that hallucinatory phenomena share many characteristics with UITs (Morrison et al., 1995). Auditory hallucinations commonly have external precipitants (Nayani & David, 1996), as do UITs (Parkinson & Rachman, 1981), and these voices often increase with stress (Nayani & David, 1996), as do UITs (Horowitz, 1975).

Like the UITs studies in other disorders (Rachman & de Silva, 1978), it is possible to conceptualize hallucinations as a variant of an essentially normal experience (Morrison, 1998a). Similarities in content are also evident between UITs and auditory hallucinations. For example, voices often comment on sexual, religious, and violent themes (Chadwick & Birchwood, 1994), which are also common themes in UITs (Rachman, 1994). Hallucinations and delusions frequently are perceived as being difficult to control (Chadwick & Birchwood, 1994; Haddock, McCarron, Tarrier, & Faragher, 1999). These psychotic symptoms are often accompanied by recurrent intrusive images, which are related to the themes of the psychotic experiences, such as the perceived source of a voice, the content of voices and delusional beliefs, and traumatic memories (Morrison et al., 2002a).

From the symptoms outlined previously, and their noted similarities with UITs, it is clear that many psychotic experiences could be conceptualized as the result of an external attribution for a UIT, image, or impulse. For example, if patients believe that they are having thoughts beamed into their head by an alien device, this could be the result of a misattributed UIT; patients who feel that their movements are controlled by God or the Devil could be misattributing intrusive impulses; and a patient who hears the voice of his or her next-door neighbor telling the patient to harm him- or herself or someone else could be externally misattributing UITs. Indeed, recent cognitive theories of psychosis explicitly suggest that such psychotic experiences occur as a result of external attributions or appraisals (Bentall, 1990; Garety, Kuipers, Fowler, Freeman, & Bebbington, 2001; Morrison et al., 1995). As mentioned earlier, the main difference between many psychotic experiences and nonpsychotic UITs is this attribution of source, which could be viewed as a distinct appraisal of the UIT rather than a defining characteristic. However, many psychotic UITs are recognized as internally generated (such as paranoid or grandiose thoughts), and are characterized by being culturally unacceptable (Morrison, 2001). Therefore, it is possible that culturally unacceptable UITs are viewed as psychotic, and that an external attribution for UITs increases the likelihood that it will be culturally unacceptable.

There is only one study that has assessed traditionally defined UITs in people with psychosis. Morrison and Baker (2000) used the Distressing Thoughts Questionnaire (Clark & de Silva, 1985) to assess the frequency and dimensions of UITs in patients with a diagnosis of schizophrenia. They found that the patients experienced more frequent anxiety-related intrusive thoughts, in comparison with a nonpatient sample. They also found that "voice hearers" experienced more frequent depression-related intrusive thoughts, and that such differences were also evident for the dimensions of disapproval and difficulty to remove and worry about the thoughts. In a study that compared obsessive–compulsive phenomena and delusional beliefs, patients with obsessional thoughts were more likely to resist their thoughts, view them as senseless, and seek reassurance in relation to them than are patients with delusions (Jakes & Hemsley, 1996).

There are several studies that have assessed the prevalence and dimensions of UITs, using the broader definition that incorporates delusional ideas and hallucinatory phenomena (i.e., UITs that are externally attributed), in people with psychosis and the general population. In studies of delusional beliefs, Verdoux et al. (1998) and Peters, Joseph, and Garety (1999) have shown that large proportions of people with no psychiatric history endorse items concerning delusional ideation. Peters et al. (1999) found that 30% of a large normal sample ($n = 470$) endorsed individual items of delusional ideation, and that a comparison group of people belonging to religious cults scored significantly higher. They report that it is not the content of delusional beliefs that distinguishes between patients with psychotic diagnoses and the general population or adherents to new religious movements as the range in frequency of delusional ideation had considerable overlap between the groups. Rather, it appears that it is the degree of conviction, distress, and preoccupation with the delusional belief that distinguishes clinical and nonclinical samples. This is strikingly similar to the differentiation between individuals with obsessive–compulsive disorder from nonclinical individuals who report unwanted ego-dystonic intrusive thoughts with very similar content (Rachman & de Silva, 1978; Salkovskis & Harrison, 1984).

Studies of hallucinatory phenomena also suggest that such experiences are common within the general population. Student samples frequently report relatively high rates (24–49%) of experiences such as hearing voices or their thoughts being spoken aloud (Barrett & Etheridge, 1992; Morrison, Wells, & Nothard, 2000; Posey & Losch, 1983). The annual prevalence of auditory hallucinations in community samples is approximately 5% (Johns, Nazroo, Bebbington, & Kuipers, 1998; Tien, 1991), and lifetime prevalence estimates range between 10 and 25% (Johns & van Os, 2001). Statistically, it would appear that the experience of hallucinations is normal following certain life experiences, such as the death of a spouse (Grimby, 1993, 1998; Reese, 1971).

It has been shown that patients' beliefs about their voices are associated with affective and behavioral responses (Chadwick & Birchwood, 1994). For example, if patients believe that their voices are powerful and malevolent, they are likely to become distressed and try to resist or suppress their voices, whereas if they believe their voices to be benevolent, they are likely to experience positive affect and engage with their voices. Similarly, patients' interpretations of their voices are associated with elevations in subjective distress, and these interpretations are a better predictor of distress than the actual frequency of the hallucinations (Morrison & Baker, 2000). These studies suggest that "psychotic" intrusive phenomena can occur as normal phenomena, but it is how these intrusions are interpreted, and responded to, that differentiates between psychotic patients and the general population. As with UITs in other disorders, the distress associated with unwanted intrusive psychotic experiences is mediated by its appraisal.

It has been suggested that cultural acceptability may play a critical role in whether interpretations are classified as psychotic symptoms, or nonpsychotic phenomena (Morrison, 2001). For example, if someone was to experience an intrusive impulse to throw his child across the room but viewed it as a product of being tired and stressed and dismissed it, it is unlikely to result in any mental health problems. If the person had the same impulse and recognized it as a product of his own mind but worried that this meant that he was going to act on it, and therefore tried to suppress the experience, it might contribute to the development of obsessive–compulsive disorder (OCD). However, if the person appraised the impulse as being sent from beyond the grave by a dead relative who is trying to control him and responded by engaging in behavior designed to prevent it from happening, it might contribute to the person being perceived as psychotic. Similarly, if someone interpreted an intrusive thought about harm to her family in a car accident as meaning that she has to perform rituals in order to prevent it from happening, it would be seen as a symptom of OCD. If, however, she interpreted the thought as having been put in her mind by a government agency in order to torment her, it would be seen as a psychotic symptom. Thus, in summary, it may be the appraisal (or interpretation) of, and response to, UITs that differentiates normal from abnormal in relation to psychotic experiences, and it may be the appraisal (or attribution) of source that distinguishes nonpsychotic UITs from experiences that are labeled psychotic.

THE DEVELOPMENT AND MAINTENANCE OF UNWANTED INTRUSIONS IN PSYCHOSIS

There are several theories that implicate the occurrence of UITs in the development and/or maintenance of psychosis. Morrison et al. (1995)

suggested that auditory hallucinations may occur as the direct result of an external attribution for intrusive thoughts, and that this bias is influenced by an inconsistency between the experience of UITs and metacognitive beliefs about the importance and meaning of UITs. Morrison (2001) has suggested that it is the culturally unacceptable interpretation of intrusions that characterizes psychotic phenomena. Wells and Matthews (1994) have proposed a model of cognitive self-regulation, which suggests that there is a cognitive-attentional syndrome associated with psychological dysfunction that includes self-focused attention, monitoring of threat, and unhelpful self-regulation strategies that are driven by positive and negative beliefs. Recent applications of this model to an understanding of psychotic experience also suggest that appraisals of intrusive phenomena, and the strategies that are adopted to control them, are implicated in psychotic experiences such as hallucinations (Morrison et al., 2000; Morrison, Wells, & Nothard, 2002c) and delusions (Freeman & Garety, 1999).

UITs and the Development of Psychosis

There is some evidence to suggest that UITs may have a direct influence on the development of psychotic experiences. To test the hypothesis that auditory hallucinations occur as the result of externally attributed UITs, Baker and Morrison (1998) compared groups of patients with a diagnosis of schizophrenia with and without voices and nonpatients on a source monitoring task involving word association. They found that voice hearers perceived that they had significantly less control over the thoughts that came to mind and perceived these thoughts to be more unwanted in comparison with both control groups. This study also demonstrated that negative metacognitive beliefs about the uncontrollability and danger of UITs were a significant predictor of hallucinatory status (i.e., whether the person heard voices); thus, the more strongly a person believed that UITs in general were uncontrollable and dangerous, the more likely he or she was to be a voice hearer. It has also been shown that negative metacognitive beliefs about uncontrollability and danger of UITs are associated with an external attributional bias (Baker & Morrison, 1998).

Research interest has recently focused on the prediction and prevention of psychotic episodes in high-risk populations. An Australian study suggests that it is possible to identify a group of people at ultra high risk of developing a first episode of psychosis, approximately 40–50% of whom will become psychotic in a 12-month period (Yung et al., 1996;

Yung et al., 1998). Evidence from a recent randomized controlled trial of cognitive therapy for the prevention of psychosis in such a high-risk population has shown that people at ultra high risk score significantly higher on worry about controllability and negative beliefs about UITs than do nonpatients (Morrison et al., 2002b).

There is clearly some evidence that is consistent with the idea that UITs may be related to the development and onset of psychosis, although this remains speculative at present. However, several areas of research also suggest that factors associated with the maintenance of UITs may too be involved in the persistence of psychosis.

UITs and the Maintenance of Psychosis

It is apparent that there are many similarities in the processes that have been shown to contribute to the maintenance of UITs and psychotic experiences. Such processes include safety behaviors, dysfunctional thought control strategies (including suppression), unhelpful appraisals, metacognitive beliefs, mood, and physiology. Each of these processes is considered in relation to the maintenance of culturally unacceptable UITs (i.e., psychotic experiences).

A common interpretation of UITs across different psychological disorders is one of impending madness or loss of mental control (e.g., in OCD, panic disorder, posttraumatic stress disorder, and generalized anxiety disorder). Negative social stereotypes of madness portray people with serious mental disorders as incomprehensible, out of control, and threatening to society; patients with psychotic diagnoses share such views of themselves (Birchwood, Mason, MacMillan, & Healy, 1993). Some 70% of those with psychotic diagnoses report a "fear of going crazy" as the most common prodromal symptom (Hirsch & Jolley, 1989). In a recent study of 19 first-episode patients with a diagnosis of schizophrenia, it was noted that 8 reported concerns about loss of mental control as early prodromal signs (Moller & Husby, 2000). Therefore, appraisals of loss of control appear to be implicated in the maintenance of psychotic experiences.

Safety behaviors (behaviors designed to prevent a feared outcome that may contribute to the maintenance of distressing appraisals by preventing disconfirmation) and dysfunctional thought control strategies have been identified in relation to psychotic experiences. Morrison (1998a) suggested that people who hear voices adopt safety behaviors in order to prevent feared outcomes associated with the idiosyncratic meaning of their hallucinations. A recent study has shown that safety behaviors are identifiable (and operationalizable) in people who hear distressing voices (Nothard, Morrison, & Wells, 2003). Similarly, safety behaviors have been shown to be present in patients experiencing persecutory delusions (Freeman, Garety, & Kuipers, 2001). Such safety behaviors could include adopting a disguise or taking specific routes to avoid being attacked in patients experiencing persecutory ideas and adopting idiosyncratic strategies (such as praying, thinking good thoughts, distraction, and avoidance) to avoid obeying command hallucinations in patients who hear voices.

Several studies have examined control strategies for UITs, in relation to psychosis, using the Thought Control Questionnaire (Wells & Davies, 1994). Morrison et al. (2000) found that nonpatients who scored higher on predisposition to hallucination used significantly more punishment and reappraisal thought control strategies in comparison with participants of low predisposition. Freeman and Garety (1999) compared thought control strategies in patients with persecutory delusions and patients with generalized anxiety disorder and found no significant differences between the two groups. In another study, patients with a diagnosis of schizophrenia used significantly more worry and punishment-based control strategies and less distraction-based strategies than did nonpatients (Morrison & Wells, 2000).

The paradoxical effects of thought suppression on UITs have been discussed at length (Wegner, 1994). However, little research has specifically examined the effects of suppression on the occurrence of psychotic experiences such as hallucinations and delusions, despite suggestions that suppression may be involved in the maintenance of such symptoms (Morrison et al., 1995). However, a recent study examined the effects of thought suppression on the vividness of auditory illusions in a nonclinical population (Garcia-Montes, Perez-Alvarez, & Fidalgo, 2003). They reported that repeated suppression of self-discrepant (or ego-dystonic) thoughts increased the vividness of illusions. This is consistent with the view that suppression of UITs may be involved in the development and maintenance of hallucinatory phenomena.

Another common maintenance factor for UITs in other disorders is selective attention. Research on patients with psychosis has demonstrated that they do exhibit high levels of self-consciousness and awareness of UITs. For example, patients who experience auditory hallucinations score higher than control groups on a measure of private self-consciousness (Morrison & Haddock, 1997b), and adopting an internal focus of attention increases their tendency to make external attributions for their thoughts (Ensum & Morrison, 2003). Several studies have also demonstrated high levels of self-consciousness and hypervigilance toward threatening information in patients with persecutory delusions (Bentall & Kaney, 1989; Freeman, Garety, & Phillips, 2000; Smari, Stefansson, & Thorgilsson, 1994).

Mood and physiological factors can also contribute to the development and maintenance of unwanted psychotic experiences. It has been suggested that anxiety is central to the formation of persecutory delusions (Freeman et al., 2002), and Freeman and colleagues clearly incorporate anticipation of danger (Freeman & Garety, 2000). Hallucinations are exacerbated by stress (Slade, 1972), and emotional salience of thoughts increases the external attributional bias of patients experiencing hallucinations (Morrison & Haddock, 1997a). A comprehensive review of the direct influence of emotion on delusions and hallucinations can be found in Freeman and Garety (2003). Emotional processes clearly correlate with physiological processes. Several studies have shown associations between physiological arousal and psychotic experiences (Tarrier & Turpin, 1992; Toone, Cooke, & Lader, 1981).

Metacognitive beliefs (beliefs about the meaning and operation of cognitive products and processes such as thoughts, images, memory, and attention), which influence plans for information processing and strategy selection (Wells & Matthews, 1994), have also been examined in patients with psychotic diagnoses and in nonpatient populations (in relation to measures of psychosis-proneness), mostly using the Meta-Cognitions Questionnaire (MCQ; Cartwright Hatton & Wells, 1997). People with a high predisposition to hallucinations exhibit higher levels of beliefs about the uncontrollability and danger associated with UITs and cognitive self-consciousness, in comparison with those of low predisposition (Morrison et al., 2000). Patients with a diagnosis of schizophrenia who experience auditory hallucinations have been shown to score higher on positive beliefs about worry and negative beliefs about uncontrollability and danger than did the nonpatient group (Baker & Morrison, 1998). This study also demonstrated that patients with a diagnosis of schizophrenia (both with and without voices) scored higher than nonpatients on cognitive confidence and negative beliefs including superstition, punishment, and responsibility.

Freeman and Garety (1999) found that the majority of a sample of people with persecutory delusions experienced "metaworry" (i.e., worry about worry [Wells, 1995]), over the control of delusional thoughts. Lobban, Haddock, Kinderman, and Wells (2002) found that patients with a diagnosis of schizophrenia (both with and without voices) scored significantly higher than both a nonpatient group and a group of patients with anxiety disorders on their strength of belief that their unwanted thoughts should be consistent with each other. A recent study examined metacognition in patients who met criteria according to the fourth edition, text revision of *Diagnostic and Statistical Manual of Mental Disorders* (DSM-IV-TR; American Psychiatric Association, 2000) for schizophrenia spectrum disorders with auditory hallucinations, for schizophrenia spectrum disorders with persecutory delusions, and for panic disorder and in nonpatients (Morrison & Wells, 2003). They found that psychotic patients who experience auditory hallucinations tended to exhibit higher levels of dysfunctional metacognitive beliefs than did other patient groups, scoring significantly higher than at least two of the three comparison groups on positive beliefs about worry, negative beliefs about uncontrollability and danger, cognitive confidence, and negative beliefs including superstition, punishment, and responsibility. They also found that the metacognitive beliefs of patients with persecutory delusions and panic patients were often similar to each other, and elevated in comparison to nonpatients, suggesting that, as the self-regulatory executive functioning (S-REF) model predicts, such beliefs are generic vulnerability factors. In addition to such generic metacognitive beliefs, there are also such beliefs that appear specific to psychosis; for example, recent research suggests that positive beliefs about paranoia (e.g., "being paranoid keeps you from being harmed") may be predictive of persecutory ideation, and negative beliefs about paranoia (e.g., "my paranoia gets out of control") may be predictive of distress associated with such ideation (Morrison et al., 2003a).

It would appear that there is some evidence that is consistent with a role for UITs in the development and maintenance of psychosis. It would appear that UITs share the same characteristics as many psychotic experiences, and that other psychotic experiences may be the result of external attributions for nonpsychotic UITs. Unhelpful beliefs about the meaning of UITs are found in patients with psychotic diagnoses, and such beliefs also characterize patients at high risk of developing psychosis. There is also evidence that the processes involved in the maintenance of other clinical disorders are similar to the appraisals of and responses to UITs that are also implicated in psychosis (e.g., safety behaviors, suppression, thought control strategies, and selective attention). It has been suggested that UITs and their appraisals, which are culturally unacceptable in content, give rise to cognitive, behavioral, emotional, and physiological responses that maintain the distress and disability associated with psychotic experiences (Morrison, 2001). However, much additional research is required before any conclusions can be reached about the causal nature of UITs in psychosis; at present, it would appear that it is the culturally unacceptable appraisal of UITs that is most significant in relation to psychotic experiences and any resulting distress.

DIAGNOSTIC STATUS OF UITS

When considering the diagnostic status of UITs in psychosis, it would appear that cultural unacceptability is the central feature, as discussed earlier. However, it is common for people with psychosis to report UITs that are related to anxiety and depression as well (Morrison & Baker, 2000). It is also common for patients with a diagnosis of schizophrenia to meet criteria for other disorders such as depression (Birchwood, Iqbal, Chadwick, & Trower, 2000), anxiety disorders (Cosoff & Hafner, 1998), and posttraumatic stress disorder (PTSD) (Frame & Morrison, 2001; McGorry et al., 1991). Indeed, the content of depressive and posttraumatic intrusions in patients with schizophrenia is related to the psychosis itself (Birchwood et al., 2000), often taking the form of intrusive memories of their psychotic episodes (Frame & Morrison, 2001).

ASSESSMENT OF INTRUSIONS IN PSYCHOSIS

The clinical assessment of intrusions in psychosis should be incorporated within a standard cognitive-behavioral assessment (Morrison, 1998b). Clinical assessment should include the generation of a problem list, the gathering of information to facilitate the development of a formulation, a problem history, a focus on current problems, and an analysis of recent incidents. These should be analyzed in order to identify environmental, cognitive, behavioral, emotional, and physiological factors that might be involved in the pathogenesis of psychotic symptoms.

Certain aspects of the assessment will be particularly relevant to UITs. Cognitive variables that should be assessed include the intrusions themselves; the immediate appraisal of the intrusions; underlying metacognitive beliefs about the meaning, importance, and expected consequences of having UITs; any associated cognitive control strategies (such as suppression, distraction, rumination, punishment, and worry); and information-processing biases (such as selective attention). Other phenomena that should be assessed in relation to UITs are safety behaviors, behavioral control strategies, emotional consequences, physiological correlates, and environmental triggers and consequences. In addition, any reciprocal relationships between these variables should be specified. Other comorbid disorders should be considered, and UITs in relation to these conditions should also be assessed. This information can then be used to develop a case conceptualization, based on a cognitive model of intrusions in psychosis (Morrison, 2001), which will then direct the selection of treatment strategies.

Assessment can be performed using clinical interview, questionnaires and rating scales, self-monitoring tasks and diaries, and behavioral tests and observation. Detailed guidance regarding the content of clinical interviews for psychotic patients (Morrison, Renton, Dunn, Williams, & Bentall, 2003b) and UITs (Wells, 2000) can be found elsewhere. However, there are some useful standardized measures for the assessment of unwanted psychotic phenomena and the appraisal of such experiences that are available to the clinician. Delusional ideation and associated dimensions (such as conviction, distress, and preoccupation) can be assessed using a semistructured interview (Psychotic Symptoms Rating Scales [PSYRATS]; Haddock et al., 1999) and a self-report measure (Peters Delusions Inventory [PDI]; Peters et al., 1999). Auditory hallucinations and their dimensions can also be assessed with a semistructured interview (PSYRATS; Haddock et al., 1999), and predisposition to hallucinations can be assessed using several self-report measures (Launay & Slade, 1981; Morrison et al., 2002c; Posey & Losch, 1983). Appraisals of hallucinations can be assessed using self-report measures (Beliefs about Voices Questionnaire; Chadwick, Lees, & Birchwood, 2000; Interpretations of Voices Inventory [IVI]; Morrison et al., 2002c) and a measure of appraisals of paranoid ideas was recently developed (Beliefs about Paranoia Scale; Morrison et al., 2003a). In addition, standardized measures for the assessment of intrusions and their appraisals (e.g., Obsessive Compulsive Cognitions Working Group, 2001), metacognition (e.g., MCQ: Cartwright Hatton & Wells, 1997) and control strategies (e.g., Thought Control Questionnaire; Wells & Davies, 1994) can be useful for the psychotic disorder itself or for comorbid conditions. The development of similar measures for the assessment of unwanted psychotic experiences would certainly improve our ability to assess UITs in psychosis.

It is worth noting that the assessment process itself can be beneficial in reducing the occurrence of UITs and associated distress. There is some evidence that self-monitoring of UITs using diaries and rating scales can reduce the frequency of such symptoms. For example, patients with PTSD who monitored their intrusions experienced a significant decrease in intrusive symptomatology (Reynolds & Tarrier, 1996). Focusing approaches that have been used with auditory hallucinations can be viewed as a therapeutic application of self-monitoring of unwanted intrusive experiences (Haddock, Slade, Bentall, & Faragher, 1998). However, it remains to be seen whether self-monitoring measures can significantly reduce unwanted intrusive thoughts, images, or impulses that characterize psychotic states.

INTERVENTION STRATEGIES FOR UNWANTED INTRUSIONS IN PSYCHOSIS

Treatment strategies for UITs in people with psychosis are similar to those for other disorders. Much of the focus of intervention strategies is on the appraisal of UITs, rather than on the UIT itself. Initially, it is useful to provide information regarding the prevalence of unwanted psychotic experiences in the general population, emphasizing the fact that many people experience delusional ideas and hear voices without ever requiring contact with mental health services. Written normalizing information summarizing this research and the epidemiology of such experiences can be helpful. The normalizing approach to psychosis was pioneered by Kingdon and Turkington (1991), and there is evidence to support such an approach from randomized controlled trials (Sensky et al., 2000; Turkington, Kingdon, & Turner, 2002). Information on UITs in other disorders, such as obsessional thoughts, can also be used to normalize the experience of UITs for individuals in a psychotic state.

The provision of normalizing information represents one way of decatastrophizing the experience of UITs and can help to modify distressing appraisals regarding the meaning and significance of UITs (e.g., normalizing information can be used to counter dysfunctional appraisals, such as that UITs are a sign of going mad, losing control, persecution or alien insertion). The standard cognitive therapy techniques that have been developed for other disorders (Beck, Rush, Shaw, & Emery, 1979; Wells, 1997) are also applicable to the treatment of distressing unwanted psychotic experiences. It is often helpful to begin with a consideration of the advantages and disadvantages of such experiences, as psychotic phenomena are often maintained by their functional status. For example, voices often provide company and advice (Miller, O'Connor, & DiPasquale, 1993) and paranoia can be useful as a survival strategy in a hostile environment (Morrison et al., 2003a). In addition, theoretical and empirical work suggests that persecutory delusions may serve to protect self-esteem under some circumstances, making a person feel special and blameless for negative events (Bentall, Kinderman, & Kaney, 1994). If significant benefits are identified, negotiation should take place about alternative ways of achieving such advantages, with a cost-benefit analysis examined for maintaining psychotic symptoms.

Following agreement that psychotic UITs should be targeted for intervention, several strategies can be effective in reducing the distress and disability that may be associated with the appraisal of such thoughts. Verbal reattribution strategies, such as generating alternative appraisals, examining the evidence for and against each of the interpretations, and reviewing ongoing and historical factors that relate to the appraisals can be helpful. Behavioral experiments to test the accuracy of the different possible appraisals can also be a very powerful way of dealing with problematic interpretations and evaluations.

Other factors can also be useful to manipulate in treatment. If the formulation suggests it will be useful, safety behaviors and control strategies such as suppression and rumination can be examined in a behavioral experiment, and the effects on distress, belief in the appraisals, and frequency of UITs can be recorded. It may be important to consider environmental change if factors in the social context are implicated as triggers or maintenance factors (i.e., family relationships, social networks, cultural factors, or specific factors related to the local neighborhood or geography). It may be necessary to identify and evaluate metacognitive beliefs about the meaning and mechanisms of mental processes in order to facilitate change, and attentional style may also require a therapeutic intervention. The meaning of UITs in psychosis should also be considered in the relapse prevention process. These issues are more fully illustrated with a case example, and Table 7.1 shows a summary of treatment strategies.

Recent studies examining cognitive therapy (CT) for schizophrenia-like psychoses, which typically includes the aforementioned strategies, have shown it to be effective in reducing residual positive symptoms on an outpatient basis, and in maintaining these gains at follow-up (Chadwick & Birchwood, 1994; Garety, Kuipers, Fowler, Chamberlain, & Dunn, 1994; Kuipers et al., 1998; Kuipers et al., 1997; Sensky et al., 2000; Tarrier et al., 1993; Turkington et al., 2002). CT has been shown to be superior to other psychological treatments such as supportive counseling (Tarrier et al., 1998) and to treatment as usual involving case management and antipsychotic medication (Kuipers et al., 1997) and routine psychiatric care (Tarrier et al., 1998). A reduced stay in the hospital (by 54% in comparison with control group) has also been shown for cognitive-behavioral treatment of patients with a diagnosis of schizo-

TABLE 7.1. A Summary of Treatment Strategies

Treatment target	Strategy
UITs	• Attentional manipulation (e.g., internal vs. external focus) • Behavioral experiments comparing thought control strategies (e.g., suppression vs. Acceptance) • Arousal reduction • Manipulation of triggers • Exploration and modification of positive beliefs about UITs and their consequences
Distress resulting from UITs or appraisals	• Generation of alternative explanations • Normalizing information • Collaborative development of cognitive-behavioral case

phrenia in acute settings (Drury, Birchwood, Cochrane, & MacMillan, 1996), and recovery time for symptom reduction was also improved suggesting that CT is of benefit for inpatients as well as outpatients. Sensky et al. (2000) have demonstrated that both befriending and cognitive therapy produced significant reductions in positive symptoms, negative symptoms, and depression at end of treatment in patients with a diagnosis of schizophrenia and persistent positive symptoms. However, at 9-month follow-up, patients who received cognitive therapy continued to improve whereas those who received befriending did not; this is consistent with the aim of CT, which is to help patients to become their own therapists, learning a process of identifying and challenging their beliefs. Recent meta-analyses have concluded that CT is an effective treatment for persistent psychotic symptoms, that the effects of CT are robust over time, and that dropout rates are low (Gould, Mueser, Bolton, Mays, & Goff, 2001; Pilling et al., 2002). Therefore, it appears that CT methods can be used to promote symptom reduction and reduce time spent in the hospital, as well as promoting relapse prevention.

A CASE EXAMPLE

Jim, a 23-year-old male, believed that his UITs were the result of telepathic insertion from hostile people who lived in his community (a gang of young men who were well-known troublemakers). The intrusions were a combination of verbal thoughts and images that concerned harm happening to him and his family, and he believed that the gang members were doing this to him either to drive him mad or to make him aware of their planned actions. Assessment and formulation helped to identify maintenance cycles and factors that contributed to the distress associated with such experiences. Jim believed that these UITs were likely to happen in real life, and all these appraisals seemed to contribute to his distress (mainly fear, with occasional anger and helplessness). Jim dealt with these intrusions by trying to suppress them and trying to avoid the gang, and occasionally he would report his telepathic premonitions to the police, which at times resulted in unwanted contact with mental health services. He also spent a lot of time trying to "secure" his mind by focusing on his mental processes, but at times he worried that he would miss out on a vital premonition by doing so. It was important to check out whether these experiences had any advantages for Jim, in addition to the obvious distress that they caused him. Questioning revealed that Jim did feel special as a result of this, and he felt that the vigilance for threat served an important function in keeping him and his family safe.

We agreed to explore alternative ways of making Jim feel special, using positive data logs and continua that defined different dimensions of specialness, and to evaluate whether or not his telepathy did provide safety and whether such vigilance was required. We reviewed the evidence to date regarding the accuracy of the telepathic predictions and found that they were extremely unlikely to occur (they had only been correct on two occasions, both of which concerned his younger brother being assaulted at school). These incidents were examined in discussion with his brother, and Jim decided that they were not specifically related to his fears about the gang. An exploration of Jim's life history suggested that he had good reasons to be vigilant for threat and concern for his family's safety. Frequently he had been bullied at school and his family home had been burgled many times in recent years, which had led to an exacerbation of his mother's anxiety. He did live in a neighborhood that was generally agreed to be unsafe, with an extremely high rate of crime and interpersonal violence.

Jim's evidence concerning his UITs being telepathically delivered from the gang members related to past incidents of violence and his current fears. He believed that the reason that many of the other incidents that had been predicted did not occur was because his advance knowledge had allowed him to prevent the feared outcome, by either changing his behavior or that of his relatives. At times he would stay at home all day to avoid the perceived threatening situations. When asked how he knew that these were not his own thoughts, he laughed, saying that he loved his family a great deal and certainly wouldn't be having these kinds of thoughts about them. Provision of normalizing information about intrusive thoughts and the frequency of paranoia and unusual beliefs in the general population helped Jim to construct an alternative explanation for his experiences. As an alternative to his dysfunctional belief that he was receiving telepathic messages, it was proposed that in reality the intrusions were his own thoughts that he misinterpreted in a threatening way. This misinterpretation is understandable because the thoughts were unacceptable to him and he had good reason to be preoccupied with safety given his living circumstances.

A series of behavioral experiments and homework tasks were conducted in order to help Jim examine these possible explanations for the intrusive "threatening gang" thoughts. He conducted a survey of family and friends of the family regarding UITs and found that the majority of people reported such experiences but dismissed them as meaningless. He then tried varying his use of suppression and found a relationship between increased suppression and increased frequency of the UITs, which was not especially consistent with his gang theory (although he did suggest that they may try harder when he resisted). Following several sessions of verbal reattribution and some behavioral experiments, Jim felt sufficiently safe to try going out with his family on a day when disaster was predicted, and he was encouraged to drop all of his safety behaviors (e.g., trying to modify his families behavior, taking "safe" routes, and leaving escape routes). A series of these experiments allowed Jim to evaluate the accuracy of his concerns, and he concluded that he was misinterpreting normal UITs as being telepathically transmitted with an intention to harm him. He also concluded that this had served a purpose of making him feel safer (for himself and his family), which made sense given his own experiences and those of his family. The difficult environment in which he lived had also contributed to his need for perceived safety. Jim decided that a more useful approach to this dilemma would be to learn self-defense and to try to get his family rehoused (making functional use of his label of schizophrenia to become a priority on the housing list).

At the end of this phase of treatment, Jim still had some anxieties concerning social situations and leaving his house. He responded positively to standard CT for social phobia and panic disorder with agoraphobia and was able to go back to college to study. In the relapse prevention phase of treatment, some time was spent reiterating the work regarding the normality of UITs and the importance of appraisal in determining distress, in order to minimize the likelihood of Jim's interpreting an increase in UITs as being a sign of impending madness (or relapse of his schizophrenia), which would likely lead to an increase in stress and use of suppression and other control strategies that may precipitate a vicious circle.

CONCLUSIONS

It is clear that the phenomenon of UITs is helpful in understanding the development and maintenance of psychotic experiences. Some psychotic experiences may be the result of culturally unacceptable appraisals of UITs (e.g., some delusional beliefs), whereas others, such as hallucinations, appear to be UITs misattributed to an external source. Unhelpful beliefs about the meaning of UITs are found in patients with psychotic diagnoses and in patients at high risk of developing psychosis. Similarly, the processes involved in the maintenance of psychosis can be conceptualized as appraisals of and responses to UITs. It has been suggested that UITs and their appraisals, which are culturally unacceptable in content, give rise to cognitive, behavioral, emotional, and physiological responses that maintain the distress and disability associated with psychotic experiences (Morrison, 2001). However, much additional research is required before any conclusions can be reached about any causal nature of UITs in psychosis; at present, it would appear that it is the culturally unacceptable appraisal of UITs that is most significant in relation to psychotic experiences and any resulting distress. Issues regarding causality, specificity to psychosis, and the relation of UITs to other psychotic symptoms and the course of the disorder remain to be fully determined.

It is possible that, in the future, our understanding of UITs may contribute to the conceptualization of other psychotic phenomena, such as formal thought disorder. It has been observed that the content of incoherent speech often reflects the intrusion or "intermingling" of highly salient personal information into the ongoing conversation (Harrow & Prosen, 1979); thus it is possible that thought disorders characterized by loose associations may be related to UITs and metacognitive beliefs about speech. Other future directions for research and treatment in psychosis should include a more detailed examination of the relationships between psychotic experiences and factors such as thought suppression and mental control and a thorough analysis of the different dimensions of unwanted psychotic experiences, such as controllability, intrusiveness, and acceptability.

REFERENCES

American Psychiatric Association. (2000). *Diagnostic and statistical manual of mental disorders* (4th ed., text rev.). Washington, DC: Author.

Baker, C. A., & Morrison, A. P. (1998). Cognitive processes in auditory hallucinations: Attributional biases and metacognition. *Psychological Medicine, 28,* 1199–1208.

Barrett, T. R., & Etheridge, J. B. (1992). Verbal hallucinations in normals: I. People who hear voices. *Applied Cognitive Psychology, 6,* 379–387.

Beck, A. T., Rush, A. J., Shaw, B. F., & Emery, G. (1979). *Cognitive therapy of depression.* New York: Guilford Press.

Bentall, R. P. (1990). The syndromes and symptoms of psychosis: Or why you can't play 20 questions with the concept of schizophrenia and hope to win. In R. P. Bentall (Ed.), *Reconstructing schizophrenia* (pp. 23–60). London: Routledge.

Bentall, R. P., & Kaney, S. (1989). Content-specific information processing and persecutory delusions: An investigation using the emotional Stroop test. *British Journal of Medical Psychology, 62,* 355–364.

Bentall, R. P., Kinderman, P., & Kaney, S. (1994). The self, attributional processes and abnormal beliefs: Towards a model of persecutory delusions. *Behaviour Research and Therapy, 32,* 331–341.

Birchwood, M., Iqbal, Z., Chadwick, P., & Trower, P. (2000). Cognitive approach to depression and suicidal thinking in psychosis: 1. Ontogeny of post-psychotic depression. *British Journal of Psychiatry, 177,* 516–521.

Birchwood, M., Mason, R., MacMillan, F., & Healy, J. (1993). Depression, demoralization and control over psychotic illness: A comparison of depressed and non-depressed patients with a chronic psychosis. *Psychological Medicine, 23,* 387–395.

Cartwright Hatton, S., & Wells, A. (1997). Beliefs about worry and intrusions: The Meta-Cognitions Questionnaire and its correlates. *Journal of Anxiety Disorders, 11*(3), 279–296.

Chadwick, P., & Birchwood, M. (1994). The omnipotence of voices: A cognitive approach to auditory hallucinations. *British Journal of Psychiatry, 164,* 190–201.

Chadwick, P., Lees, S., & Birchwood, M. (2000). The revised Beliefs about Voices Questionnaire (BAVQ-R). *British Journal of Psychiatry, 177,* 229–232.

Clark, D. A., & de Silva, P. (1985). The nature of depressive and anxious depressive thoughts: Distinct or uniform phenomena? *Behaviour Research and Therapy, 23,* 383–393.

Cosoff, S. J., & Hafner, R. J. (1998). The prevalence of comorbid anxiety in schizophrenia, schizoaffective disorder and bipolar disorder. *Australian and New Zealand Journal of Psychiatry, 32,* 67–72.

Drury, V., Birchwood, M., Cochrane, R., & MacMillan, F. (1996). Cognitive therapy and recovery from acute psychosis: I. Impact on psychotic symptoms. *British Journal of Psychiatry, 169,* 593–601.

Ensum, I., & Morrison, A. P. (2003). The effects of focus of attention on attributional bias in patients experiencing auditory hallucinations. *Behaviour Research and Therapy, 41*, 895–907.

Frame, L., & Morrison, A. P. (2001). Causes of posttraumatic stress disorder in psychotic patients. *Archives of General Psychiatry, 58*, 305–306.

Freeman, D., & Garety, P. A. (1999). Worry, worry processes and dimensions of delusions: An exploratory investigation of a role for anxiety processes in the maintenance of delusional distress. *Behavioural and Cognitive Psychotherapy, 27*, 47–62.

Freeman, D., & Garety, P. A. (2000). Comments on the contents of persecutory delusions: Does the definition need clarification? *British Journal of Clinical Psychology, 39*, 407–414.

Freeman, D., & Garety, P. A. (2003). Connecting neurosis and psychosis: the direct influence of emotion on delusions and hallucinations. *Behaviour Research and Therapy, 41*, 923–947.

Freeman, D., Garety, P. A., & Kuipers, E. (2001). Persecutory delusions: developing the understanding of belief maintenance and emotional distress. *Psychological Medicine, 31*, 1293–1306.

Freeman, D., Garety, P. A., Kuipers, E., Fowler, D., & Bebbington, P. E. (2002). A cognitive model of persecutory delusions. *British Journal of Clinical Psychology, 41*(4), 331–347.

Freeman, D., Garety, P. A., & Phillips, M. L. (2000). An examination of hypervigilance for external threat in individuals with generalized anxiety disorder and individuals with persecutory delusions using visual scan paths. *Quarterly Journal of Experimental Psychology, 53*, 549–567.

Garcia-Montes, J. M., Perez-Alvarez, M., & Fidalgo, A. M. (2003). Influence of the suppression of self-discrepant thoughts on the vivdness of perception of auditory illusions. *Behavioural and Cognitive Psychotherapy, 31*, 33–44.

Garety, P. A., & Hemsley, D. R. (1994). *Delusions*. London: Psychology Press.

Garety, P. A., Kuipers, L., Fowler, D., Chamberlain, F., & Dunn, G. (1994). Cognitive behavioural therapy for drug-resistant psychosis. *British Journal of Medical Psychology, 67*, 259–271.

Garety, P. A., Kuipers, E., Fowler, D., Freeman, D., & Bebbington, P. E. (2001). A cognitive model of the positive symptoms of psychosis. *Psychological Medicine, 31*, 189–195.

Gould, R. A., Mueser, K. T., Bolton, E., Mays, V., & Goff, D. (2001). Cognitive therapy for psychosis in schizophrenia: an effect size analysis. *Schizophrenia Research, 48*, 335–342.

Grimby, A. (1993). Bereavement among elderly people: Grief reactions, post-bereavement hallucinations and quality of life. *Acta Psychiatrica Scandinavica, 87*, 72–80.

Grimby, A. (1998). Hallucinations following the loss of a spouse: Common and normal events among the elderly. *Journal of Clinical Geropsychology, 4*, 65–74.

Haddock, G., McCarron, J., Tarrier, N., & Faragher, E. B. (1999). Scales to measure dimensions of hallucinations and delusions: The psychotic symptoms rating scales (PSYRATS). *Psychological Medicine, 29,* 879–889.

Haddock, G., Slade, P. D., Bentall, R. P., & Faragher, B. F. (1998). Cognitive-behavioural treatment of auditory hallucinations: A comparison of the long-term effectiveness of two interventions. *British Journal of Medical Psychology, 71,* 339–349.

Harrow, M., & Prosen, M. (1979). Schizophrenic thought disorders: Bizarre associations and intermingling. *American Journal of Psychiatry, 136,* 293–296.

Hirsch, S. R., & Jolley, A. G. (1989). The dysphoric syndrome in schizophrenia and its implications for relapse. *British Journal of Psychiatry, 5*(Suppl.), 46–50.

Horowitz, M. (1975). Intrusive and repetitive thoughts after experimental stress. *Archives of General Psychiatry, 78,* 86–92.

Jakes, I. C., & Hemsley, D. R. (1996). The characteristics of obsessive–compulsive experience. *Clinical Psychology and Psychotherapy, 3,* 93–102.

Johns, L. C., Nazroo, J. Y., Bebbington, P. E., & Kuipers, E. (1998). Occurrence of hallucinations in a community sample. *Schizophrenia Research, 29,* 23.

Johns, L. C., & van Os, J. (2001). The continuity of psychotic experiences in the general population. *Clinical Psychology Review, 21*(8), 1125–1141.

Kingdon, D. G., & Turkington, D. (1991). Preliminary report: The use of cognitive behaviour therapy and a normalizing rationale in schizophrenia. *Journal of Nervous and Mental Disease, 179,* 207–211.

Kuipers, E., Fowler, D., Garety, P., Chizholm, D., Freeman, D., Dunn, G., et al. (1998). London-East Anglia randomised controlled trial of cognitive-behavioural therapy for psychosis III: Follow-up and economic considerations. *British Journal of Psychiatry, 173,* 61–68.

Kuipers, E., Garety, P., Fowler, D., Dunn, G., Bebbington, P., Freeman, D., et al. (1997). The London–East Anglia randomised controlled trial of cognitive-behaviour therapy for psychosis I: Effects of the treatment phase. *British Journal of Psychiatry, 171,* 319–327.

Launay, G., & Slade, P. D. (1981). The measurement of hallucinatory predisposition in male nd female prisoners. *Personality and Individual Differences, 2,* 221–234.

Lobban, F., Haddock, G., Kinderman, P., & Wells, A. (2002). The role of metacognitive beliefs in auditory hallucinations. *Personality and Individual Differences, 32*(8), 1351–1363.

McGorry, P. D., Chanen, A., McCarthy, E., van Riel, R., McKenzie, D., & Singh, B. S. (1991). Post traumatic stress disorder following recent onset psychosis. *Journal of Nervous and Mental Disease, 179,* 253–258.

Miller, L. J., O'Connor, E., & DiPasquale, T. (1993). Patients' attitudes to hallucinations. *American Journal of Psychiatry, 150,* 584–588.

Moller, P., & Husby, R. (2000). The initial prdodrome in schizophrenia: searching for naturalistic core dimensions of experience and behaviour. *Schizophrenia Bulletin, 26,* 217–232.

Morrison, A. P. (1998a). A cognitive analysis of the maintenance of auditory hallucinations: Are voices to schizophrenia what bodily sensations are to panic? *Behavioural and Cognitive Psychotherapy, 26,* 289–302.

Morrison, A. P. (1998b). Cognitive behaviour therapy for psychotic symptoms of schizophrenia. In N. Tarrier, A. Wells, & G. Haddock (Eds.), *Treating complex cases: The cognitive behavioural therapy approach* (pp. 195–216). London: Wiley.

Morrison, A. P. (2001). The interpretation of intrusions in psychosis: An integrative cognitive approach to hallucinations and delusions. *Behavioural and Cognitive Psychotherapy, 29,* 257–276.

Morrison, A. P., & Baker, C. A. (2000). Intrusive thoughts and auditory hallucinations: A comparative study of intrusions in psychosis. *Behaviour Research and Therapy, 38,* 1097–1106.

Morrison, A. P., Beck, A. T., Glentworth, D., Dunn, H., Reid, G., Larkin, W., et al. (2002a). Imagery and Psychotic Symptoms: A Preliminary Investigation. *Behaviour Research and Therapy, 40,* 1063–1072.

Morrison, A. P., Bentall, R. P., French, P., Walford, L., Kilcommons, A., Knight, A., et al. (2002b). A randomised controlled trial of early detection and cognitive therapy for preventing transition to psychosis in high risk individuals: Study design and interim analysis of transition rate and psychological risk factors. *British Journal of Psychiatry, 181*(Suppl. 43), 78–84.

Morrison, A. P., Gumley, A. I., Schwannauer, M., Campbell, M., Gleeson, A., Griffin, E., et al. (2003a). *The beliefs about paranoia scale: Preliminary validation of a metacognitive approach to conceptualising paranoia.* Manuscript submitted for publication.

Morrison, A. P., & Haddock, G. (1997a). Cognitive factors in source monitoring and auditory hallucinations. *Psychological Medicine, 27,* 669–679.

Morrison, A. P., & Haddock, G. (1997b). Self-focused attention in schizophrenic patients with and without auditory hallucinations and normal subjects: A comparative study. *Personality and Individual Differences, 23,* 937–941.

Morrison, A. P., Haddock, G., & Tarrier, N. (1995). Intrusive thoughts and auditory hallucinations: a cognitive approach. *Behavioural and Cognitive Psychotherapy, 23,* 265–280.

Morrison, A. P., Renton, J. C., Dunn, H., Williams, S., & Bentall, R. P. (2003b). *Cognitive Therapy for Psychosis: a Formulation-based Approach.* London: Psychology Press.

Morrison, A. P., & Wells, A. (2000). Thought control strategies in schizophrenia: A comparison with non-patients. *Behaviour Research and Therapy, 38,* 1205–1209.

Morrison, A. P., & Wells, A. (2003). Metacognition across disorders: Comparisons of patients with hallucinations, delusions, and panic disorder with non-patients. *Behaviour Research and Therapy, 41,* 251–256.

Morrison, A. P., Wells, A., & Nothard, S. (2000). Cognitive factors in predisposition to auditory and visual hallucinations. *British Journal of Clinical Psychology, 39*, 67–78.

Morrison, A. P., Wells, A., & Nothard, S. (2002c). Cognitive and emotional factors as predictors of predisposition to hallucinations. *British Journal of Clinical Psychology, 41*, 259–270.

Nayani, T. H., & David, A. S. (1996). The auditory hallucination: a phenomenological survey. *Psychological Medicine, 26*, 177–189.

Nothard, S., Morrison, A. P., & Wells, A. (2003). *The role of safety behaviours in the maintenance of negative beliefs and distress associated with the experience of hearing voices.* Manuscript submitted for publication.

Obsessive Compulsive Cognitions Working Group. (2001). Development and initial validation of the Obsessive Beliefs Questionnaire and the Interpretations of Intrusions Inventory. *Behaviour Research and Therapy, 39*, 987–1006.

Parkinson, L., & Rachman, S. J. (1981). The nature of intrusive thoughts. *Advances in Behaviour Research and Therapy, 3*, 101–110.

Persons, J. (1986). The advantages of studying psychological phenomena rather than psychiatric diagnoses. *American Psychologist., 41*, 1252–1260.

Peters, E. R., Joseph, S. A., & Garety, P. A. (1999). Measurement of delusional ideation in the normal population: Introducing the PDI (Peters et al. Delusions Inventory). *Schizophrenia Bulletin, 25*, 553–576.

Pilling, S., Bebbington, P. E., Kuipers, E., Garety, P. A., Geddes, J., Orbach, G., et al. (2002). Psychological treatments in schizophrenia: I. Meta-analysis of family intervention and cognitive behaviour therapy. *Psychological Medicine, 32*, 763–782.

Posey, T. B., & Losch, M. E. (1983). Auditory hallucinations of hearing voices in 375 normal subjects. *Imagination, Cognition and Personality, 2*, 99–113.

Rachman, S. J. (1981). Unwanted intrusive cognitions. *Advances in Behaviour Research and Therapy, 3*, 89–99.

Rachman, S. J. (1994). Pollution of the mind. *Behaviour Research and Therapy, 32*, 311–314.

Rachman, S. J., & de Silva, P. (1978). Abnormal and normal obsessions. *Behaviour Research and Therapy, 16*, 233–238.

Reese, W. D. (1971). The hallucinations of widowhood. *British Medical Journal, 210*, 37–41.

Reynolds, M., & Tarrier, N. (1996). Monitoring of intrusions in post-traumatic stress order: A report of single case studies. *British Journal of Medical Psychology, 69*, 371–379.

Salkovskis, P. M., & Harrison, J. (1984). Abnormal and normal obsessions: A replication. *Behaviour Research and Therapy, 22*(5), 549–552.

Sensky, T., Turkington, D., Kingdon, D., Scott, J. L., Scott, J., Siddle, R., et al. (2000). A randomized controlled trial of cognitive-behavioral therapy for persistent symptoms in schizophrenia resistant to medication. *Archives of General Psychiatry, 57*, 165–172.

Slade, P. D. (1972). The effects of systematic desensitization on auditory hallucinations. *Behaviour, Research and Therapy, 10,* 85–91.

Smari, J., Stefansson, S., & Thorgilsson, H. (1994). Paranoia, self-consciousness and social cognition in schizophrenics. *Cognitive Therapy and Research, 18,* 387–399.

Tarrier, N., Beckett, R., Harwood, S., Baker, A., Yusupoff, L., & Ugarteburu, I. (1993). A trial of two cognitive-behavioural methods of treating drug-resistant residual psychotic symptoms in schizophrenic patients: I: Outcome. *British Journal of Psychiatry, 162,* 524–532.

Tarrier, N., & Turpin, G. (1992). Psychosocial factors, arousal and schizophrenic relapse: The physiological data. *British Journal of Psychiatry, 161,* 3–11.

Tarrier, N., Yusupoff, L., Kinner, C., McCarthy, E., Gladhill, A., Haddock, G., et al. (1998). A randomized controlled trial of intense cognitive behaviour therapy for chronic schizophrenia. *British Medical Journal, 317,* 303–307.

Tien, A. Y. (1991). Distribution of hallucinations in the population. *Social Psychiatry and Psychiatric Epidemiology, 26,* 287–292.

Toone, B. K., Cooke, E., & Lader, M. H. (1981). Electrodermal activity in the affective disorders and schizophrenia. *Psychological Medicine, 11,* 497–508.

Turkington, D., Kingdon, D., & Turner, T. (2002). Effectiveness of a brief cognitive-behavioural therapy intervention in the treatment of schizophrenia. *British Journal of Psychiatry, 180,* 523–527.

Verdoux, H., Maurice-Tison, S., Gay, B., Van Os, J., Salamon, R., & Bourgeois, M. L. (1998). A survey of delusional ideation in primary-care patients. *Psychological Medicine, 28,* 127–134.

Wegner, D. M. (1994). *White bears and other unwanted thoughts: Suppression, obsession, and the psychology of mental control.* New York: Guilford Press.

Wells, A. (1995). Meta-cognition and worry: A cognitive model of generalised anxiety disorder. *Behavioural and Cognitive Psychotherapy, 23,* 301–320.

Wells, A. (1997). *Cognitive therapy for anxiety disorders.* London: Wiley.

Wells, A. (2000). *Emotional disorders and metacognition: Innovative cognitive therapy.* New York: Wiley.

Wells, A., & Davies, M. I. (1994). The Thought Control Questionnaire: A measure of individual differences in the control of unwanted thoughts. *Behaviour Research and Therapy, 32*(8), 871–878.

Wells, A., & Matthews, G. (1994). *Attention and emotion.* London: Erlbaum.

Yung, A., McGorry, P. D., McFarlane, C. A., Jackson, H., Patton, G. C., & Rakkar, A. (1996). Monitoring and care of young people at incipient risk of psychosis. *Schizophrenia Bulletin, 22,* 283–303.

Yung, A., Phillips, L. J., McGorry, P. D., McFarlane, C. A., Francey, S., Harrigan, S., et al. (1998). A step towards indicated prevention of schizophrenia. *British Journal of Psychiatry, 172*(Suppl. 33), 14–20.

CHAPTER 8

UNWANTED THOUGHTS AND FANTASIES EXPERIENCED BY SEXUAL OFFENDERS

Their Nature, Persistence, and Treatment

W. L. MARSHALL
CALVIN M. LANGTON

Sexual offending is unfortunately far more widespread in our communities than most people would like to believe (Freeman-Longo & Blanchard, 1998; Marshall & Barrett, 1990), and the consequences for victims and their families are frequently severe and a burden on health services (Conte, 1988; Koss & Harvey, 1991). Clearly, enhancing understanding of these offenders is important, particularly the clinical issues that might elucidate both why such individuals engage in sexually abusive behavior and how treatment might reduce the likelihood of sexual reoffending. In the relative absence of significant previous work on the occurrence of unwanted intrusive thoughts in this population (see Johnston, Ward, & Hudson, 1997, for a notable exception), the present discussion is intended to identify key issues of concern relevant to treatment providers concerning such thoughts among sexual offenders.

In the broad literature on intrusive thoughts among clinical and

nonclinical samples, the term *unwanted intrusive thoughts* refers to repetitive thoughts, images, and impulses that the individual attributes to
an internal origin and experiences as unacceptable or personally distressing, difficult to control, and disruptive to ongoing cognitive activity
(American Psychiatric Association, 1994; Clark & Purdon, 1995; Rachman, 1981). Such a definition includes both content and process elements. Unwanted intrusive thoughts have been implicated in the etiology
and maintenance of a wide range of clinical problems, including obsessive–compulsive disorder (Wang & Clark, 2002), posttraumatic stress
disorder (Falsetti, Monnier, Davis, & Resnick, 2002), and depression
(Wenzlaff, 2002). Furthermore, from the research it is clear that nonclinical samples also experience unwanted intrusive thoughts that are similar
in content to those experienced by clinical patients (Purdon & Clark,
1993), although differences in the appraisals (misappraisals in the case
of clinical samples) associated with these unwanted intrusive thoughts
are implicated in the escalation of such thoughts to clinical obsessions
(Obsessive Compulsive Cognitions Working Group, 1997). Despite the
relative lack of research on unwanted thoughts among sexual offenders,
intrusive thoughts of a sexual nature among nonoffending clinical (e.g.,
Gordon, 2002) and nonclinical groups (e.g., Byers, Purdon, & Clark,
1998) have received attention. Here we draw on the wider literature as it
relates to our discussion of intrusive thoughts in sexual offenders.

With the aforementioned general definition in mind, one of the
problems that faced us in writing this chapter is that a significant proportion of sexual offenders are not obviously distressed by their crimes
except insofar as their acts may get them into trouble. Thus deviant sexual thoughts rarely trouble these particular offenders, partly at least because they do not believe their offenses cause harm to the victims. This
may seem to be such an absurd viewpoint that most people might want
to claim that it is simply an attempt by the offenders to protect
themselves from the negative image of being a person who, out of self-
interest, hurts others. Perhaps this is true, but for whatever reason, a
number of sexual offenders do significantly minimize victim harm and,
as a consequence, are not typically distressed by thoughts of sexually
abusing someone. For example, research has shown that some child molesters believe that children (or at least their particular victims) are interested in having sex with an adult and enjoy such sexual encounters
(Langton & Marshall, 2000; Segal & Stermac, 1990). Similarly, some
rapists believe that women fantasize being raped and cannot be raped
unless they want to be abused (Fernandez, Anderson, & Marshall, 1999;
Marshall & Hambley, 1996; Segal & Stermac, 1990). Exhibitionists

consider their offenses to be not only nonharmful, because they do not attempt physical contact, but actually enjoyable to the victim (Ball & Seghorn, 1999). Thus, we cannot expect many sexual offenders to be troubled by deviant thoughts (at least not until they develop the motivation to stop offending) except for the possible consequences to themselves of being caught.

After considering the possibility that at least some sexual offenders may have unwanted thoughts over which they can exercise only limited control at best, discussing the issue with colleagues, surveying the literature, and reflecting on our clinical experience, we were able to identify three major areas where such unwanted thoughts may be intrusive and related to offending and possible treatment: (1) negative self-appraisals, (2) ruminations about detection, and (3) deviant sexual thoughts. Our hope is that by addressing these possibilities we will have made some progress toward clarifying the problem of unwanted thoughts in sexual offenders and that this will enhance the treatment of these offenders.

NEGATIVE SELF-APPRAISALS

There are two classes of negative self-appraisals among sexual offenders: general self-denigrating thoughts and specific negative self-appraisals that follow a lapse.

General Self-Appraisals

Given the extremely derogatory nature of media accounts of sexual offending, the widespread abhorrence of such crimes, the punitive responses meted out by society, and the humiliating aspects of the investigative and prosecutorial processes, it is perhaps no surprise that by the time sexual offenders arrive at a treatment program their self-esteem is quite low. There is now considerable evidence of self-deficits among these offenders and the relationship between these deficits and other dysfunctional features of sexual offenders (Marshall, Anderson, & Champagne, 1997).

In a series of studies of nonoffenders, we (Marshall & Christie, 1982; Marshall, Christie, Lanthier, & Cruchley, 1982) found that people low in self-esteem, compared to those high in self-esteem, emit far more derogatory self-statements both throughout each day and in response to specific social interactions. Similar observations have been made by others (see Baumeister, 1993, for details) and our clinical experience indicates that sexual offenders characteristically engage in similar, if not more extreme, negative self-appraisals (Marshall, 1996).

For some of these sexual offenders (e.g., those 40–50% whose self-esteem score is more than 1 standard deviation below the normative mean), negative self-appraisals occur at quite high frequencies and are particularly noticeable when they are under stress. At these times, negative self-statements serve to induce gloom and feelings of helplessness. This is problematic because evidence shows that when sexual offenders are in a negative mood state they are more likely to resort to deviant fantasies (Looman, 1995; McKibben, Proulx, & Lusignan, 1994; Proulx, McKibben, & Lusignan, 1996) and more likely to reoffend sexually (Hanson & Harris, 2000; Pithers, Beal, Armstrong, & Petty, 1989). Providing sexual offenders with ways to deal with distressing thoughts that lead to negative mood states can be a valuable treatment component, and teaching them better ways to manage stress in their lives and to cope more appropriately should also be a component of treatment. Wenzlaff (Chapter 3, this volume) offers helpful advice on these matters. When sexual offenders do engage in negative self-appraisals, these appraisals are of themselves as a whole person rather than of specific aspects of their behavior. In this respect they view themselves as unworthy, incapable, and unattractive "monsters" (Marshall, 1996). This induces a state of hopelessness and helplessness, as a result of which it is very difficult to engage them in treatment.

As noted, these negative self-appraisals are, in many of these offenders, triggered constantly throughout each day, and they are seen by the offenders as unbidden and unwanted thoughts they cannot resist. Due to the association in sexual offenders between such thoughts and offense proclivities, we consider it essential to eliminate the tendency to negatively self-appraise. In addition, persistent negative self-appraisals erode a sense of self-efficacy which Bandura (1977) has repeatedly shown to be essential in order for clients of all kinds to benefit from treatment. There is also other research evidence (see Marshall, Anderson, et al., 1997, for a review of this research) showing that unless self-esteem is enhanced, progress in treatment will be slow and posttreatment relapses will be high. Thus the enhancement of self-worth, or the reduction of negative self-statements, appears to be an essential feature of effective treatment.

Thought-stopping procedures (Wolpe, 1958) would not be expected to inhibit these unwanted negative self-appraisals. Research with a wide range of populations has shown that such techniques lead to greater accessibility to the very thoughts over which control is attempted (Wegner, 1994). In the single experimental study published to date on thought suppression among sexual offenders, Johnston, Hudson, and Ward (1997) found that although offenders against children appeared able to suppress sex-related words when instructed, in a postsuppression test sex-related and child-related words were more accessible for preferential child molesters compared with situational child molesters or nonsexual offenders. Theoretical work would suggest that among certain subtypes of rapists this hyperaccessibility or "rebound" effect might also be evident (Langton & Marshall, 2001). These results, then, indicate that thought stopping would be a counterproductive intervention strategy to deal with unwanted intrusive thoughts in sexual offenders. Fortunately, our research suggests that emphasizing an increase in positive self-appraisals may be effective in reducing unwanted intrusive thoughts among sexual offenders. In nonoffending subjects low in self-esteem, we (Marshall & Christie, 1982; Marshall et al., 1982) demonstrated that increasing the range and frequency of both social interactions and mildly pleasurable activities, as well as increasing the clients' focus on these interactions and activities, markedly enhanced self-esteem; these procedures also reduced the frequency and intensity of negative self-thoughts and increased clients' control over them. An additional component that required subjects to list and then repeatedly rehearse several positive self-statements produced even greater increases in self-esteem and control over negative self-appraisals (Marshall & Christie, 1982). Combining these techniques into a treatment package for sexual offenders led to significant and clinically meaningful enhancements of their self-image (Marshall, Champagne, Sturgeon, & Bryce, 1997).

In a related vein, greater emphasis on the preparation and maintenance of social supports for sexual offenders may lessen the impact of intrusive negative self-appraisals or of intrusive reoffense-related self-appraisals (to which we turn in a moment). This idea is based on the encouraging work on social support and intrusive thoughts among other populations. Lewis et al. (2001) found that social support moderated the relationship between cancer-related intrusive thoughts and quality of life in their sample of breast cancer survivors. Among bereaved mothers, Lepore, Silver, Wortman, and Wayment (1996) reported a positive relationship between intrusive thoughts at first interview and depressive symptoms over time for socially constrained mothers (i.e., those who construed their social relationships as strained and felt constrained in discussing their thoughts and feelings with others), while the reverse was found for unconstrained mothers. Certainly, sexual offenders can be expected to experience social constraints in the form of reduced access to nonoffending adults who might otherwise provide acceptance and support. Without the provisions of alternative interpretations and challenges from selected others, we might expect sexual offenders to have greater difficulty processing their intrusive thoughts and impulses, resulting in attempts to conceal these thoughts and urges (Newth & Rachman, 2001).

Lapse-Related Self-Appraisals

In the early forms of the application of relapse prevention approaches to treating sexual offenders (Pithers, Marques, Gibat, & Marlatt, 1983), the so-called *abstinence violation effect* (AVE) played a prominent role. The AVE is best described by reference to cigarette smokers. When a smoker attempts to quit and remains abstinent for, say, 4 weeks only to succumb to temptation and have a cigarette at a party (a lapse), he or she is said to automatically entertain thoughts that depict him- or herself as a failure. This catastrophizing is then said to trigger feelings of helplessness and hopelessness which, in turn, facilitate a return to prior levels of smoking (a relapse). In sexual offenders, a lapse into deviant thoughts occurring after several months of effective functioning was said by Pithers et al. (1983) to trigger a similar AVE leading to an increased probability of offending. Although recent research and theoretical analyses have made it clear that such a straightforward and automatic sequence does not always unfold (Laws, Hudson, & Ward, 2000; Ward, Hudson, & Marshall, 1994), it is equally clear that the AVE does occur in some sexual offenders (Marques, Nelson, Alarcon, & Day, 2000; Ward, Hudson, & Keenan, 1998). When it does occur, sexual offenders attribute their lapse to stable, internal factors beyond their control, and this attribution is thought to strengthen their negative self-schema by focusing attention on their failings (Langton & Marshall, 2000).

Interestingly, in the quite distinct literature on obsessive–compulsive disorder, research has concentrated on a particular type of cognitive bias, *thought–action fusion* (TAF), which is said to be important in the etiology and maintenance of pathological obsessions. In essence, TAF involves the self-appraisal of intrusive thoughts as equivalent to unwanted action (Rachman, 1993; Shafran, Thordarson, & Rachman, 1996). Such an overevaluation of the personal significance of the intrusive thoughts is characterized by an inflated sense of responsibility for these thoughts as well as greater distress, and an enhanced desire to suppress them, which in turn is said to increase the salience and frequency of the intrusions. Correlational data indicate that TAF and thought suppression tendencies do correlate with severity of psychopathology among obsessive–

compulsive patients (Rassin, Diepstraten, Merckelbach, & Muris, 2001). Similarly, results from structural equation modeling with university undergraduates suggest that TAF triggers suppression, which in turn promotes obsessive–compulsive symptoms (Rassin, Muris, Schmidt, & Merckelbach, 2000). More specifically, among undergraduates, ratings of TAF likelihood (i.e., how likely it is that the thought/image/impulse itself will be actualized in real life) and perceived arousal predicted perceived controllability of their most upsetting sexually intrusive thought, with higher ratings on both indicating reduced control (Clark, Purdon, & Byers, 2000).

Certainly TAF represents a plausible cognitive mechanism through which the AVE might operate in sexual offenders. Informing theoretical models of sexual offending with the advances made in this wider literature also has implications for practical interventions. Results from studies of cognitive-behavioral therapy with both obsessive–compulsive and anxiety patients (Rassin et al., 2001) and a psychoeducational intervention with university students (Zucker, Craske, Barrios, & Holguin, 2002) suggest that TAF and thought suppression tendencies are susceptible to change.

With sexual offenders, the goal in attempts to modify the AVE reaction to a lapse includes apprising the offenders of the fact that lapses are to be expected (akin to the "spontaneous recovery" of extinguished conditioned responses), engaging cognitive restructuring procedures to alter their attributions for a lapse, and enhancing their more general sense of self-worth. To date there is no evidence bearing on the value of these procedures with sexual offenders, but they seem logical and are well-grounded in research from other areas. For example, among former smokers who had successfully maintained abstinence, cognitive restructuring was more commonly employed than thought suppression, but this was not true of former smokers who had relapsed (Haaga & Allison, 1994). Our clients have reported positive results from the use of the foregoing three procedures (expect lapses, use cognitive restructuring, and enhance self-worth), but their reports are a dubious source given their vested interest in presenting themselves as no longer at risk.

RUMINATIONS ABOUT DETECTION

While fears of being detected as abusers appear from clinical work to be common among sexual offenders, there is little or no literature on the subject and certainly no empirical studies have examined this issue. As a consequence, our comments here derive entirely from our clinical experience. Ruminations about detection occur prior to an offense being reported, but there are also ruminations about being identified in the community after release from prison or discharge from treatment.

Worries about being reported, identified, prosecuted, and imprisoned seem to be most evident early in the career of a sexual offender. With repeated offending these worries, and associated ruminations concerning catastrophic consequences of being identified, gradually dissipate presumably as a result of desensitization in the absence of negative consequences. The processes associated with repeated offending and the avoidance of detection not only reduce fears and ruminations but also appear to embolden the offenders. A brief case summary illuminates these changes.

Eddie was 32 years old when he first presented at our community clinic. He had been referred for treatment for his persistent exhibitionistic acts. Eddie reported that the first several occasions of exposing occurred in a park located in a town some 30 miles from the city in which he lived. Although he offered no account of the origin of his behavior, Eddie said that he initially drove to the nearby town then left his car and walked some distance to the park, as a strategy to avoid detection. If a victim reported him, the police would be unlikely to identify him and he would not be accidentally seen later because he did not live in the town where he exposed. Clearly Eddie was very concerned from the outset of his offending to avoid detection.

Eddie indicated that after his first offense he immediately became obsessed with the idea that somehow he would be identified. He could not stop thinking about this possibility and repeatedly entertained catastrophic thoughts about the consequences of being caught. These thoughts were associated with upsetting high arousal states which bordered on panic responses and caused Eddie considerable grief. Try as he might he could not make the thoughts stop. The content of the thoughts focused on being arrested in front of his wife and child, being spoken to in a disparaging way by the arresting officers, being placed in a holding cell with nonsex offenders who would beat him, being identified in the local newspaper as a sexual offender, losing his job, being rejected by his family and friends, and receiving a long sentence. Embarrassment and humiliation were central to Eddie's distressing thoughts, as were the loss of his status, security, and family. Eddie reported that after his first exposure these thoughts persisted over a 3- to 4-week period and initially occupied almost every waking moment. They were experienced as very intense, extremely distressing, and uncontrollable. Over repeated occasions of his exhibitionistic behaviors, Eddie said the intensity, and most particularly the persistence, of these intrusive thoughts was reduced, but the thoughts never went away entirely.

We have had numerous other clients (including child molesters and rapists) who report experiences similar to those described by Eddie. Again, the pattern seems to be that catastrophizing about the consequences of detection is most persistent, intense, and experienced as unwanted after the initial offenses. Once offending becomes entrenched, the strength of these distressing thoughts diminishes and in some these thoughts are so reduced as to no longer be experienced as troublesome. However, in many sexual offenders these unwanted, catastrophic thoughts remain, albeit in a somewhat attenuated form. They are, therefore, experienced as problematic by the client. It is, perhaps, not at all surprising that sexual offenders view the prospect of detection as extremely aversive, as indeed it must be. Sexual offenders are acutely aware that the rest of society views sexual offending as abhorrent or, more to the point, they are aware that society views sexual offenders (rather than just their behavior) as repulsive. When they ruminate about the consequences of detection, the focus, as we have noted, is more on the humiliating aspects and loss of status than it is on the possibility of imprisonment, although this is also present. Thus, thoughts of these possible consequences unsettle sexual offenders because they are afraid of losing status with their friends, family, and coworkers. In addition, they threaten the offenders' views of themselves as good persons, a belief they attempt to maintain in spite of their awareness that their offending is viewed as abhorrent by others.

No doubt many people would be pleased to learn that even if a sexual offender does not get caught, at least the offender suffers after each offense. The majority of people would not, therefore, see such ruminations as problematic. While we might share the feeling that these catastrophizing ideas are not a problem that calls for a treatment intervention, still such thoughts do seem to meet criteria as unwanted, intrusive, and distressing to the person. Offenders typically report that such thoughts come unbidden, that they are unable to control or dismiss them, and that they produce considerable distress.

It may seem surprising that such catastrophic, unwanted thoughts have little impact on the offending behavior. However, there is a solid body of evidence indicating that when punishing events follow a series of strongly reinforced behaviors (e.g., sexual acts associated with highly pleasurable sexual feelings), punishment effects are markedly reduced or eliminated (Domjan, 1998). For punishment (in this case the covert rehearsal of catastrophic consequences) to be effective it needs to occur in immediate temporal contiguity with the behavior as well as early in the sequence that leads to the final consumatory response (in this case the actual sexual assault) and to be of sufficient intensity (Barker, 2001). Castastrophizing thoughts that sexual offenders have after an offense may be intense enough but they do not meet the other two criteria for effective punishment. It is, as a consequence, not unexpected that such thoughts would do little to reduce the likelihood of offending behavior, particularly given the demonstrated association between negative mood states and deviant sexual fantasies (Proulx et al., 1996) and between negative mood states, sexually deviant thoughts, and reoffending (Hanson & Harris, 2000). In addition, of course, sexual offenders do attempt to distract themselves so that these negative thoughts are excluded from awareness. They appear to be successful at this task except in the period after an offense when efforts to suppress catastrophizing thoughts are unsuccessful, or at other times of cognitive overload (e.g., when a series of unpleasant events occur). Given that sexual offenders can successfully banish these thoughts from awareness most of the time, it is little wonder that these thoughts of detection and its consequences have no effect on inhibiting their offensive behaviors.

Like most other sexual offenders, Eddie reported that he did not repeat his offending behavior for several weeks after the initial offense due to the profound immediate impact of his catastrophizing. In fact, Eddie believed he would never offend again. Unfortunately, as the weeks passed, the repeated evocation of these thoughts seemed to attenuate their impact—a process akin to "flooding" (Marshall, Gauthier, & Gordon, 1979) or "desensitization" (Marshall & Segal, 1988), and consistent with the habituation of intrusive thoughts noted by Parkinson and Rachman (1980). While the result of this process was to make Eddie's fear of detection reduce to a level that allowed him to contemplate, plan, and enact another offense, it did not eliminate his tendency to respond to each new offense by catastrophizing. However, the persistence of his unwanted ruminations about being detected was progressively reduced over some 30 repeated offenses such that by the time he was caught these thoughts lasted only a matter of 1 or 2 days, and then at a lower intensity. Note, however, that the distressing thoughts never disappeared.

After only three interviews Eddie did not return to the clinic until 18 months later after being caught again. At that time Eddie reported that he still catastrophized immediately after an offense although this was short-lived on most occasions. Interestingly, Eddie said that the response was variable. On those occasions when he offended at a time at which he was otherwise distressed, Eddie said the intensity and duration of his postoffense catastrophizing was far greater than following an offense committed when he was feeling in good spirits. Although many sexual offenders, including Eddie, report they are more likely to offend when in a negative mood state (Pithers et al., 1989), offending also occurs for some offenders when they are in a positive mood (Ward & Hudson, 2000).

It seems clear that these thoughts of undesirable consequences of being detected are characteristic of sexual offenders and are unwanted, intrusive, and distressing. Salkovskis (1989) has suggested that intrusive thoughts can become obsessional only when the thoughts pose a threat for which the individual holds him- or herself personally responsible. The postoffense catastrophizing engaged by sexual offenders clearly meets this criterion, but unlike obsessions these unwanted thoughts are of limited duration and are almost entirely triggered by a highly specific type of event. Furthermore, unlike most obsessions, ruminations about the consequences of detection are not unrealistic, if somewhat exaggerated. Wegner (1994) has shown that attempts to suppress unwanted thoughts in fact lead to an increase in their persistence, and this is consistent with the reports of sexual offenders concerning their attempts to shut out fears of detection.

The presence of these unwanted thoughts among sexual offenders is not seen as justifying the introduction of interventions aimed at reducing their intensity and frequency. Indeed, quite the contrary effect is aimed for in treating these men. Therapists working with sexual offenders typically require these clients to provide a detailed, written cost-benefit analysis of both abstaining from future offending or continuing to offend. The aim of this is to entrench the idea of negative consequences to continued offending and to highlight the advantages of an offense-free life. Thus, in the treatment of sexual offenders one goal is to increase the salience as well as intensity and frequency of unpleasant thoughts whenever the client contemplates reoffending. This is quite unlike the approach taken with the majority of non-sexual offender clients, as the other chapters in this book clearly illustrate. By these procedures, therapists working with sexual offenders hope to "recastrophize" the notion of detection. This is particularly essential in those cases in which the actuality of detection and prosecution did not generate the humiliating and other devastating consequences they previously imagined would occur.

Of course, treatment providers would not attempt to help sexual offenders reduce these thoughts. If treatment is effective, which it is in most cases (Hanson et al., 2000), this problem of unwanted thoughts about the consequences of detection would necessarily disappear. But this would only happen if the offender had admitted to, and paid the price for, *all* of his offenses. Otherwise he might be repeatedly haunted by the prospect of a past unreported offense being belatedly identified. A persuasive argument for confessing to all their crimes can, as a result, be presented to sexual offenders during treatment. Sometimes such an argument can be successful and the relief associated with such admissions is significant. Certainly such catastrophizing thoughts could conceivably recur even after the offender has been detected and convicted of some but not all his offenses.

Ruminations after Release

One other aspect to disturbing and intrusive thoughts about detection concerns the possibility that on release back into the community, someone may discover that the man has a history of committing sexual offenses. Where there are systematic procedures for community notification, as there are in many cities in the United States, these fears and the associated ruminations about the consequences of exposure are obviously realistic. In those circumstances there is the continual fear of an endless succession of new people becoming aware of the offending. Unlike the catastrohpizing thoughts that occur prior to the original detection, these fears and the associated unwanted brooding about the consequences of more widespread awareness of his crimes can undermine a treated sexual offender's determination to remain offense free.

As noted earlier, research has shown that negative mood states, some of which may be in response to fears of exposure as a sexual offender, frequently precede, and presumably trigger, an offense (Hanson & Harris, 2000; Pithers et al., 1989). Accordingly, these intrusive thoughts about the possibility of being exposed as a sexual offender present a problem that needs to be addressed in treatment. Offenders can adopt various tactics to reduce the chance that others will learn about their offense history—for example, informing only those who need to know and can be relied on to keep it confidential; seeking jobs, accommodation, and leisure activities where their history is unlikely to be raised; and generally maintaining a low profile. In addition, sexual offenders need to understand that it is likely, and perhaps even inevitable, that their past history will come to the attention of people who will respond negatively. They need to learn to accept this and respond appropriately. Discussions of these issues need to be part of sexual offender treatment, and most programs address this topic. Particular interventions aimed at strengthening offenders' sense of self-worth and desensitizing them to the negative responses of others can also be helpful.

DEVIANT SEXUAL THOUGHTS

The problem with sexual thoughts, deviant or otherwise, as far as control over their occurrence is concerned is that they generate pleasurable sensations even in the absence of acting on these thoughts (either by masturbating or engaging in sexual contact). As Singer (1975) notes, sexual fantasies are associated with very strong pleasurable emotions, and this makes them difficult to control. In general, sexual thoughts can be construed as generating at least momentary positive affect, even if their occurrence is subsequently distressing (Davidson & Hoffman, 1986; Zimmer, Borchardt, & Fischle, 1983). Such an association between sexual thoughts and pleasure replicates the procedures essential for conditioning and we might, as a consequence, expect a subsequent increase in the probability of similar thoughts. By their nature, sexual thoughts and fantasies can be expected to present difficulties in control. Fortunately, while sexually deviant fantasies are reported by nonoffending samples (Crepault & Couture, 1980), most people do not experience unwanted intrusive sexual thoughts as persistent, distressing, or uncontrollable, even sexual thoughts that would be considered deviant (Byers et al., 1998).

The exception to this general rule is that people with obsessive–compulsive disorder (OCD) frequently report intrusive sexual thoughts that are distressing to them (see Clark & O'Connor, Chapter 6, this volume). For clients with OCD, the first step in treatment is to help them recognize that unlike sexual offenders they do not enjoy these thoughts. With sexual offenders the first step is to get them to change their view of the deviant thoughts to seeing them as unacceptable. Perhaps the most obvious difference between clients with OCD and sexual offenders, in terms of their response to intrusive sexual thoughts, is that clients with OCD catastrophize about these thoughts whereas sexual offenders enjoy them. Sexual offenders typically rationalize these thoughts in one way or another. They may convince themselves that having deviant thoughts will not only not lead to offending, it will reduce their need to offend because, they persuade themselves, fantasizing alone will be satisfying. Others modify the content of the deviant fantasies so that the victim is

perceived as enjoying being abused. Unfortunately, some quite dangerous sexual offenders do the opposite and include humiliating elements in
their fantasies as well as depictions of victim suffering. These latter offenders are typically quite resistant to the idea of eliminating their deviant thoughts.

Among both offenders and nonoffenders who have deviant sexual
thoughts, some make no attempt to control them while others struggle
to inhibit such thought. It is those sexual offenders who are unconcerned
about their deviant thoughts who pose the greatest difficulties on treatment. Fortunately, at least after detection and prosecution, some sexual
offenders realize the danger to themselves of continuing to indulge in
their deviant fantasies. For most of the rest, motivational strategies
readily secure their cooperation in treatment procedures aimed at reducing deviant thoughts. A few, as noted, resist efforts to persuade them to
attempt to eliminate deviant thoughts.

As Hudson, Ward, and McCormack (1999) observe, some sexual
offenders view their offending positively. These offenders dismiss the
possibility that they have harmed their victims, or they consider society's
prohibitions to be inappropriate, or they are simply entirely focused on
their own satisfaction and pleasure. For these offenders, deviant sexual
thoughts are neither intrusive nor unwanted; they deliberately initiate
deviant thoughts and enjoy them. However, some sexual offenders are
clearly bothered by deviant sexual thoughts and some of them strive des-
perately, but unsuccessfully, to inhibit these fantasies. Such thoughts and
fantasies may be fleeting and occur in response to some specific event or
state, or they may be persistent and self-generated.

Specific Triggers

For some sexual offenders, unwanted deviant ideas occur during unanticipated encounters with potential victims or by unexpected scenes in
media depictions (i.e., movies, television, newspapers, advertisements,
and cybersex sites). However, for many sexual offenders deviant sexual
thoughts are triggered by an upsetting event or distressing mood state, or
by a self-induced altered state (e.g., intoxication).

Among those offenders for whom deviant sexual thoughts are triggered by unanticipated encounters or scenes, these thoughts are typically
only seen as unwanted quite early in their offending careers. For example, a man may be surprised and repulsed by having sexual feelings and
thoughts about a child he has unexpectedly witnessed changing into a
bathing costume. For some incest offenders, it may be that a change in

circumstances affecting the relations in the family precipitates a change in the way the father appraises his child's behavior. Unexpected intrusive sexual thoughts triggered by normal child care activities such as bathing may become distressing, at least initially. As a consequence these individuals may attempt to suppress these thoughts. Some may successfully suppress these thoughts while others may feel they cannot control them. These latter individuals may, for at least a short time, continue to have deviant thoughts only in response to contacts with potential victims (or images of such persons), but most are likely to develop persistent and more pervasive deviant thoughts; we discuss these latter individuals in more detail when we turn to those having self-generated and persistent deviant fantasies.

Numerous sexual offenders claim that they only entertain deviant thoughts or engage in deviant acts when they are intoxicated (Valliere, 1997). This, of course, may simply be an attempt to divert responsibility, but the fact is that intoxication is an altered state during which various atypical behaviors can emerge. In an examination of the effects of alcohol intoxication on the sexual responses of healthy (and putatively "normal") male university students, Barbaree, Marshall, Yates, and Lightfoot (1983) found unsettling results. Selecting subjects who had previously demonstrated high arousal to consenting sex and low arousal to rape, Barbaree et al. (1983) then had one group drink an alcoholic beverage (half were told it was alcohol, half were told it was soda) that increased their blood alcohol level to the legal limit for driving; the remainder drank soda (half were told it was soda, half were told it was alcohol). Those who drank alcohol (regardless of instructions) subsequently showed markedly increased levels of sexual arousal to rape and somewhat attenuated responses to consenting sex. Expectancy effects were not apparent in this study. Clearly alcohol intoxication does increase the propensity to respond sexually to deviant stimuli that were not provocative when the subjects were sober. There may, therefore, be some truth to the claim by sexual offenders that intoxication alters their propensity to respond in deviant ways. This, however, does not absolve them from responsibility as it is always their choice to become intoxicated and they are clearly aware of its effects.

Of course, these observations have implications for treatment (i.e., use of intoxicants must be addressed) and they have relevance for our current concerns. Obviously most men do not have deviant sexual thoughts when intoxicated, but apparently some men do. The question is, Are these latter individuals unable to control deviant tendencies when intoxicated? Presumably Barbaree et al.'s university students did not want to appear deviant and some did indicate they were surprised by their responses. This does suggest reduced levels of control over responding, and likely over thoughts. No one has yet examined whether sexual offenders who attribute some responsibility for their crimes to an intoxicated state experience greater difficulty in controlling their thoughts when intoxicated than when they are sober. However, Wormith, Bradford, Pawlak, Borzecki, and Zohar (1988) observed more strongly deviant responses to rape and child molestation when offenders were intoxicated. Thus, like nonoffender males, it appears that sexual offenders' control over deviant tendencies is reduced when they are intoxicated. In any event, attempts to reduce future intoxication would be helpful and most programs address this issue (Marshall, Anderson, & Fernandez, 1999).

In their examination of psychiatric patients, Zelin et al. (1983) reported a strong relationship between fantasies and negative affect. When these patients engaged in fantasies they claimed they felt better and experienced less frustration. Wilson and Barber (1983) found that fantasy-prone adults had lonely, unhappy childhoods during which time they learned to use fantasies to relieve feelings of isolation. Marshall and Marshall (2000), in their accounts of the origins of sexual offending, provide evidence suggesting that as children sexual offenders employ sexual fantasies and masturbation as a way of coping with similar feelings of loneliness, abuse, and neglect. Recent evidence indicates that deviant sexual thoughts are increased and experienced as irresistible by sexual offenders when they are having problems or when they are in a negative mood. Several studies have directly addressed this issue and the results are consistent.

For example, Yates, Barbaree, and Marshall (1984), in a study similar to their examination of the effects of alcohol intoxication, demonstrated that anger induced by a woman generated surprisingly strong arousal to rape in otherwise normal men. This suggests that mood states may facilitate deviant responding, and other researchers have found exactly that. Wilson and Lang (1981) found that the frequency and intensity of sadistic and masochistic fantasies in nonoffender males increased during periods of dissatisfaction with relationships. McKibben et al. (1994) had sexual offenders keep a personal "fantasy report" which recorded, throughout every second day for 2 months, their deviant and nondeviant sexual thoughts and associated masturbatory activities. They were also required to record their interpersonal conflicts and emotional states. McKibben et al. found that conflicts and negative mood states (feelings of loneliness, inadequacy, humiliation, and anger) were followed by overwhelming and irresistible deviant sexual fantasies and re-sultant masturbation to these fantasies. No relationship was observed between conflicts or mood states and nondeviant fantasies. In a follow-up to this study using larger samples, Proulx et al. (1996) essentially replicated these findings. In addition, Proulx et al. found that conflict and negative moods actually decreased the frequency and intensity of appropriate sexual fantasies and associated masturbation. Perhaps the most important finding from their two studies for the current issue was that the deviant fantasies triggered by the conflicts and negative moods were overwhelming; that is, the sexual offenders experienced them as irresistible.

Looman (1995; Looman, Serran, & Marshall, 2003) reported two studies that similarly revealed a relationship between deviant fantasies and feelings of loneliness, inadequacy, and humiliation and the experi-ence of rejection. Most important, Looman's (1995) child molesters re-ported feeling scared and guilty while fantasizing about sex with a child. On the other hand, the child molesters said they felt comfortable and pleased when having fantasies of sex with an adult.

These studies by Looman and those by Proulx and McKibben indicate that a significant number of sexual offenders escape distressing feelings and problems by engaging in sexual activities and that these sexual activi-ties are typically deviant. Directly relevant to this issue, Cortoni and Mar-shall (2001) reported that when sexual offenders had problems (e.g., rela-tionship difficulties, disappointing news, feeling taken advantage of, and feeling threatened), their rates of sexual activity (i.e., fantasizing, mastur-bating, or overt sexual acts) markedly increased. These changes, unlike what was observed in the studies by Looman and Proulx and McKibben, reflected increases in normative as well as deviant themes. Across all these studies, sexual offenders responded to stress by engaging in sexual activi-ties. As we noted earlier, sexual activity generates pleasure (i.e., is posi-tively reinforced), which can be thought of as providing the conditioning basis for subsequent increases in arousal to whatever sexual themes were present (Abel & Blanchard, 1974; McGuire, Carlisle, & Young, 1965). When sex is coupled with escape from an aversive state, as was shown by the aforementioned series of studies, such behaviors will also be associated with negative reinforcement. Behaviors that are both positively and nega-tively reinforced at the same time can be expected to increase in frequency and intensity and become progressively more persistent over time (Laws & Marshall, 1990). Thus, the responses of sexual offenders to stress may serve to increase their deviance. This obviously is a serious problem, par-ticularly when deviant thoughts come unbidden and are experienced as unwanted. As we have seen, voluntary attempts to suppress such thoughts typically lead to their increase.

On the basis of these studies we suggest that for some sexual offenders (e.g., 61% of Looman's child molesters), the experience of negative mood states and/or conflict in relationships triggers unwanted and irresistible deviant sexual thoughts. Having these fantasies further adds to their distress, which in turn likely decreases their sense of control over these thoughts. Thus addressing these issues in a comprehensive treatment program needs to be a priority. This is particularly the case when we consider that research has consistently found poor relationship skills and marked loneliness in sexual offenders (Marshall, 1993; Ward, Hudson, & McCormack, 1997) as well as problems in emotional regulation (Ward & Hudson, 2000).

The standard treatment approach to dealing with the occurrence of deviant sexual fantasies is to either implement behavioral procedures or administer a pharmacological agent. Antiandrogens (Bradford, 1990) and selective serotonin reuptake inhibitors (Greenberg & Bradford, 1997) have been effectively employed to reduce deviant fantasies, but they are typically used in conjunction with psychological treatment so it is difficult to infer their specific effects. While some procedures such as covert sensitization have been reportedly successful in changing deviant fantasies and arousal (Maletzky, 1991), the evidence for the effectiveness of most behavioral interventions is less than satisfying (Laws & Marshall, 1991; Quinsey & Earls, 1990). Even when these behavioral techniques or pharmacological interventions are effective in reducing self-reported deviant sexual thoughts, the precipitating factors such as relationship problems, loneliness, rejection, and negative mood states remain unaddressed. Fortunately, effective procedures are available to attenuate mood states, decrease loneliness, and increase relationship skills (Marshall et al., 1999). There are also effective ways to enhance the ability of offenders to cope with problematic life events. Given that preliminary evidence suggests that social skills training alone does not reduce the frequency of self-reported deviant thoughts among sexual offenders (Kempf, 1994), interventions should focus on these precipitating factors, as well as more directly address the (re-)appraisal and management of the deviant sexual thoughts themselves.

Pervasive Deviant Thoughts

A relatively small proportion of sexual offenders report experiencing intrusive and unwanted deviant sexual thoughts repeatedly throughout each day, with these thoughts typically involving elaborated and detailed sexual fantasies. Jones and Barlow (1990) found that among non-offending males, those whose rates of sexual activity were high (more overt acts, higher rates of masturbating) also engaged more frequently in sexual fantasies, and Giambra and Martin (1977) report that the frequency of sexual fantasies varies with the intensity of sexual drive. We can, therefore, expect sexual offenders who report persistent deviant fantasies also to be strongly sexually driven, which may increase their risk to reoffend. Ward and Hudson (2000) point to problems of sexual self-regulation being related to the likelihood that sexual offenders will continue to offend, and Hanson and Harris (2000) provide evidence that this is indeed true. Those offenders who report a bothersome rate of deviant fantasies and are distressed by these fantasies typically make repeated but unsuccessful attempts to rid themselves of these thoughts. Unfortunately, this distress, and the associated failed attempts to suppress the fantasies, appears to increase rather than decrease the thoughts (Johnston et al., 1997).

Such high rates of deviant fantasizing, particularly when they are reported as uncontrollable, cause alarm among those who must make release decisions concerning these offenders. It is assumed, not unreasonably, that high rates of uncontrollable deviant fantasizing indicate a high risk to reoffend. Such a view is consistent with the evidence reported previously from studies by Jones and Barlow (1990) and by Giambra and Martin (1977). Direct evidence indicating a link between elevated levels of deviant sexual fantasizing and repeated sexual offending comes from two studies. The first, using a small sample of very serious offenders, found that a significantly higher percentage of serial (i.e., three or more victims) sexual murderers self-reported deviant fantasies compared with single victim sexual murderers (Prentky et al., 1989). Using a much larger sample of sexual offenders, Hanson and Harris (2000) identified a range of dynamic factors that distinguished those offenders who went on to sexually recidivate from those who did not. Among the correlates of sexual recidivism, sexual preoccupation (e.g., use of prostitutes, excessive masturbation, and self-reported deviant sexual fantasies/urges) was significant. Consequently, procedures need to be implemented to reduce the intensity and frequency of persistent deviant sexual thoughts.

Additional studies have directly examined the percentage of sexual offenders who report high-frequency deviant sexual thoughts, although these studies have typically combined sexual offenders with other paraphilics. For example, Kafka (2003) summarizes his research comparing paraphilics with individuals meeting criteria for "paraphilic-related disorder." The latter group engage in exceedingly high rates of normative sexual behaviors and feel driven to do so. Paraphilics, in Kafka's studies include some sexual offenders (i.e., only those meeting diagnostic criteria for pedophilia, voyeurism, sexual sadism, and exhibitionism) as well as nonoffending paraphilics (e.g., fetishists and transvestites). Approximately 23% of the total sample (i.e., combining the paraphilics and paraphilic-related disorders) had multiple paraphilias, were sexually preoccupied for at least 2 hours each day, and had 10 or more sexual outlets (orgasms) per week. Of these subjects, 68% were sexual offenders. Our own work on this issue (Marshall & Marshall, 2001), which is in its earliest stages, has attempted to determine the percentage of sexual offenders (only child molesters and rapists) who display signs of hypersexuality. Using measures of sexual addiction we found that 45% of sexual offenders met criteria for excessive sexual desire disorder; that is, 45% of them reported a history of preoccupation with sex that they believed they could not control and high rates (i.e., one or more times each day) of sexual outlets resulting in orgasm.

Thus, there is some limited evidence that at least a significant proportion of sexual offenders have persistent deviant sexual thoughts over which they are unable to exercise control. On the other hand, only 5–10% of our sexual offender clients over the past 34 years have requested help in dealing with overwhelming sexual urges and uncontrollable deviant sexual fantasies. Just what these discrepant results, between the research and clinical incidence of hypersexuality and troublesome sexual thoughts, indicate remains to be seen. It seems likely that the issue is, in part, one of terminology and measurement. Among sexual offenders with persistent deviant sexual thoughts, it will be important to distinguish between those who experience these thoughts as unwanted, intrusive, and ego-dystonic (those, it is hoped, who are motivated to avoid reoffending) and those who actively foster such thoughts and experience them as positive and ego-syntonic. Regardless, there is a problematic group of sexual offenders who complain of unwanted and persistent deviant sexual thoughts. Oddly enough not all these men display abnormal or even high normal levels of plasma testosterone. For those who do have high testosterone (or any of the other sexually activating steroids), the administration of an antiandrogen appears to lower the intensity, frequency, and duration of deviant thoughts and create feelings of control in the client (Bradford, 1997). In addition, some behavioral procedures have proved effective with some of these clients (Marshall, in press-a, in press-b).

CONCLUSIONS

We have seen that sexual offenders may have unwanted, intrusive, and distressing thoughts in several areas of functioning. Negative self-appraisals among sexual offenders are experienced as pervasive, undermine self-efficacy, and serve to block treatment progress. Those self-appraisals related to the likelihood or imminence of relapse represent especially important treatment targets given the relationship between deviant sexual thoughts, affective intensity, and reoffense. While ruminations about detection, prior to initial identification as an offender, are experienced as intrusive and unwanted, they do not represent suitable targets for treatment. Nevertheless, increasing both the intensity and the likely occurrence of these thoughts among sexual offenders participating in treatment might be useful in reinforcing their desire to avoid future incarcerations and harm to victims, at least among those with sufficient self-esteem. As a strategy for self-monitoring, it would be necessary to effect a shift in the occurrence of such thoughts from postoffense to an earlier stage in an unfolding offense chain. Certainly we would want to reduce unwanted thoughts about being identified as an offender by other community citizens when a sexual offender is released from prison or discharged from treatment. The unfortunate and ill-informed programs of aggressive community notification in the United States can only serve to increase rather than decrease the risk sexual offenders pose to society.

Deviant sexual thoughts and fantasies have long been implicated in the etiology and maintenance of sexually abusive behavior. Further research is needed to determine whether, and when, these thoughts are experienced by sexual offenders as wanted or unwanted, positive or negative, and internally or externally generated. Interventions can then be refined to more effectively address these differing characteristics of this important treatment target. Unwanted deviant sexual thoughts or fantasies are problematic, whether triggered by specific unexpected experiences or pervasively unbidden, and procedures need to be adopted to reduce the frequency, duration, and intensity of these thoughts.

REFERENCES

Abel, G. G., & Blanchard, E. B. (1974). The role of fantasy in the treatment of sexual deviation. *Archives of General Psychology, 30,* 467–475.

American Psychiatric Association. (1994). *Diagnostic and statistical manual of mental disorders* (4th ed.). Washington, DC: Author.

Ball, C. J., & Seghorn, T. K. (1999). Diagnosis and treatment of exhibitionism and other sexual compulsive disorders. In B. K. Schwartz (Ed.), *The sex offender: Theoretical advances, treating special populations, and legal developments* (pp. 28-1–28-16). Kingston, NJ: Civic Research Institute.

Bandura, A. (1977). Self-efficacy: Toward a unifying theory of behavior change. *Psychological Review, 84,* 191–215.

Barbaree, H. E., Marshall, W. L., Yates, E., & Lightfoot, L. O. (1983). Alcohol intoxication and deviant sexual arousal in male social drinkers. *Behaviour Research and Therapy, 21,* 365–373.

Barker, L. M. (2001. *Learning and behavior: Biological, psychological, and social perspectives* (3rd ed.). Upper Saddle River, NJ: Prentice-Hall.

Baumeister, R. F. (1993). *Self-esteem: The puzzle of low self-regard.* New York: Plenum Press.

Bradford, J. M. W. (1990). The antiandrogen and hormonal treatment of sex offenders. In W. L. Marshall, D. R. Laws, & H. E. Barbaree (Eds.), *Handbook of sexual assault: Issues, theories, and treatment of the offender* (pp. 297–310). New York: Plenum Press.

Bradford, J. M. W. (1997). Medical interventions in sexual deviance. In D. R.Laws & W. O'Donohue (Eds.), *Sexual deviance: Theory, assessment, and treatment* (pp. 449–464). New York: Guilford Press.

Byers, E. S., Purdon, C., & Clark, D. A. (1998). Sexual intrusive thoughts of college students. *Journal of Sex Research, 35,* 359–369.

Clark, D. A., & Purdon, C. L. (1995). The assessment of unwanted intrusive thoughts: A review and critique of the literature. *Behaviour Research and Therapy, 33,* 967–976.

Clark, D. A., Purdon, C., & Byers, E. S. (2000). Appraisal and control of sexual and non-sexual intrusive thoughts in university students. *Behaviour Research and Therapy, 38,* 439–455.

Conte, J. R. (1988). The effects of sexual abuse on children: Results of a research project. *Annals of the New York Academy of Sciences, 528,* 310–326.

Cortoni, F. A., & Marshall, W. L. (2001). Sex as a coping strategy and its relationship to juvenile sexual history and intimacy in sexual offenders. *Sexual Abuse: A Journals of Research and Treatment, 13,* 27–43.

Crepault, C., & Couture, M. (1980). Men's erotic fantasies. *Archives of Sexual Behavior, 9,* 565–581.

Davidson, J. K., & Hoffman, L. E. (1986). Sexual fantasies and sexual satisfaction: An empirical analysis of erotic thought. *Journal of Sex Research, 22,* 184–205.

Domjan, M. (1998). *The principles of learning and behavior* (4th ed.). Pacific Grove, CA: Brooks/Cole.

Falsetti, S. A., Monnier, J., Davis, J. L., & Resnick, H. S. (2002). Intrusive thoughts in posttraumatic stress disorder. *Journal of Cognitive Psychotherapy, 16,* 193–208.

Fernandez, Y. M., Anderson, D., & Marshall, W. L. (1999). The relationship among empathy, cognitive distortions, and self-esteem in sexual offenders. In

B. K. Schwartz (Ed.), *The sex offender: Theoretical advances, treating special populations, and legal developments* (pp. 4-1–4-12). Kingston, NJ: Civic Research Institute.

Freeman-Longo, R. W., & Blanchard, G. T. (1998). *Sexual abuse in America: Epidemic of the 21st century.* Brandon, VT: Safer Society Press.

Giambra, L. M., & Martin, C. E. (1977). Sexual daydreams and quantitive aspects of sexual activity: Some relations for males across adulthood. *Archives of Sexual Behavior, 6,* 497–505.

Gordon, W. M. (2002). Sexual obsessions and OCD. *Sexual and Relationship Therapy, 17,* 343–354.

Greenberg, D. M., & Bradford, J. M. W. (1997). Treatment of the paraphilic disorder: A review of the role of the selective serotonin reuptake inhibitors. *Sexual Abuse: A Journal of Research and Treatment, 9,* 349–360.

Haaga, D. A. F., & Allison, M. L. (1994). Thought suppression and smoking relapse: A secondary analysis of Haaga (1989). *British Journal of Clinical Psychology, 33,* 327–331.

Hanson, R. K., Gordon, A., Harris, A. J. R., Marques, J. K., Murphy, W. D., Quinsey, V. L., et al. (2000). First report of the collaborative outcome project on the effectiveness of psychological treatment for sex offenders. *Sexual Abuse: A Journal of Research and Treatment, 12,* 169–194.

Hanson, R. K., & Harris, A. J. R. (2000). Where should we intervene? Dynamic predictors of sexual offense recidivism. *Criminal Justice and Behavior, 27,* 6–35.

Hudson, S. M., Ward, T., & McCormack, J. C. (1999). Offense pathways in sexual offenders. *Journal of Interpersonal Violence, 8,* 779–798.

Johnston, L., Hudson, S. M., & Ward, T. (1997). The suppressions of sexual thoughts by child molesters: A preliminary investigation. *Sexual Abuse: A Journal of Research and Treatment, 9,* 303–319.

Johnston, L., Ward, T., & Hudson, S. M. (1997). Suppressing sex: Mental control and the treatment of sexual offenders. *Journal of Sex Research, 3,* 121–130.

Jones, J. C., & Barlow, D. H. (1990). Self-reported frequency of sexual urges, fantasies and masturbatory fantasies in heterosexual males and females. *Archives of Sexual Behavior, 19,* 269–279.

Kafka, M. P. (2003). Sex offending and sexual appetite: The clinical and theoretical relevance of hypersexual desire. *International Journal of Offender Therapy and Comparative Criminology, 47,* 439–451.

Kempf, J. L. (1994). *The effects of a social skills intervention on the sexually intrusive thoughts of male adult child molesters.* Unpublished doctoral dissertation, University of San Francisco.

Koss, M. P., & Harvey, M. R. (1991). *The rape victim: Clinical and community intervention.* (2nd ed.). Newbury Park, CA: Sage.

Langton, C. M., & Marshall, W. L. (2000). The role of cognitive distortions in relapse prevention programs. In D. R. Laws, S. M. Hudson, & T. Ward (Eds.). *Remaking relapse prevention with sex offenders: A sourcebook* (pp. 167–186). Thousand Oaks, CA: Sage.

Langton, C. M., & Marshall, W. L. (2001). Cognition in rapists: Theoretical patterns by typological breakdown. *Aggression and Violent Behavior, 6*, 499–518.

Laws, D. R., Hudson, S. M., & Ward, T. (Eds.). (2000). *Remaking relapse prevention with sex offenders: A sourcebook.* Thousand Oaks, CA: Sage.

Laws, D. R., & Marshall, W. L. (1990). A conditioning theory of the etiology and maintenance of deviant sexual preference and behavior. In W. L. Marshall, D. R. Laws, & H. E. Barbaree (Eds.), *Sexual assault: Issues, theories, and treatment of the offender* (pp. 209–229). New York: Plenum Press.

Laws, D. R., & Marshall, W. L. (1991). Masturbatory reconditioning with sexual deviates: An evaluative review. *Advances in Behaviour Research and Therapy, 13*, 13–25.

Lepore, S. J., Silver, R. C., Wortman, C. B., & Wayment, H. A. (1996). Social constraints, intrusive thoughts, and depressive symptoms among bereaved mothers. *Journal of Personality and Social Psychology, 70*, 271–282.

Lewis, J. A., Manne, S. L., DuHamel, K. N., Vickburg, S. M. J., Bovbjerg, D. H., Currie, V., Winkel, G., et al. (2001). Social support, intrusive thoughts, and quality of life in breast cancer survivors. *Journal of Behavioral Medicine, 24*, 231–245.

Looman, J. (1995). Sexual fantasies of child molesters. *Canadian Journal of Behavioural Science, 27*, 321–332.

Looman, J., Serran, G., & Marshall, W. L. (2003). *Mood, conflict and sexual fantasies: Comparisons between sexual offenders and a nonoffender comparison group.* Manuscript submitted for publication.

Maletzky, B. M. (1991). *Treating the sexual offender.* Newbury Park, CA: Sage.

Marques, J. K., Nelson, C., Alarcon, J. M., & Day, D. M. (2000). Preventing relapse in sex offenders: What we learned from SOTEP's experimental treatment program. In D. R. Laws, S. M. Hudson, & T. Ward (Eds.), *Remaking relapse prevention with sex offenders: A sourcebook* (pp. 321–340). Thousand Oaks, CA: Sage.

Marshall, L. E., & Marshall, W. L. (2001). Excessive sexual desire disorder among sexual offenders: The development of a research project. *Sexual Addiction and Compulsivity: Journal of Treatment and Prevention, 8*, 301–307.

Marshall, W. L. (1993). The role of attachment, intimacy, and loneliness in the etiology and maintenance of sexual offending. *Sexual and Marital Therapy, 8*, 109–121.

Marshall, W. L. (1996). The sexual offender: Monster, victim, or everyman? *Sexual Abuse: A Journal of Research and Treatment, 8*, 217–335.

Marshall, W. L. (in press-a). Olfactory aversion and directed masturbation in the modification of deviant preferences: A case study of a child molester. *Clinical Case Studies.*

Marshall, W. L. (in press-b). Ammonia aversion with an exhibitionist: A case study. *Clinical Case Studies.*

Marshall, W. L., Anderson, D., & Champagne, F. (1997). Self-esteem and its relationship to sexual offending. *Psychology, Crime and Law, 3*, 81–106.

Marshall, W. L., Anderson, D., & Fernandez, Y. M. (1999). *Cognitive behavioural treatment of sexual offenders.* Chichester, UK: Wiley.

Marshall, W. L., & Barrett, S. (1990). *Criminal neglect: Why sex offenders go free.* Toronto: Doubleday.

Marshall, W. L., Champagne, F., Sturgeon, C., & Bryce, P. (1997). Increasing the self-esteem of child molesters. *Sexual Abuse: A Journal of Research and Treatment, 9*, 321–333.

Marshall, W. L., & Christie, M. M. (1982). The enhancement of social self-esteem. *Canadian Counsellor, 16*, 82–89.

Marshall, W. L., Christie, M. M., Lanthier, R. D., & Cruchley, J. (1982). The nature of the reinforcer in the enhancement of social self-esteem. *Canadian Counsellor, 16*, 90–96.

Marshall, W. L., Gauthier, J., & Gordon, A. (1979). The current status of flooding therapy. In M. Hersen, R. Eisler, & P. Miller (Eds.), *Progress in behavior modification* (Vol. 7, pp. 205–275). New York: Academic Press.

Marshall, W. L., & Hambley, L. S. (1996). Intimacy and loneliness, and their relationship to rape myth acceptance and hostility toward women among rapists. *Journal of Interpersonal Violence, 11*, 586–592.

Marshall, W. L., & Marshall, L. E. (2000). The origins of sexual offending. *Trauma, Violence, and Abuse: A Review Journal, 1*, 250–263.

Marshall, W. L., & Segal, Z. V. (1988). Behavior therapy. In G. C. Last & M. Hersen (Eds.), *Handbook of anxiety disorders* (pp. 338–361). New York: Pergamon Press.

McGuire, R. J., Carlisle, J. M., & Young, B. G. (1965). Sexual deviations as conditioned behavior: A hypothesis. *Behaviour Research and Therapy, 2*, 185–190.

McKibben, A., Proulx, J., & Lusignan, R. (1994). Relationships between conflict, affect and deviant sexual behaviours in rapists and pedophiles. *Behaviour Research and Therapy, 32*, 571–575.

Newth, S., & Rachman, S. (2001). The concealment of obsessions. *Behaviour Research and Therapy, 39*, 457–464.

Obsessive Compulsive Cognitions Working Group. (1997). Cognitive assessment of obsessive–compulsive disorder. *Behaviour Research and Therapy, 35*, 667–681.

Parkinson, L., & Rachman, S. (1980). Are intrusive thoughts subject to habituation? *Behaviour Research and Therapy, 18*, 409–418.

Pithers, W. D., Beal, L. S., Armstrong, J., & Petty, J. (1989). Identification of risk factors through clinical interviews and analysis of records. In D. R. Laws (Ed.), *Relapse prevention with sex offenders* (pp. 63–72). New York: Guilford Press.

Pithers, W. D., Marques, J. K., Gibat, C. C., & Marlatt, G. A. (1983). Relapse prevention with sexual aggressors: A self-control model of treatment and maintenance of change. In J. G. Greer & I. R. Stuart (Eds.), *The sexual aggressor:*

Current perspectives on treatment (pp. 214–239). New York: Van Nostrand Reinhold.

Prentky, R. A., Burgess, A. W., Rokous, F., Lee, A., Hartman, C., Ressler, R., et al. (1989). The presumptive role of fantasy in serial sexual homicide. *American Journal of Psychiatry, 146,* 887–891.

Proulx, J., McKibben, A., & Lusignan, R. (1996). Relationships between affective components and sexual behaviors in sexual aggressors. *Sexual Abuse: A Journal of Research and Treatment, 8,* 279–290.

Purdon, C., & Clark, D. A. (1993). Obsessive intrusive thoughts in nonclinical subjects. Part 1. Content and relation with depressive, anxious and obsessional symptoms. *Behaviour Research and Therapy, 31,* 713–720.

Quinsey, V. L., & Earls, C. M. (1990). The modification of sexual preferences. In W. L. Marshall, D. R. Laws, & H. E. Barbaree (Eds.), *Handbook of sexual assault: Issues, theories, and treatment of the offender* (pp. 279–295). New York: Plenum Press.

Rachman, S. (1981). Part 1. Unwanted intrusive cognitions. *Advances in Behaviour Research and Therapy, 3,* 89–99.

Rachman, S. (1993). Obsessions, responsibility and guilt. *Behaviour Research and Therapy, 31,* 149–154.

Rassin, E., Diepstraten, P., Merckelbach, H., & Muris, P. (2001). Thought–action fusion and thought suppression in obsessive-compulsive disorder. *Behaviour Research and Therapy, 39,* 757–764.

Rassin, E., Muris, P., Schmidt, H., & Menkelbach, H. (2000). Relationships between thought-action fusion, thought suppression and obsessive–compulsive symptoms: A structural equation modeling approach. *Behaviour Research and Therapy, 38,* 889–897.

Salkovskis, P. M. (1989). Cognitive-behavioural factors and the persistence of intrusive thoughts in obsessional problems. *Behaviour Research and Therapy, 27,* 677–682.

Segal, Z. V., & Stermac, L. E. (1990). The role of cognition in sexual assault. In W. L. Marshall, D. R. Laws, & H. E. Barbaree (Eds.), *Handbook of sexual assault: Issues, theories, and treatment of the offender* (pp. 161– 174). New York: Plenum Press.

Shafran, R., Thordson, D. S., & Rachman, S. (1996). Thought-action fusion in obsessive compulsive disorder. *Journal of Anxiety Disorders, 10,* 379–391.

Serran, G. A. (2003). *Changes in coping with treatment of sexual offenders.* Unpublished doctoral thesis, University of Ottawa, Canada.

Singer, J. L. (1975). *The inner world of daydreaming.* New York: Harper & Row.

Valliere, V. N. (1997). Relationships between alcohol use, alcohol expectancies, and sexual offenses in convicted offenders. In B. K. Schwartz & H. R. Cellini (Eds.), *The sex offender: New insights, treatment innovations, and legal developments* (pp. 3-1–3-14). Kingston, NJ: Civic Research Institute.

Wang, A., & Clark, D. A. (2002). Haunting thoughts: The problem of obsessive mental intrusions. *Journal of Cognitive Psychotherapy, 16,* 193–208.

Ward, T., & Hudson, S. M. (2000). A self-regulation model of relapse prevention.

In D. R. Laws, S. M. Hudson, & T. Ward (Eds.), *Remaking relapse prevention with sex offenders: A sourcebook* (pp. 79–101). Thousand Oaks, CA: Sage.

Ward, T., Hudson, S. M., & Keenan, T. (1998). A self-regulation model of the sexual offense process. *Sexual Abuse: A Journal of Research and Treatment, 10,* 141–157.

Ward, T., Hudson, S. M., & Marshall, W. L. (1994). The abstinence violation effect in child molesters. *Behaviour Research and Therapy, 32,* 431–434.

Ward, T., Hudson, S. M., & McCormack, J. (1997). Attachment style, intimacy deficits, and sexual offending. In B. K. Schwartz & H. R. Cellini (Eds.), *The sex offender: New insights, treatment innovations, and legal developments* (pp. 2-1-2-14). Kingston, NJ: Civic Research Institute.

Wegner, D. M. (1994). Ironic processes of mental control. *Psychological Bulletin, 101,* 34–52.

Wenzlaff, R. M. (2002). Intrusive thoughts in depression *Journal of Cognitive Psychotherapy, 16,* 145–159.

Wilson, G. D., & Lang, R. J. (1981). Sex differences in sexual fantasy patterns. *Journal of Personality and Individual Differences, 2,* 143–146.

Wilson, S. C., & Barber, T. X. (1983). The fantasy-prone personality: Implications for understanding imagery, hypnosis, and parapsychological phenomena. In A. A. Sheikh (Ed.), *Imagery: Current theory, research and application* (pp. 340–387). New York: Wiley.

Wolpe, J. (1958). *Psychotherapy by reciprocal inhibition.* Stanford, CA: Stanford University Press.

Wormith, J. S., Bradford, J. M. W., Pawlak, A., Borzecki, M., & Zohar, A. (1988). The assessment of deviant sexual arousal as a function of intelligence, instructional set and alcohol ingestion. *Canadian Journal of Psychiatry, 33,* 800–808.

Yates, E., Barbaree, H. E., & Marshall, W. L. (1984). Anger and deviant sexual arousal. *Behavior Therapy, 15,* 287–294.

Zelin, M. L., Bernstein, S. B., Heijin, C., Jampel, R. M., Myerson, P. G., Adler, G., et al. (1983). The Sustaining Fantasy Questionnaire: Measurement of sustaining functions of fantasies in psychiatric patients. *Journal of Personality Assessment, 47,* 427–439.

Zimmer, D., Borchardt, E., & Fischle, C. (1983). Sexual fantasies of sexually distressed and nondistressed men and women: An empirical comparison. *Journal of Sex and Marital Therapy, 9,* 38–50.

Zucker, B. G., Craske, M. G., Barrios, V., & Holguin, M. (2002). Thought–action fusion: Can it be corrected? *Behaviour Research and Therapy, 40,* 653–664.

CHAPTER 9

UNWANTED INTRUSIVE THOUGHTS

Present Status and Future Directions

CHRISTINE PURDON

Unwanted intrusive thoughts can be a nuisance at best or a scourge of the mind at worst. In clinical states they often persist despite strenuous effort to control them, wreaking havoc on concentration and mood, and making even the simplest of tasks difficult to execute. It is no surprise that disorders characterized most prominently by the persistent recurrence of unwanted distressing thoughts are either the most difficult to treat (chronic worry, insomnia, obsessive–compulsive disorder [OCD], posttraumatic stress disorder [PTSD], schizophrenia and paraphilias) or the most vulnerable to relapse (depression). Our patients come to us with the same quandaries: How do I stop what I have not willed? What does it mean about me that my mind generates these thoughts? Why can't I control these thoughts? What can I do to stop them? Will my thoughts lead to behavior?

Over the past three decades social experimental research on consciousness and clinical research on the cognitive basis of various psychological disorders have provided some new insights into the nature of conscious thought. In fact, this volume is possible because of the knowledge base now available on one particular aspect of conscious thought: unwanted intrusive thoughts. And yet, our understanding of this cognitive phenomenon is still quite rudimentary and diverse theoretical perspectives can be found on the topic. In the psychoanalytic view, unwanted thoughts are considered manifestations of unconscious conflict (e.g., mental parapraxes), interesting only to the extent that they allude to the nature of the underlying conflict that is the root of the disorder. Proponents of positivism in science (e.g., Skinner) rejected the idea of studying thoughts because, unlike behavior, they cannot be accessed and observed directly by the researcher. Other arguments against studying thoughts have been made as well. For example, Wells (Chapter 5, this volume) reminds us chapter that until the 1980s, worry was considered simply the cognitive component of anxiety and was therefore of little interest in and of itself. Intrusive thoughts in schizophrenia (e.g., commanding voices) have been viewed as the product of a malfunctioning brain and therefore not amenable to intervention or worthy of study from a cognitive–clinical perspective.

Early behavioral views of unwanted thoughts understood them as stimuli that gave rise to an aversive response which could be extinguished through the process of reciprocal inhibition (Wolpe, 1958) or exposure (Marks, 1987). In reciprocal inhibition, a response incompatible with the emotion evoked by the thought is induced (e.g., relaxation or pain), whereas in exposure the individual holds the thought in mind until the aversive response extinguishes (Marks, 1987). This model of unwanted thoughts could be empirically tested (assuming the reliability of subjective reports of thoughts), and it certainly yielded interventions that targeted the thoughts directly. However, reasons *why* a thought might give rise to a fearful response were not systematically studied until Rachman (1971, 1976, 1981; Rachman & de Silva, 1978; Rachman & Hodgson, 1980) began examining individuals' cognitive and affective responses to obsessions. The late 1970s also saw the emergence of Beck's cognitive model of depression, which considered that negative mood does not derive from events themselves but rather from a negative appraisal or meaning of the event (e.g., Beck, Rush, Shaw, & Emery, 1979).

It is at this point that we begin to see significant interest in thoughts, appraisal, and emotion. Borkovec and his colleagues examined the role of appraisal in anxiety (e.g., Borkovec, Grayson, & Hennings, 1979), defined the construct of worry, and began to examine factors that influenced its course (e.g., Borkovec, 1985; Borkovec, Robinson, Pruzinsky, & DePree, 1983). Foa pioneered work on biased cognitive processes in

OCD (e.g., Persons & Foa, 1984) and developed her model for the mechanisms of emotional habituation, which emphasizes the role of thoughts and appraisal in the persistence of anxiety disorders (Foa & Kozak, 1986). Here were models of psychopathology that implicated cognitive appraisal as a key mechanism in the development and persistence of psychopathology, and models whose tenets, like those of behavioral approaches, lent themselves to empirical validation.

An explosion of research on cognitive appraisal followed, which in turn fostered the development of increasingly sophisticated and useful models for understanding psychopathology. Methods for studying thoughts were refined, including indirect means of assessing cognition (visual dot-probe tasks, modified Stroop tasks, etc.) and direct means (i.e., thought sampling and self-report). As a result of these efforts we began to see improvements in our ability to treat mental disorders, particularly depression and, more recently, OCD. In many ways our understanding of the relationships between thoughts, mood, and behavior has progressed. However, clinical researchers and practitioners continue to ask the same questions as do our patients; what can be done to help people who suffer from persistent, unwanted clinically relevant intrusive thoughts?

THE CENTRALITY OF APPRAISAL

Fortunately we are beginning to discover some answers to these fundamental questions about the origins, persistence, and treatment of unwanted intrusive thoughts. Each chapter in this book presents novel and exciting breakthroughs in our understanding of recurrent, unwanted thoughts and each has direct treatment implications. A review of these chapters readily yields the conclusion that what is common across the disparate types of thoughts studied is the centrality of the *appraisal* of unwanted thoughts as the driving mechanism behind the distress and ameliorative coping strategies that serve as key factors in the persistence of the disorder. Several types of appraisal are relevant. First, there is the negative appraisal of the thought's content. Second, there is the negative appraisal of what it means to have the thought in the first place. Third, appraisals may focus on the necessity and utility of using a specific ameliorative strategy to control the thoughts and their negative affect, as well as on the perceived consequences of failing to use that strategy.

In his model of generalized anxiety disorder (GAD) Wells (Chapter 5, this volume) suggests that positive beliefs about worry (e.g., "Worry helps me cope, if I don't worry I'm tempting fate") guide selection of worry as a strategy for coping with future threat. However, worry that persists becomes increasingly aversive and is perceived as uncontrollable which, in turn, leads to worry about the worry ("If I don't stop worrying I'll go crazy," "My worrying will kill me"). This increases anxiety, which in turn leads to the selection of further worry as a means of coping. The negative beliefs about worry also drive avoidance of worry triggers and suppression of worry. The latter causes individuals to be hypervigilant to worry-related cues, thereby increasing the frequency of worry and enhancing the belief that worry is uncontrollable.

In their chapter on obsessional thoughts, Clark and O'Connor (Chapter 6, this volume) argue that a number of different appraisal types contributes to the persistence of OCD. These include appraisals that the intrusion (1) has significance for some future negative action (e.g., "Having this thought makes it more likely to happen"), (2) signifies some personal immorality or irresponsibility (e.g., "Having a thought about X is as bad as doing X," "If I don't do anything to prevent potential harm caused by this thought it is the same as deliberately causing harm"), (3) indicates that the thoughts must be controlled (e.g., "Control over thoughts is an important part of self-control," "If I don't control these thoughts it means I'm crazy"), and (4) represents an inconsistency with valued aspects of the self and/or with immediate goals (e.g., "Does this thought mean I am a homicidal maniac at heart?" "Am I actually quite irrational and crazy at heart?"). These faulty appraisals create considerable distress and motivate the individual to engage in strategies to neutralize potential harm. Furthermore, the maladaptive appraisals often lead to thought suppression responses. When the individual engages in these ameliorative strategies anxiety is reduced, but the person is never able to learn that the appraisal is incorrect. Suppression also makes the individual hypervigilant for unwanted thought occurrences, and the inevitable thought recurrences further enhance the negative appraisal of the thought as important and potentially dangerous internal stimuli.

In his model of schizophrenia, Morrison (chapter 7, this volume) argues that psychotic experiences, especially hearing voices, derive from the occurrence of an unwanted intrusive thought that is attributed to an external source. Further faulty appraisal of the intrusive thoughts as dangerous and as having negative consequences leads to the use of suppression and other problematic strategies that contribute to increased frequency and intensity of the thought. Positive beliefs about the utility of certain behaviors characteristic of psychotic disorders also drive their use (e.g., "Being paranoid keeps you from being harmed"). In their comprehensive review, Falsetti, Monnier, and Resnick (Chapter 2, this volume) note that PTSD develops when individuals appraise the trauma and its sequelae (e.g., intrusive thoughts about the trauma) as having implications for current threat (e.g., "If this happened to me, the world is a dangerous place and I must be vigilant forever"), as having negative implications for the self ("I can't rely on my own judgment"), and as resulting from one's own carelessness ("I should have known better"). Erroneous conclusions about the meaning of the intrusive thought or image recurrences (e.g., "Having this thought means I'm crazy") will lead to heightened distress over the thoughts as well as greater symptom severity.

Harvey (Chapter 4, this volume) suggests that certain dysfunctional beliefs such as "not getting 'enough' sleep can be harmful to health and performance" (both while attempting to fall asleep and during the day following a "poor" night of sleep) play a key role in the persistence of insomnia. Such beliefs and appraisals may lead to behaviors that actually interfere with nighttime sleep (napping during the day) and to hypervigilance for signs that performance and well-being are impaired by the perceived lack of sleep. This will lead to the interpretation of benign events as evidence of harm due to sleep deprivation. Harvey also argues that negative appraisal of insomnia drives suppression of thoughts that interfere with sleep, which has the unintended effect of actually increasing the frequency of the unwanted mental intrusions. These faulty appraisals may be in part driven by erroneous beliefs about sleep requirements, the consequences of insomnia, and the negative effects of failing to maintain continuous nighttime sleep. Finally, Harvey observes that one feature that distinguishes individuals with insomnia is that they hold more positive beliefs about the utility of worrying in bed (e.g., "worry helps me sort out/put things in order in my mind"). Thus, like Wells's individuals with GAD, worry is selected as a strategy for removing obstacles to current goals, but one that ironically impedes the attainment of these goals.

In his work on thought suppression, dysphoric mood, and depressive relapse, Wenzlaff (Chapter 3, this volume) observes that people who have previously been depressed are vulnerable to relapse when they interpret negative thoughts as being a sign that they are becoming depressed again, and thus are motivated to suppress them. He also argues that depressed individuals suppress depressive rumination in an attempt to alleviate negative mood. Suppression is ineffective because other negative thoughts are much more accessible when mood state is low and are more likely to be used as distracters from the "to-be-suppressed" thought. Furthermore, suppression efforts are easily thwarted by cognitive load, so if the individual attempting to suppress negative thoughts is under stress, suppression efforts are more likely to fail. As a consequence, the person experiences more frequent depressotypic thoughts, a further decline in mood, and heightened accessibility of other depressotypic cognitions.

In their review of intrusive thoughts in paraphilias, Marshall and Langton (Chapter 8, this volume) note that for many offenders, the central problem in exploitative sexual behavior is the *absence* of negative appraisal of sexual thoughts (e.g., "These thoughts and acts are harmless; society overreacts") and the derivation of pleasure from the thoughts. (Even if the individual does not want to have the thoughts, they are sexually arousing and pleasurable at some level.) Deviant sexual fantasies are the first step in the chain of behavior leading to a sexual offense. Individuals who appraise their thoughts about sexual exploitation as enjoyable and harmless are more likely to generate fantasies around them and/or masturbate in response to the thoughts, the latter of which serves as positive reinforcement for having the thoughts. Concerns about acting on the thoughts and getting caught, as well as not wanting to be a sexually exploitative person, may motivate attempts to suppress deviant sexual thoughts and fantasies, but these attempts may make them more accessible later on, which also increases the potential for further sexual offenses. At the same time, negative appraisals of the self ("I am a bad, weak person") are connected with recidivism. When offenders experience negative mood they are more likely to use deviant fantasies as a means of ameliorating their bad feelings about themselves. After an offense, catastrophizing about the consequences of getting caught typically occurs and serves as a deterrent for reoffending. However, the individual gradually habituates to the fear, and it ceases to serve as a deterrent.

INFORMATION-PROCESSING BIASES

What accounts for the distorted or "unbalanced" appraisals we see in various psychological disorders? The cognitive–clinical perspective posits that individuals with psychological problems possess negative schemas relevant to the self, world, and future that subsequently guide how information is attended to, stored, and retrieved. Information consistent with the schema has higher priority for processing and is readily encoded. Information inconsistent with the schema has lower processing priority (i.e., is more likely to go unnoticed) and is ignored, discounted, or trivialized. In the chapters presented here, information-processing biases and deficits are implicated either implicitly or explicitly in the persistence of unwanted cognition.

Wenzlaff (Chapter 3, this volume) reviews a significant body of work that reveals a negative bias in attentional processes in depression, such that negative stimuli relevant to self, world, and future are given higher processing priority. This processing bias will serve to maintain negative mood and may cause it to become worse. Morrison (Chapter 7, this volume) suggests that individuals prone to psychotic disorders tend to be selectively attentive to threatening information (as in persecutory delusions) and to internal events such as intrusive thoughts (as in auditory delusions). Harvey (Chapter 4, this volume) observes that individuals with insomnia tend to hold positive beliefs about the utility of worrying in bed, despite the fact that their worry is seldom productive. She suggests that schema relevant to the utility of worry guide the processing of information about worry such that times when worry is productive are stored in memory and readily recalled, whereas incidents in which worry is unproductive are not accurately encoded in memory.

Clark and O'Connor (Chapter 6, this volume) note that one important factor in the escalation of a normal intrusive thought into an obsession is the experience of the thought as being inconsistent with existing schema about the self (e.g., a loving parent has a thought of harming his child). Most individuals would assimilate the obsessional thought into their existing schema (e.g., "Even a person like me can have thoughts like this"), whereas those prone to developing obsessions may actually change their schema to accommodate the thought (e.g., "Maybe I am a homicidal maniac at heart"). Once the self-schema is questioned or altered, schema-congruent information is recalled and elaborated ("there was that time in grade school when I pushed that kid to the ground") and schema-incongruent information is ignored. This has the cumulative effect of strengthening an emerging negative self-schema.

In addition to the selective processing of OCD-related schematic information, Clark and O'Connor note that individuals with OCD also engage in a faulty inferential process that will further contribute to a tendency toward information processing bias. In OCD a primary inference of doubt develops from faulty deductive reasoning characterized by a selective use of factual information, categorization errors, and the creation of an imaginary sequence of possible events. This inverse inference process generates a state of *inferential confusion* in which an imaginary discourse of doubt is confused with reality. In this formulation of OCD, then, biased information processing plays a key role in the pathogenesis of obsessional thinking, in terms of both schema-driven processing and faulty inferential thinking.

Falsetti et al. (Chapter 2, this volume) note that there is some evidence to suggest that individuals with PTSD process information about the trauma in a more rudimentary, "data driven" manner rather than at a higher-order conceptual level. That is, sensory and perceptual information is stored without being processed at a more abstract, conceptual level. This interferes with the ability to process the meaning of the event and is associated with the development of disorganized memories of the event. Negative appraisal of the experience of having fragmented, or disorganized memories (e.g., "There is something wrong with me that I can't remember this better") is associated with an escalation in PTSD symptomatology. Falsetti et al. suggest that this "data driven" processing may occur because the individual has no existing schema capable of processing the event conceptually. The traumatic event may be so inconsistent with existing schema of self, world, and future that it cannot be processed in accordance with the person's internal representation of experience. Individuals prone to developing PTSD may accommodate to the traumatic event by changing schema ("The world is dangerous," "I cannot trust my judgment," "I am a bad person deserving of this," "Worse things could happen at any moment"), which in turn will bias one's appraisal of specific events.

Other types of information processing biases have also been implicated in the persistence of intrusive thoughts. Harvey (Chapter 4, this volume) concluded that individuals with insomnia also tend to overestimate the amount of time it takes to fall asleep and underestimate how much sleep is obtained. She notes that time estimates increase with the number of information units an individual is processing. Individuals who worry in bed are processing a significant number of information units. Thus, they overestimate the amount of time it has taken to fall asleep. As noted earlier, Clark and O'Connor emphasize the role of faulty inferential processes in the persistence of obsessional doubt. They argue that individuals with OCD experience a doubt but behave as if the doubt is actually a truth (e.g., "Maybe my hands are dirty" becomes "My hands are dirty"), even in the absence of any information to the contrary (e.g., that the hands had just been thoroughly washed minutes earlier and nothing dirty touched since). For the person with OCD, the premise is "guilty until proven innocent," except that information that may establish "innocence" (or, evidence of no serious contamination) is not noticed or is trivialized or discounted.

DEFINING MENTAL INTRUSIONS

What is an intrusive thought? Clark and Rhyno (Chapter 1, this volume) offer a detailed discussion on the nature of unwanted intrusive thoughts, concluding that mental intrusions are commonplace in nonclinical and clinical samples and are characteristic of a wide variety of psychological disorders. Are all intrusive thoughts alike? Common elements include intrusiveness (i.e., they take attentional priority and are difficult to discount or ignore), unwantedness, and an association with negative mood. All unwanted thoughts can be internally or externally triggered. However, there are key distinctions between unwanted intrusive thoughts with similar content and/or process that can give rise to quite different symptom profiles. Harvey (Chapter 4, this volume) comments that important distinctions can be made between worry, rumination, and intrusive thoughts, especially in terms of the temporal orientation (e.g., rumination involves thoughts about past events, worry about future events). She argues that clarity on these distinctions would contribute to a better understanding of different clinical disorders. For example, depressive rumination tends to be characterized by thoughts about *perceived* past failures and tends to be actively generated, except during remission, when individuals try to suppress such thoughts (Wenzlaff, Chapter 3, this volume).

On the other hand, worries that are characteristic of GAD and thoughts reported by people with insomnia tend to reflect concerns about current and future problems. They tend to be actively generated, at least initially, but lead to active attempts at control when their costs are perceived to outweigh the benefits. Wells (Chapter 5, this volume) also notes that the content of worries tends to be more commonplace than that of obsessions. Obsessions are more strongly disapproved of than worry and are perceived as threatening because of their inconsistency with important self-views. The unwanted intrusive thoughts characteristic of PTSD are distinct in that they involve memories, impressions, or thoughts about an actual event that took place in the past. These thoughts are always strenuously resisted. The unwanted intrusions experienced by sex offenders are thoughts about engaging in sexual activity that is desirable but could result in prison and social ostracization. These thoughts may be actively generated (e.g., when the individual's mood is low) or suppressed (e.g., when the individual truly desires not to act out on the thoughts). Obsessional thoughts are unusual thoughts that do not make much sense and may be at total odds with one's personality, morals, values, and goals (especially in the case of repugnant obsessions). Obsessions give rise to active resistance and are rarely, if ever, actively generated (note that even if an individual "gives in" to the compulsion the moment the thought is experienced, he or she typically engages in strenuous attempts to avoid having the thought in the first place).

Unwanted intrusive thoughts, then, can vary in terms of content and process. One difficulty with categorizing on the basis of content alone is that the unwanted intrusions characteristic of one disorder can have content that is somewhat similar to the unwanted intrusions evident in another disorder. For example, unwanted thoughts about illness can be characteristic of OCD or GAD (or, for that matter, health anxiety). Unwanted thoughts about harming others can occur in OCD as well as in psychotic disorders, as Morrison points out. Thoughts about engaging in sexually exploitative behavior can be a characteristic of OCD or of a paraphilia. Process characteristics alone may not always distinguish between disorder-relevant intrusions, given that all unwanted intrusions can be internally or externally triggered and most are actively generated or suppressed depending on circumstances. To understand the nature of unwanted intrusive thoughts in any psychological disorder, it is important to take into account the thought content, process characteristics or properties, appraisal patterns, and functional responses to the mental intrusion.

EGO-DYSTONICITY: A DEFINING FEATURE OF UNWANTED INTRUSIVE THOUGHTS

Clark and O'Connor, Wenzlaff, and Wells (Chapters 6, 3, and 5, respectively, this volume) all suggest that one key distinguishing feature of unwanted intrusive thoughts may be the extent that the thought is consistent or inconsistent with an individual's morals, values, goals, and preferences. If one values being a loving parent, the thought of sexually molesting one's child is alarming because it is unexpected and repugnant. The thought is actively resisted because its content and the fact of its presence are so disturbing. The thought is, then, obsessional in nature. Individuals vulnerable to developing psychotic problems may experience such a thought as wholly ego alien but reconcile this dissonance by interpreting the thought as being externally imposed. The thought, then, is a psychotic delusion. However, if an individual is sexually attracted to children, the thought of molesting a child is sexually arousing and may be actively generated and elaborated. The thought, then, is a key feature of pedophilia.

As another example, consider the thought that maybe a loved one has been hurt in an accident. Concern over the safety of loved ones is ego-syntonic. However, if the thought is experienced as being ego-dystonic—that is, outside the realm of thoughts one would expect oneself to have, given the circumstances—the individual may begin to search for reasons for the occurrence of the thought. One interpretation is that the thought is a prophetic warning sign. This could lead to high anxiety and a perceived need to "undo" the harm potentiated by the thought (e.g., thinking a good thought about the person) and attempts not to have the thought again. On the other hand, if the person experiences the thought as ego-syntonic—that is, as rational under the circumstances and as a thought well within the realm of what he or she might expect—there is no search for an explanation as to why the thought occurred but, rather, a search for solutions to problems ensuing from the event represented in the thought. In the former case, we have symptoms of OCD; in the latter case, symptoms of GAD will emerge. Similarly, if one is facing a stressful day, thoughts about that day while attempting to fall asleep will be evaluated as entirely expected under these circumstances. Resolution lies not in determining the origins of the thoughts but, rather, in solving the real-life problems they represent. In PTSD, one major concern is why the thoughts of such a horrific event returns; although there is an historical context for the thought, the cognitions are wholly unwanted and unacceptable. Again, the individual searches for explanations, leading to consideration of the possibility that her or his mind is "breaking."

This construct of ego-dystonicity may be valuable in understanding why thoughts of the same content evoke quite different pathological responses. However, it too is complicated. Purdon and colleagues have attempted to operationalize and assess the construct of ego-dystonicity. They defined as ego-dystonic a thought that "is perceived as having little or no context within one's own sense of self or personality. That is, the thought is perceived as occurring outside the context of one's morals, attitudes, beliefs, preferences, past behaviour and/or one's expectations about the kinds of thoughts one would experience" (Cripps, 2000, p. 14). They are currently working on the development of a measure of ego-dystonicity. This self-report measure shows some ability to distinguish between thoughts characteristic of worry and of obsessions (Cripps, 2000). This approach is a beginning, but there are numerous difficulties inherent in assessing ego-dystonicity that still need to be resolved. First, over time a thought initially appraised as irrational and unexpected can begin to feel quite rational and comes to be expected. Second, if Purdon and Clark are correct, the individual may begin to accommodate the thought by altering the self-view; hence the thought becomes less ego-dystonic. Third, a thought may be ego-dystonic in that it is unwanted but ego-syntonic in that it has a context within the individual's sense of self (e.g., the pedophile who does not want to be a pedophile). Fourth, a thought may be ego-syntonic during one phase of a disorder (e.g., suicidal thoughts during severe depression) but more ego-dystonic during the recovery phase (e.g., suicidal thoughts after depression has remitted). Thus, ego-dystonicity fluctuates over time and course of a psychological problem.

It is important to note that ego-dystonicity is actually one form of thought appraisal. This returns us to the notion that it is not thought content or process that best distinguishes unwanted intrusive thoughts characteristic of one disorder versus another but, rather, the pattern of appraisal. Appraisal not only determines whether a "normal" unwanted intrusive thought becomes a clinically significant symptom but also appears to determine what kind of symptom profile will develop.

CONTROL OF UNWANTED COGNITIONS

Thought suppression is viewed as a central factor in thought persistence by all authors. Again, it is the appraisal of the thought as requiring conscious control that drives suppression in all cases. Interest in the role of suppression in the persistence of unwanted intrusions was sparked by Wegner's (1994) seminal paper that suggested that suppression leads to an ironic increase in the frequency of the to-be-suppressed thought once suppression efforts have ceased. These findings and the model for the ironic effect of suppression are reviewed thoroughly by Wenzlaff (Chapter 3, this volume). Suppression is insidious for three reasons. First, it may actually lead to an increase in unwanted thoughts. Second, suppression uses attentional resources because individuals must be vigilant to thought cues and be ready to distract themselves from the target thought. Thus, when people suppress, they are less able to concentrate on other relevant stimuli and their suppression efforts are readily disrupted with the introduction of competing attentional demands. Third, it is significantly more difficult to suppress mood-congruent than -incongruent thoughts because the controlled distracter search is much more likely to detect other mood-congruent thoughts as distracters. This will paradoxically lead to enhanced cueing of the unwanted target thought.

In his analysis of the persistence of unwanted thoughts in depression, Wenzlaff (Chapter 3, this volume) presents a series of studies examining the effects of suppression on depressive rumination. He first establishes that a negative bias in information processing is characteristic of depression, noting that depressed mood evokes processing biases and heightens accessibility to negative memories and thoughts, which in turn intensifies negative mood (associative network theory). Individuals who are depressed often will use suppression as a strategy to manage their mood. However, depressed individuals are highly susceptible to experiencing the ironic effects of suppression because they are more likely to choose distracters that have an emotional association to the material they are trying to suppress. This biased selection of mood-congruent distractors occurs because negative mood and stress drain cognitive resources, thereby making it difficult to generate distracters. Furthermore, inevitable failures in thought control may be attributed to personal inadequacy, leading to a renewal of mental control efforts. Wenzlaff (Chapter 3, this volume) also found that individuals who were previously depressed actually engaged in fairly consistent efforts at suppressing negative thoughts, efforts that are readily thwarted when a competing attentional demand is introduced. This helps explain why depressive relapse is more likely to occur in times of stress; stress is the "cognitive load" that thwarts suppression efforts.

It is important to note that the ironic effect of suppression has not been consistently replicated, with many studies finding no effect of suppression on frequency and some consistently finding it only with specific kinds of thoughts (see Purdon, 1999, 2004, for reviews). Falsetti et al. (Chapter 2, this volume) note that studies on suppression of trauma-related thoughts in PTSD have consistently found an ironic effect of suppression on frequency and the suppression of trauma-related thoughts in the immediate posttrauma period and this was associated with a greater likelihood of the development of PTSD. On the other hand, suppression of obsessional thoughts in clinical samples, of worry, or of cognitive intrusions during sleep onset, does not have an ironic effect on frequency. However, Purdon, Antony, and Rowa (in press) found that inevitable failures in thought control while suppression efforts are in operation are associated with more negative appraisal of the thought's meaning, more negative mood state, and escalating attempts at thought control, findings consistent with those reported by Wenzlaff. Similarly, Harvey (Chapter

4, this volume) found that suppression of cognitive intrusions while trying to sleep did not increase the number of unwanted intrusions, but it was associated with later sleep onset and poorer sleep quality. Even if suppression does not lead to a paradoxical increase in unwanted thought frequency, it is clear that it has other insidious effects on mood and thought appraisal.

Finally, the act of intentional suppression assumes that the to-be-suppressed thought is dangerous or harmful and so must be controlled; a faulty assumption that must be overcome if the disorder is to be successfully treated. Even in the case of sex offenders, where the thought itself actually is dangerous (in that it is the first step in the chain of behavioral actions leading to offending), suppression is unlikely to be useful because it may lead to a greater frequency of thoughts. (There is not enough empirical evidence to draw conclusions about the effect of suppression on frequency of sexual thoughts in sexual offenders.) Furthermore, suppression does not provide the offender the opportunity to evaluate the danger represented by the thought in an appropriate manner. Marshall and Langton (Chapter 8, this volume) suggest that the sequence of behavior leading to offenses is best interrupted by a full, balanced appraisal of the thought, the actions it represents, the impact on the victim, and the generation of alternative coping strategies.

TREATMENT IMPLICATIONS

These chapters contribute substantially to the arsenal of resources clinicians can use to treat persistent, unwanted negative thoughts. It is apparent from the reviews of different disorders that in addition to addressing negative appraisal, the assessment of beliefs (appraisals) about the efficacy of problematic coping strategies such as suppression, distraction, and worrying must be considered. Information-processing biases are present, such as time estimations based on information units processed rather than actual passage of time and the faulty deductive reasoning and inverse inferences evident in OCD. Erroneous beliefs about thoughts and thought processes should also be assessed and corrective intervention strategies instituted to bring about schematic change. Recognition of the centrality of unwanted negative intrusions in the phenomenology of these various disorders makes "third wave" cognitive therapies, such as mindfulness-based cognitive therapy, more attractive. As Harvey (Chapter 4, this volume) notes, interventions that teach clients to develop a detached awareness from their thoughts (e.g., watching their thoughts float by without acting on or reacting to them) might prove especially helpful in treating disorders characterized by persistent unwanted thoughts. This has obvious implications for correcting faulty appraisals of the meaning of different kinds of thoughts, as well as implicitly helping clients learn that their strategies for coping with the thoughts are not necessary; that is, that unwanted intrusive thoughts appear and disappear on their own if left alone.

FUTURE DIRECTIONS

The chapters reviewed here make a convincing argument for the importance of unwanted intrusions as cardinal characteristics of major mental illness. Many questions remain. What is the mechanism by which normal unwanted thoughts become clinically significant symptoms; that is, what drives the specific appraisal that contributes to symptom formation? What is the effect of thought suppression on thought frequency, appraisal, and mood state across disorders?

Examination of unwanted thoughts presents numerous challenges to researchers. First, what is a thought? Take the example of obsessional doubt as to whether an appliance has been turned off. A typical sample of the chain of thoughts would be, "Maybe I didn't really turn the stove off, maybe I just thought I did. I'd better go back and check it. I don't really want to check because I'm running late. But, if I don't check and the stove is left on, a scrap of paper could blow onto the burner and cause a fire and it will be all my fault. I'd better go back and check." Is that one thought or five thoughts? Are all the thoughts obsessional or do they represent a mix of obsession and worry? Both Harvey and Wells suggest that unwanted intrusive thoughts typically trigger worry. In this case, we could consider the first thought to be the obsession and the rest a worry episode.

Most research on unwanted intrusive thoughts has not attempted to define what a "thought occurrence" is, typically leaving it up to participants to tell us when they have had a particular type of thought. Some studies use "stream-of-consciousness verbalization" in which participants say their thoughts aloud into a tape recorder. The stream of verbalization is then coded for content (e.g., directly related to a specific thought, indirectly related to a specific thought, and unrelated to a specific thought) as in Wegner's work or in research by Roemer and Borkovec (1994). Another means of assessing thought frequency is to assess the proportion of time spent on a particular content area or theme (D. A. Clark, personal communication, December, 2003).

There is some evidence to suggest that the methodology employed to record thought occurrences has an impact on the number of cognitive events reported by participants when the thought is considered "forbidden." For example, in their meta-analysis of experimental investigations of thought suppression Abramowitz, Tolin, and Street (2001) found that studies that used thought expression instructions (i.e., instructions to actively generate the thought) as opposed to "think anything" instructions (i.e., think anything you like, including the target thought) had a greater rebound effect. Studies in which thought frequency was assessed by overt means (e.g., stream of consciousness reporting and ringing a bell when the thought occurred) exhibited a greater rebound effect than did studies that used more covert means (e.g., pressing a key when the thought occurs). The rebound effect was stronger for studies in which participants were suppressing thoughts about an entire story rather than suppressing a specific, discrete thought.

Another problem for research on unwanted intrusive thoughts is that thought frequency is confounded by duration (see Purdon, 2004; Purdon et al., in press). If participants are instructed to record how often a thought occurs in a given period, someone with three thought occurrences would appear to have less control than the person who reports one thought occurrence. However, in the latter case, the one thought occurrence may have lasted the entire duration of the interval, whereas in the former case the thoughts were readily dismissed. The person who has more thought occurrences but who is able to dismiss them may subjectively suffer considerably less than the person who simply cannot dismiss the thought at all.

Finally, given that unwanted intrusive thoughts have distinct characteristics, it is critical that researchers clearly define the cognitive phenomenon under investigation. For example, in pilot research, we found that individuals who are "normal worriers" (i.e., who score within a half standard deviation of the nonclinical mean on diagnostic measures of worry) will, when asked, "worry" about a problem. However, unlike high worriers (those scoring within half a standard deviation of the clinical mean on diagnostic measures of worry), normal worriers remained focused on the immediate problem (as opposed to the problems generated in the negative catastrophic fantasy) and generated practical solutions, thereby resolving the matter quite readily. Their worry led to a reduction in anxiety. Regardless, they described this process as "worry" and found it a stressful process. The "worry" of high worriers was characterized by a much higher ratio of catastrophizing to problem solving. This begs the question as to whether the positive beliefs about "worry" reported by "normal" worriers are actually quite realistic; their worry does indeed help them cope and reduce anxiety but at an apparent high personal cost (i.e., elevated stress). Although "normal worriers" and "clinical worriers" use the same label (i.e., worry) for an intrusive thought process, nevertheless the actual properties and outcomes associated with self-labeled worry were quite different.

When we attempt to assess unwanted obsessional thoughts in nonclinical samples, participants often end up reporting on worries—that is, commonplace problems that are ego-syntonic in nature. Different approaches have been taken to rectify this problem. Purdon and Clark (1993, 1994) developed an inventory of obsessional thoughts (i.e., Revised Obsessional Intrusions Inventory; ROII) for use in nonclinical samples. The ROII was based on structured interviews with a large sample of nonclinical individuals in which obsessional thoughts were defined in accordance with criteria for obsessions according to the third edition, revised of *Diagnostic and Statistical Manual of Mental Disorders* (DSM-III-R; American Psychiatric Association, 1987). The advantage of this measure is that items were restricted to content that was clearly obsessional in nature. The disadvantage is that obsessional thoughts are highly idiosyncratic and the items in the ROII may not represent a specific individual's obsession-relevant concerns.

The Obsessive Compulsive Cognitions Working Group (1997, 2001) developed the Interpretation of Intrusions Inventory to assess appraisal of obsessional thoughts. It relies on a verbal definition of the phenomenon, a list of examples, and a definition of what kinds of thoughts are *not* of interest (i.e., worries). However, research from our lab and others indicates that despite the caveats in the instructions, nonclinical individuals still tend to report thoughts that appear more representative of worry than OCD (e.g., "Thoughts that my boyfriend will leave me").

Falsetti et al. also emphasize that in PTSD, thoughts about the trauma can take various forms, including intrusive memories of the event itself; thoughts about the unfairness and injustice of the trauma; thoughts about the event's meaning for the self, world, and future; and thoughts about the trauma sequelae. When investigating unwanted intrusions in PTSD, then, it may be important to specify the different types of unwanted trauma-related intrusions and the appraisal associated with each. As mentioned previously, intrusive memories about the event itself may well be experienced as ego-dystonic, leading to active resistance, whereas thoughts about the event's meaning for self, world, and future may be entirely ego-syntonic, leading to active elaboration and generation.

Each of the contributors to this edited book have grappled with the phenomenon of unwanted intrusive thoughts, images, and impulses in the pathogenesis of various clinical disorders. Each of the contributors has offered a clearer specification of this cognitive phenomenon. In this regard, progress has been made in our knowledge of the nature and treatment of unwanted intrusive thoughts. The research literature reviewed in the preceding chapters provides a base for a more informative conceptualization of unwanted intrusive cognition. However, much more needs to be learned in order to more effectively alleviate persistent unwanted mental intrusions in distressed individuals.

REFERENCES

Abramowitz, J. S., Tolin, D. F., & Street, G. P. (2001). Paradoxical effects of thought suppression: A meta-analysis of controlled studies. *Clinical Psychology Review, 21*, 683–703.

American Psychiatric Association. (1987). *Diagnostic and statistical manual of mental disorders* (3rd ed., rev.). Washington, DC: Author.

Beck, A. T., Rush, A. J., Shaw, B. F., & Emery, G. (1979). *Cognitive therapy of depression*. New York: Guilford Press.

Borkovec, T. D. (1985). Worry: A potentially valuable concept. *Behaviour Research and Therapy, 23*, 481–482.

Borkovec, T. D., Grayson, J. B., & Hennings, B. L. (1979). Mitigation of false physical feedback effects on anxiety via cognitive appraisal. *Cognitive Therapy and Research, 3*, 381–387.

Borkovec, T. D., Robinson, E., Pruzinsky, T., & DePree, J. A. (1983). Preliminary exploration of worry: some characteristics and processes. *Behaviour Research and Therapy, 21*, 9–16.

Cripps, E. (2000). *Ego-dystonicity: Assessment and relationship to thought control strategies*. Unpublished master's thesis, University of Waterloo, Ontario, Canada.

Foa, E. B., & Kozak, M. J. (1986). Emotional processing of fear: Exposure to corrective information. *Psychological Bulletin, 99*, 20–35.

Marks, I. (1987). *Fears, phobias and rituals*. Oxford, UK: Oxford University Press.

Obsessive Compulsive Cognitions Working Group. (1997). Cognitive assessment of obsessive compulsive disorder. *Behaviour Research and Therapy, 35*, 667–681.

Obsessive Compulsive Cognitions Working Group. (2001). Development and initial validation of the obsessive beliefs questionnaire and the interpretation of intrusions inventory. *Behaviour Research and Therapy, 39*, 987–1006.

Persons, J. B., & Foa, E. B. (1984). Processing of fearful and neutral information by obsessive compulsives. *Behaviour Research and Therapy, 22*, 259–265.

Purdon, C. (1999). Thought suppression and psychopathology. *Behaviour Research and Therapy, 37*, 1029–1054.

Purdon, C. (2004). Empirical investigations of thought suppression in OCD. *Journal of Behaviour Therapy and Experimental Psychiatry, 35*, 121–136.

Purdon, C., & Clark, D. A. (1993). Obsessional intrusive thoughts in nonclinical subjects. Part I. Content and relation with depressive, anxious and obsessional symptoms. *Behaviour Research and Therapy, 31*, 713–720.

Purdon, C., & Clark, D. A. (1994). Perceived control and appraisal of obsessional intrusive thoughts: A replication and extension. *Behavioural and Cognitive Psychotherapy, 22*, 269–286.

Purdon, C., Faull, M., Cripps, E., & Rowa, K. (2004). *Development of a measure of ego dystonicity.* Manuscript in preparation.

Purdon, C., Rowa, K., & Antony, M. M. (in press). Thought supression and its effects on thought frequency, appraisal and mood state in individuals with obsessive–compulsive disorder. *Behaviour Research and Therapy.*

Rachman, S. (1971). Obsessional ruminations. *Behaviour Research and Therapy, 9*, 229–235.

Rachman, S. (1976). The modification of obsessions: A new formulation. *Behaviour Research and Therapy, 14*, 437–443.

Rachman, S. (1981). Part I. Unwanted intrusive cognitions. *Advances in Behaviour Research and Therapy, 3*, 89–99.

Rachman, S., & de Silva, P. (1978). Abnormal and normal obsessions. *Behaviour Research and Therapy, 16*, 233–248.

Rachman, S., & Hodgson, R. J. (1980). *Obsessions and compulsions.* Englewood Cliffs: Prentice Hall.

Roemer, L., & Borkovec, T. D. (1994). Effects of suppressing thoughts about emotional material. *Journal of Personality and Social Psychology, 103*, 467–474.

Wegner, D. M. (1994). Ironic processes of mental control. *Psychological Review, 101*, 34–52.

Wolpe, J. (1958). *Psychotherapy by reciprocal inhibition.* Stanford, CA: Stanford University Press.

INDEX

f indicates a figure; *t,* a table.

Abstinence violation effect, 204–205
Active memory, 22–23. *See also*
    Memory
Alcohol use, sexual thoughts and, 213–
    214
Anxiety
    depression and, 56
    development of obsessions and, 150,
        151*f,* 152
    inference-based treatment and, 167
    learning theory and, 31
    obsessions and, 147, 160
    worry and, 120–121, 124, 137–138,
        227, 229
Anxiety disorders
    compared to depressive intrusions,
        57–59
    emotional habituation model of, 228
    insomnia and, 87
Anxious thoughts, in nonclinical
    individuals, 8–10
Appraisal theory, 150, 151*f*
Appraisals. *See also* Beliefs
    assessment and, 185
    centrality of, 228–231
    cognitive-behavioral treatment and,
        164*t*
    description, 10–11
    development of obsessions and, 151*f*

primary, 156–158
psychosis and, 177, 192
secondary, 158–159, 161–163, 168–
    169
of sexual offenders, 201–205, 219
theories of, 228
treatment and, 187, 239–240
of worry, 15, 121–122, 124
Assessment
    description, 240–243
    Interpretations of Intrusions
        Inventory, 161–162
    Metacognitions Questionnaire, 128
    Obsessive Beliefs Questionnaire,
        161–162
    posttraumatic stress disorder and,
        39–41
    psychosis and, 185–187
    Sleep Disturbance Questionnaire, 90
    Thought Control Questionnaire, 105
    Utility of Pre-sleep Worry
        Questionnaire, 102–103
    White Bear Suppression Inventory,
        56–57, 58*t*
    of worry, 123
Attention
    cognitive interference to, 6
    controlling intrusive thoughts and,
        11

Attentional bias, depression and, 60–61
Attributions
    depression and, 67–68
    development of intrusions and, 180
    psychosis and, 177
Autobiographical memory. *See also*
        Memory
    posttraumatic stress disorder and, 33
    trauma-related intrusions and, 37
Autogenous intrusive thoughts, 10–11
Automatic negative thoughts, 17–18,
        55–56
Automatic thoughts, 17–18
Avoidance behaviors
    learning theory and, 31
    obsessive–compulsive disorder and,
        164t
    posttraumatic stress disorder and, 47
    trauma-related intrusions and, 38,
        40–41
    worry as, 121, 124

B

Behavior, inferences and, 155–156
Behavioral experiments
    beliefs regarding sleep and, 108
    case example of, 191
    metacognitive therapy for GAD and,
        137–138
    obsessive–compulsive disorder and,
        164t
    psychosis and, 188
    regarding sleep, 110–111
Behavioral responses, worry and, 123
Behaviors, avoidance
    learning theory and, 31
    obsessive–compulsive disorder and, 164t
    posttraumatic stress disorder and, 47
    trauma-related intrusions and, 38,
        40–41
    worry as, 121, 124
Behaviors, safety
    assessment and, 185
    development of intrusions and, 181–
        182
    treatment and, 188

Beliefs. *See also* Appraisals
    appraisals and, 228–231
    case conceptualization and, 135
    development of obsessions and, 152
    generalized anxiety disorder and, 141
    hallucinations, 178–179
    metacognitive therapy for GAD and,
        136–139
    secondary appraisals of control and,
        162–163
    sleep, 101–102, 108
    treatment and, 239–240
    worry, 133
Biases, cognitive
    depression and, 54, 59–61, 64, 77
    information processing and, 231–233
Biological impact of trauma, 37–38
Brain structure, 37–38
Brainstorming, 18–19
Broadcast, thought, 176

C

Case conceptualization. *See also*
        Treatment
    assessment and, 186
    in metacognitive therapy for GAD,
        134–136
Catastrophizing
    abstinence violation effect, 204
    faulty appraisals and, 157–158
    insomnia and, 99, 100f
    metacognitive therapy for GAD and,
        139
    regarding detection by sexual
        offenders, 206–211
    worry and, 121–122, 242
Category errors, obsessions and, 152–
        153t
Checking behaviors, 126–127. *See also*
        Obsessive–compulsive disorder
Choice, 75
Clinician Administered PTSD Scale. *See*
        also Assessment
    description, 39
    multiple channel exposure therapy
        and, 44

Cognitive attentional syndrome, 139
Cognitive-behavioral model
    of obsessive–compulsive disorder,
        146, 169–170
    of posttraumatic stress disorder, 33–
        34
Cognitive-behavioral therapy. *See also*
        Treatment
    obsessive–compulsive disorder, 163,
        164*t*, 165–169
    posttraumatic stress disorder and,
        41–46
    thought–action fusion and, 205
Cognitive biases
    depression and, 54, 59–61, 64, 77
    information-processing and, 231–233
Cognitive integrative model, 33
Cognitive interference, 6
Cognitive model of depression, 69–71,
        227
Cognitive processes, in the development
        of obsessions, 150, 151*f*, 152–
        159, 153*t*
Cognitive processing therapy, 41, 42.
        See also Treatment
Cognitive resources
    mood-related depletion of, 65–66
    stress-related depletion of, 66–67
Cognitive restructuring. *See also*
        Treatment
    abstinence violation effect and, 205
    obsessive–compulsive disorder and,
        164*t*
    posttraumatic stress disorder and,
        42, 45–46
Cognitive self-regulation model,
        psychosis and, 180
Cognitive therapy, psychosis and, 187,
        188–189
Cognitive vulnerability to depression,
        69–71, 227
Compulsions. *See also* Obsessive-
        compulsive disorder
    appraisals and, 156–157
    obsessions and, 147, 154–155
Concentration, insomnia and, 87

Confusion, inferential
    inference-based treatment and, 166–
        167
    obsessions and, 153–154
    obsessive–compulsive disorder and,
        155–156
Constructivist theory of posttraumatic
        stress disorder, 32
Content-specific hypothesis, 5
Control. *See also* Thought suppression
    appraisals and, 156–157
    assessment and, 185
    depression and, 57
    description, 11, 237–239
    development of obsessions and,
        151*f*
    generalized anxiety disorder and,
        131–132
    goal framing and, 71–73
    insomnia and, 103–107
    metacognition and, 128–129
    metacognitive therapy for GAD and,
        133–139
    posttraumatic stress disorder and,
        40–41
    secondary appraisals of, 158–159,
        161–163, 168–169
    treatment and, 109–110, 188
    of worry, 15, 121–122
Conviction, inference-based treatment
        and, 167
Coping strategies
    metaworry and, 131
    trauma-related intrusions and, 38
    worry as, 121, 229
Correlates of intrusive thoughts, 10–
        12
Current concern concept, 20–21. *See
        also* Origin of intrusive
        thoughts

D

Danger, challenging beliefs about, 137–
        138
Data-driven processing, posttraumatic
        stress disorder and, 47

Daytime intrusive thoughts
    description, 98–99, 100*f*, 101
    insomnia and, 112
Definitions of intrusive thoughts, 3–7,
    5*t*, 88–89, 175–176, 200, 234–
    235, 240–241
Delusions. *See also* Psychosis
    description, 176
    metaworry and, 183–184
    self-esteem and, 187–188
Depression
    appraisals and, 230–231
    cognitive processing therapy and, 42
    description, 77
    information-processing biases and,
      232
    insomnia and, 87, 89
    negative automatic thoughts and, 17
    obsessions and, 147
    role of intrusive thoughts in, 55–59,
      58*t*, 68–71
    rumination and, 16, 234
    thought suppression and, 64–68, 238
    treatment of, 71–76
    worry and, 124
Depressive thoughts, in nonclinical
    individuals, 9–10
Desensitization, 208
Diagnosis
    of clinical insomnia, 87
    of posttraumatic stress disorder, 46
    psychosis and, 176, 185
Disclosure, depression and, 73–74
Distraction
    assessment and, 185
    insomnia and, 104–105
    ironic process theory and, 63
    thought suppression and, 65–66
    worry as, 125–127
Distress levels
    posttraumatic stress disorder and, 47
    trauma-related intrusions and, 35–36
Domestic violence, 47
Doubt, inference of
    obsessions and, 149, 152–154
    treatment and, 165–168

Doubt, obsessions and, 148–149, 152–
    153, 160–161*f*
Duration, confusing with frequency,
    241
Dysfunctional attitudes, 54–55

E

Ego-dystonic intrusive thoughts. *See*
    also Obsessive–compulsive
    disorder
    description, 59, 235–237
    obsessions and, 123, 148
Emotional habituation model, 228
Emotional response. *See also*
    Emotions
    case conceptualization and, 134
    description, 6–7
    development of obsessions and, 150,
      151*f*, 152
    frequency of intrusive thoughts and,
      10
    and the origin of intrusive thoughts,
      21–22
Emotions. *See also* Emotional
    response
    metaworry and, 131
    mood-congruent thought, 62
    theories of, 227–228
Expectations, depression and, 55
Experiences, life, 32, 64
Exposure and response prevention. *See*
    also Exposure therapy;
    Treatment
    obsessive–compulsive disorder and,
      163
    secondary appraisals of control and,
      168–169
Exposure therapy. *See also* Exposure
    and response prevention;
    Treatment
    multiple channel exposure therapy
      and, 43
    posttraumatic stress disorder and,
      41–42
Expressive writing, depression and, 73–
    74

F

Fantasy
    description, 219
    sexual thoughts and, 214–216
Fear, learning theory and, 31
Flashbacks, 46
Flooding, 208
Frequency of intrusive thoughts
    assessing, 240–241
    emotions and, 10
    posttraumatic stress disorder and,
        35–36
    thought suppression and, 238–239
Functioning
    cognitive interference to, 6
    daytime intrusive thoughts and, 98–
        99
    insomnia and, 87
    worry and, 15, 121, 123
Fusions, 156

G

Generalized anxiety disorder
    appraisals and, 228–229
    compared to nonclinical individuals,
        12
    description, 141, 235
    ego-dystonicity and, 236
    imagery control and, 106
    insomnia and, 88–89
    metacognitive model of, 129–132,
        130*f*, 132–133
    metacognitive therapy for, 133–139
    worry and, 13–14, 119, 121, 122,
        124, 126–127, 234
Goal framing, 71–73. *See also*
    Treatment

H

Hallucinations
    assessment of, 186
    case example of, 189–192
    description, 176–179, 192
    development of intrusions and, 180,
        180–185

Hopelessness, 55
Horowitz's formulation, 22–23. *See
    also* Origin of intrusive
    thoughts
Hypnosis, posttraumatic stress disorder
    and, 41

I

Idiosyncratic meanings, 36–37
Imagery
    control, 105–107
    distraction, 104–105
    obsessions and, 152–153*t*
    worry and, 122
Imagery control, 105–107. *See also*
    Control
Imagery distraction, 104–105. *See also*
    Control; Distraction
Imaginal activity, 121
Imaginal exposure, 41, 42
Impact of Event Scale. *See also*
    Assessment
    description, 39
    multiple channel exposure therapy
        and, 44
Incidence of intrusive thoughts, 7–10
Inductive idiosyncratic narrative, 152
Inference-based treatment, 165–168.
    See also Treatment
Inference model, 155–156, 169–170
Inference of doubt
    obsessions and, 149, 152–154
    treatment and, 165–168
Inferences, empirical support for, 160–
    161*f*
Inferential confusion
    inference-based treatment and, 166–
        167
    model of, 150
    obsessions and, 153–154
    obsessive–compulsive disorder and,
        155–156
Inferential confusion model, 150
Information-processing
    assessment and, 185
    metacognition and, 154

Information-processing biases, 231–233
Information-processing theories
  depression and, 238
  description, 231–233
  metacognitive therapy for GAD and,
    139
  of posttraumatic stress disorder, 32,
    33
Insertion, thought, 176
Insomnia
  appraisals and, 230
  clinical implications, 108–111
  daytime intrusive thoughts and, 98–
    99, 100f, 101
  description, 86–88
  future directions and, 111–112
  information-processing biases and,
    232, 233
  intrusive thoughts and worry and,
    89–90, 91t–92t, 93–98
  theories of, 101–108
  thought suppression and, 239
Integrated model
  empirical support for, 159–163, 161f
  treatment implications of, 163, 164t,
    165–169
Interference, cognitive, 6
Interpretations of Intrusions Inventory,
  161–162. See also Assessment
Intrusive Thoughts Questionnaire, 39–
  40. See also Assessment
Ironic process theory, 63, 103–104,
  238–239. See also Thought
  suppression

K

Knowledge
  inference-based treatment and, 165–
    166
  metacognition and, 128–129

L

Learning theory, 31
Levels of intrusiveness, 56–57
Life experiences, 32, 64

Locus of control, 75
Loss of control experiment, 137. See
  also Treatment

M

Medication, depression and, 68
Memory
  autobiographical, 33
  depression and, 61
  information-processing biases and,
    233
  insomnia and, 87
  metacognition and, 129
  and the origin of intrusive thoughts,
    22–23
  stress and, 66–67
  trauma-related intrusions and, 30–
    31, 35, 37
Mental control. See Control
Mental representations
  constructivist theory and, 32
  depression and, 59–61
  information-processing biases and,
    231–232
  and the origin of intrusive thoughts,
    22–23
  posttraumatic stress disorder and,
    32, 47
Metacognition
  assessment and, 185
  control of intrusive thoughts and,
    128–129
  development of intrusions and,
    180
  development of obsessions and,
    152
  insomnia and, 102–103
  obsessive–compulsive disorder and,
    154, 164t
  posttraumatic stress disorder and,
    125
  psychosis and, 183–184
  treatment and, 108–109
  worry and, 124
Metacognitions Questionnaire, 128. See
  also Assessment

Metacognitive model
  application of, 139–140
  empirical support for, 132–133
  of generalized anxiety disorder, 129–132, 130*f*
Metacognitive therapy, 133–139. *See also* Treatment
Metaworry. *See also* Worry
  description, 131, 141
  metacognitive model of GAD and, 132–133
  psychosis and, 183–184
Mindfulness. *See also* Treatment
  depression and, 74–76
  insomnia and, 109–110
Modified PTSD Symptom Scale, 44. *See also* Assessment
Mood-congruent thought, 61–62
Mood state
  appraisals and, 230–231
  depressive thoughts and, 64, 230–231
  frequency of intrusive thoughts and, 10
  information-processing biases and, 232
  sexual thoughts and, 212, 214–215
  theories of, 227–228
Mood-state hypothesis, 69
Motivation, 21–22
Multiple channel exposure therapy, 41–46. *See also* Treatment

N

Narratives
  inference-based treatment and, 165–168
  obsessive–compulsive disorder and, 152–154, 153*t*
Nature of intrusive thoughts, 55–59, 58*t*
Negative automatic thoughts, 17–18, 55–56
Nighttime intrusive thoughts. *See also* Insomnia
  description, 89–90, 91*t*-92*t*, 93–98

future directions and, 111–112
theories of, 101–108
Nonclinical individuals
  compared to clinical samples, 11–12, 241–242
  compared to depressed individuals, 56–57
  obsessive thoughts in, 145–146, 147–148
  stress-related thoughts in, 9–10

O

Obsessions. *See also* Obsessive–compulsive disorder
  assessing, 242
  compared to ruminations by sexual offenders, 209
  compared to worry, 122–123
  description, 13, 14*t*, 145–146, 146–149, 234–235, 240
  development of, 150, 151*f*, 152–159, 153*t*
  information-processing biases and, 232
  integrated model of, 159–163, 161*f*
  in nonclinical individuals, 7–10
  theories of, 19–23
  worry and, 126–127
Obsessive Beliefs Questionnaire, 161–162. *See also* Assessment
Obsessive Compulsive Cognitions Working Group, 158, 242
Obsessive–compulsive disorder. *See also* Obsessions
  appraisals and, 229
  compared to depression, 59
  compared to nonclinical individuals, 12
  content-specific hypothesis and, 5
  description, 145–146, 235
  development of obsessions and, 150, 151*f*, 152–159, 153*t*
  ego-dystonicity and, 123, 148, 236
  future directions and, 169–170
  information-processing biases and, 232–233

Obsessive–compulsive disorder
    (*continued*)
    integrated model of, 159–163, 161*f*
    metacognitive model of, 129, 139–
        140
    obsessions and, 146–149
    research regarding, 7–8
    sexual thoughts and, 211–212
    theories of, 227–228
    thought–action fusion and, 204–205
    treatment and, 163, 164*t*, 165–169
    worry and, 123, 124, 126–127
Origin of intrusive thoughts
    ability to identify as internal, 5–6
    depression and, 59–64
    theories of, 18–23

P

Panic attacks. *See also* Anxiety
    generalized anxiety disorder, 131
    multiple channel exposure therapy
        and, 43
Paraphilia. *See* Sexual offenders
Personality, 150, 151*f*, 152
Persuasion, depression and, 76
Physiological arousal, 35, 38
Pleasure, sexual thoughts and, 211,
    215
Positivism, 227
Posttraumatic Cognitions Inventory, 40.
    See also Assessment
Posttraumatic stress disorder
    appraisals and, 230
    assessment and, 39–41, 242–243
    description, 30–31
    ego-dystonicity and, 236
    future directions and, 46–48
    information-processing biases and,
        233
    insomnia and, 87–88
    metacognitive model of, 125, 139–
        140
    psychopathology of trauma-related
        intrusions and, 34–39
    theories of, 31–34
    thought suppression and, 238–239

treatment of unwanted intrusions
        and, 41–46
    worry and, 124, 234
Presleep thoughts. *See* Nighttime
        intrusive thoughts
Problem solving, brainstorming and,
        18–19
Prolonged exposure, 41. *See also*
        Treatment
Psychoanalytic view, 227
Psychoeducation, 164*t*
Psychological disorders
    compared to nonclinical individuals,
        11–12
    content-specific hypothesis of, 5
    targeting intrusive thoughts and, 7
Psychopathology, 34–39
Psychosis
    appraisals and, 229
    assessment and, 185–187
    case example of, 189–192
    description, 192
    development of intrusions and, 179–
        185
    information-processing biases and,
        232
    nature of intrusive thoughts in, 175–
        179
    treatment and, 187–189*t*
Punishment
    assessment and, 185
    sexual offenders and, 207–208

R

Rachman's account, 19–20. *See also*
        Origin of intrusive thoughts
Reality "sensing", 167–168
Reasoning errors, 166–167
Reattribution strategies, verbal, 188.
        See also Treatment
Rebound effect, 241
Reciprocal inhibition, 227
Relapse prevention
    case example of, 191–192
    cognitive-behavioral treatment and,
        164*t*

metacognitive therapy for GAD and, 139

Relaxation training, 42. *See also* Treatment

Resources, cognitive
 mood-related depletion of, 65–66
 stress-related depletion of, 66–67

Responsibility for thoughts
 depression and, 75
 obsessions and, 157
 in psychotic disorders, 176
 thought–action fusion and, 204–205

Restructuring, cognitive. *See also* Treatment
 abstinence violation effect and, 205
 obsessive–compulsive disorder and, 164t
 posttraumatic stress disorder and, 42, 45–46

Risk perception, 166

Ruminations
 assessment and, 185
 compared to disclosure, 73–74
 depression and, 230–231, 238
 description, 16–17, 88–89, 234
 metacognition and, 102–103
 in obsessional disorders, 127
 obsessions and, 154–155
 regarding detection by sexual offenders, 205–211, 219
 treatment and, 188

S

Safety behaviors
 assessment and, 185
 development of intrusions and, 181–182
 treatment and, 188

Schemas
 constructivist theory and, 32
 depression and, 59–61
 information-processing biases and, 231–232
 and the origin of intrusive thoughts, 22–23

posttraumatic stress disorder and, 32, 47

Schizophrenia. *See also* Psychosis
 appraisals and, 229
 cognitive therapy and, 188–189
 description, 176
 metacognitive beliefs and, 183–184

Self-appraisals, 201–205, 219. *See also* Appraisals

Self-concept, worry and, 123

Self-critical thoughts, 59

Self-determination, 75–76

Self-esteem
 depression and, 58–59
 psychosis and, 187–188
 of sexual offenders, 202–203

Self-image, 152

Self-referent theme, 166

Self-regulatory executive functioning, 184

Self-relevance of thoughts, 57–59

Self-statements, 202

Self-worth, depression and, 59

Sexual abuse, 47

Sexual offenders
 appraisals and, 231
 description, 199–201, 219
 ego-dystonicity and, 235–236
 ruminations about detection by, 205–211
 self-appraisals of, 201–205
 sexual thoughts by, 211–218, 234
 thought suppression and, 239

Sexual thoughts
 appraisals and, 231
 description, 219
 rationalization of by offenders, 200–201
 by sexual offenders, 211–218

Sleep. *See also* Insomnia
 beliefs regarding, 101–102, 108
 perceptions of, 107–108, 110–111

Sleep Disturbance Questionnaire, 90. *See also* Assessment

Socialization, to the metacognitive model, 136

Socratic method, 76
Sodium lactate infusion, 35
Stopping, thought
    depression and, 76
    by sexual offenders, 202–203
Stream-of-consciousness verbalization,
    240–241
Stress
    cognitive resources and, 66–67
    depression and, 238
    management of by sexual offenders,
        202, 215–216
    mindfulness and, 74
    in nonclinical individuals, 9–10
    and the origin of intrusive thoughts,
        22–23
    worry and, 125–126, 138
Stress inoculation therapy, 41. See also
    Treatment
Stress-related thoughts, in nonclinical
    individuals, 9–10
Structured Clinical Interview for DSM-
    IV. See also Assessment
    description, 39
    multiple channel exposure therapy
        and, 44
Substance use
    insomnia and, 87
    sexual thoughts and, 213–214
Suppressed biases, 70–71
Suppression of thoughts. See also
    Control
    appraisals and, 230–231
    assessment and, 56–57, 58t, 185
    depression and, 62–64, 64–68, 76
    description, 237–239
    disclosure and, 73–74
    generalized anxiety disorder and,
        131–132, 133, 133–139
    insomnia and, 103–105
    posttraumatic stress disorder and, 47
    psychosis and, 182
    research regarding, 11
    secondary appraisals of control and,
        158–159, 162
    by sexual offenders, 216

    thought–action fusion and, 205
    treatment and, 109–110, 188

T

Task performance, interference to, 6
Thought-action fusion bias
    description, 158
    sexual offenders and, 204–205
Thought broadcast, 176
Thought Control Questionnaire. See
    also Assessment
    description, 128
    insomnia and, 105
    worry and, 125–126
Thought insertion, 176
Thought-shifting theory, 20–22. See
    also Origin of intrusive
    thoughts
Thought stopping
    depression and, 76
    by sexual offenders, 202–203
Thought suppression. See also Control
    appraisals and, 230–231
    assessment and, 56–57, 58t, 185
    depression and, 62–64, 64–68, 76
    description, 237–239
    disclosure and, 73–74
    generalized anxiety disorder and,
        131–132, 133, 133–139
    insomnia and, 103–105
    posttraumatic stress disorder and,
        47
    psychosis and, 182
    research regarding, 11
    secondary appraisals of control and,
        158–159, 162
    by sexual offenders, 216
    thought–action fusion and, 205
    treatment and, 109–110, 188
Thought withdrawal, 176
Trauma-related intrusions. See also
    Posttraumatic stress disorder
    description, 30–31
    future directions and, 46–48
    information-processing biases and,
        233

psychopathology of, 34–39
treatment of, 41–46
worry and, 125–126
Traumatic experiences, 32. *See also*
    Posttraumatic stress disorder
Treatment
    depression, 68, 71–76
    for generalized anxiety disorder,
        133–139
    implications to, 239–240
    insomnia and, 108–111
    obsessive–compulsive disorder, 140,
        163, 164*t*, 165–169
    posttraumatic stress disorder and,
        41–46, 47, 140
    of psychotic disorders, 187–189*t*
    ruminations by sexual offenders and,
        209–210
    sexual fantasies and, 216
    targeting intrusive thoughts and, 7

U

Utility of Pre-sleep Worry
    Questionnaire, 102–103. *See
    also* Assessment

V

Verbal reattribution strategies, 188. *See
    also* Treatment
Verbal thought, worry and, 121

W

Warning signal hypothesis, 33
White bear experiment, 109
White Bear Suppression Inventory, 56–
    57, 58*t*. *See also* Assessment
Withdrawal, thought, 176
Worry
    appraisals and, 228–231
    assessment and, 185, 241–242
    compared to other intrusions, 122–
        124
    during the day, 98–99, 100*f*, 101
    description, 88–89, 119, 227, 234,
        240
    effect of on other intrusions, 125–
        127
    generalized anxiety disorder and, 141
    imagery control and, 106
    insomnia and, 111–112
    metacognition and, 102–103, 129–
        139, 130*f*
    nature of, 120–122
    during the night, 89–90, 91*t*-92*t*,
        93–98
    in nonclinical individuals, 8–10, 12
    schizophrenia and, 183
    versus unwanted intrusive thoughts,
        13–16
Worry postponement experiment, 137.
    See also Treatment

Y

Yohimbine-induced panic attacks, 35